KU-133-025

ATLAS OF

Benign Gynecologic *and* *Obstetric* *Surgery*

THOMAS G STOVALL MD

Associate Professor
Section Head Section on Gynecology
Department of Obstetrics and Gynecology
Bowman Gray School of Medicine of Wake Forest University
Winston-Salem, North Carolina, USA

FRANK W LING MD

Professor and Chairman
Department of Obstetrics and Gynecology
University of Tennessee
Memphis, Tennessee, USA

M Mosby-Wolfe

London Baltimore Bogotá Boston Buenos Aires Caracas Carlsbad, CA Chicago Madrid Mexico City Milan Naples, FL New York Philadelphia St. Louis Sydney Tokyo Toronto Wiesbaden

Project Manager:	Linda Kull
Developmental Editor:	Lucy Hamilton
	Claire Hooper
Designer:	Pete Wilder
	Mark Howard
Cover Design:	Ian Spick
Illustration:	Marion Tasker
Production:	Jane Tozer
Index:	Nina Boyd
Publisher:	Geoff Greenwood

Copyright © 1995 Times Mirror International Publishers Limited

Copyright © 1995 Illustrations Chapter 9 David Muram

Published in 1995 by Mosby, an imprint of Times Mirror International Publishers Limited

Printed by Grafos S.A. Arte sobre papel, Barcelona, Spain

ISBN 0 7234 2017 3

All rights reserved. No reproduction, copy or transmission of this publication may be made without written permission.

No part of this publication may be reproduced, copied or transmitted save with written permission or in accordance with the provisions of the Copyright Act 1988, or under the terms of any licence permitting limited copying issued by the Copyright Licensing Agency, 33–34 Alfred Place, London, WC1E 7DP.

Any person who does any unauthorised act in relation to this publication may be liable to criminal prosecution and civil claims for damages.

Permission to photocopy or reproduce solely for internal or personal use is permitted for libraries or other users registered with the Copyright Clearance Center, provided that the base fee of $4.00 per chapter plus $.10 per page is paid directly to the Copyright Clearance Center, 21 Congress Street, Salem, MA 01970. This consent does not extend to other kinds of copying, such as copying for general distribution, for advertising or promotional purposes, for creating new collected works, or for resale.

For full details of all Times Mirror International Publishers Limited titles, please write to Times Mirror International Publishers Limited, Lynton House, 7–12 Tavistock Square, London WC1H 9LB, England.

A CIP catalogue record for this book is available from the British Library.

Library of Congress Cataloging-in-Publication Data applied for.

DEDICATION

We wish to dedicate this book to our wives, Donna and Janis, and to our children, Elliott, Mandy and Trevor.

CONTENTS

PREFACE

It has often been said that a picture is worth a thousand words. At no time is this more true than when one surgeon tries to describe to another how to perform a surgical procedure. In addition to drawings and illustrations, this book primarily uses photographs taken at the time of surgery to illustrate procedures in a step-by-step fashion. While not every obstetrical and gynecologic operation has been included, a wide range of procedures for noncancerous conditins has laparoscopic and hysteroscopic procedures. The photographs, tables and illustrations for each procedure were specifically created for uuse in this text.

This textbook was written by obstetrician/gynecologists who are regularly involved in the performance and teaching of surgery in residency training programs. Each author is a recognized teacher and expert with surgical experience and scientific publications related to the subjects on which they have written. The emphasis in this text is on the actual procedure itself. The description follows a similar outline in an effort to make this text user friendly. While technique is the emphasis, each procedure is accompanied by a discussion of the indications, alternative procedures and potential complications of the procedure being discussed.

We would like to express our appreciation to each of the contributors who have made this project a success along with the countless individuals and professors who have played a part in our teaching and current understanding of obstetrical and gynecologic surgery. We hope that it will add to your library and understanding of those procedures that are commonly done by practising obstetricians and gynecologists.

Thomas G. Stovall, M.D.
Frank W. Ling, M.D.

LIST OF CONTRIBUTORS

Thomas G Stovall, MD
Associate Professor and Head
Section on Gynecology
Department of Obstetrics and Gynecology
Bowman Gray School of Medicine of Wake Forest University
Winston-Salem, North Carolina

Frank W Ling, MD
Professor and Chairman
Department of Obstetrics and Gynecology
University of Tennessee
Memphis, Tennessee

Lee P Shulman, MD
Associate Professor and Director
Division of Reproductive Genetics
University of Tennessee
Memphis, Tennessee

Robert L Summitt, Jr, MD
Associate Professor, Division of Gynecology
Chief, Section of Urogynecology
University of Tennessee
Memphis, Tennessee

Gary H Lipscomb, MD
Assistant Professor
Division of Gynecology
University of Tennessee
Memphis, Tennessee

David Muram, MD
Professor and Director
Division of Gynecology
Department of Obstetrics and Gynecology
University of Tennessee
Memphis, Tennessee

David C Shaver, MD
Director of Maternal–Fetal Medicine
Presbyterian Hospital
Charlotte, North Carolina

Marian L McCord, MD
Assistant Professor
Division of Gynecology
University of Tennessee
Memphis, Tennessee

Javier F Magrina, MD
Section Head, Gynecologic Surgery and Oncology
Mayo Clinic
Scottsdale, Arizona

Brian M Cohen, MB ChB MD
Clinical Professor
Department of Obstetrics and Gynecology
University of Texas
Dallas, Texas

James G Blythe, MD
Chairman, Department of Obstetrics and Gynecology
Chief, Section of Gynecological Oncology
St John's Mercy Medical Center
St Louis, Missouri

Peter Casson, MD
Assistant Professor
Department of Obstetrics and Gynecology
Baylor College of Medicine
Houston, Texas

Thierry Vancaillie, MD
San Antonio, Texas

Barbara R Hostetler, MD
Instructor
Division of Gynecology
Department of Obstetrics and Gynecology
University of Tennessee
Memphis, Tennessee

Claudette E Jones, MD
Assistant Professor
Division of Gynecology
Department of Obstetrics and Gynecology
University of Tennessee
Memphis, Tennessee

Fredrick J Rau, MD
Assistant Clinical Professor
Department of Obstetrics, Gynecology and Pediatrics
University of Connecticut School of Medicine
Farmington, Connecticut

1

Lesions of the Vulva

Gary H. Lipscomb

Thomas G. Stovall

VULVAR BIOPSY

In 50% of patients with invasive carcinoma of the vulva, long-standing pruritus or a mass has been present for months. After seeking medical attention, it is not uncommon for patients to receive medical treatment for a year or more before diagnosis of the cancer. Fortunately, vulvar carcinoma is frequently a slow-growing, indolent lesion that undergoes metastasis late in its clinical course. Early diagnosis and cure are possible only with aggressive biopsy of all suspicious lesions of the vulva as well as of any condition that does not respond promptly to treatment.

SURGICAL INDICATIONS

Any pigmented lesion or non-healing area of the vulva is an indication for vulvar biopsy. Likewise, any condition that does not respond promptly to appropriate therapy should be biopsied to rule out preinvasive or invasive vulvar carcinoma. Small lesions such as nevi and true neoplastic areas are best excised completely. Vulvar intraepithelial neoplasia (VIN), particularly in hair-bearing areas of the vulva, are often also best treated with total excision.

SURGICAL PROCEDURE
Step 1
The abnormal area is identified (*Fig. 1.1*) and the surgical field prepped with povidone–iodine solution. The skin around the lesion is infiltrated with 1% lidocaine. Pain from infiltration can be minimized by using 30-gauge dental needles and avoiding rapid injection of the anesthetic solution.

Step 2
The vulvar skin is fixed in position with the hand and a dermatologic punch biopsy is twisted in a circular fashion until loss of resistance is met (*Fig. 1.2*).

Step 3
The disk of tissue is lifted with small tissue forceps and removed by incising the base with scissors (*Figs 1.3, 1.4*).

Step 4
If the defect is small, hemostasis can be obtained with a silver nitrate applicator. Larger defects can be closed with an interrupted stitch of #3-0 or #4-0 absorbable suture (*Fig. 1.5*).

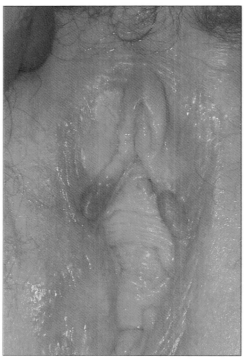

1.1 Identification of the abnormal lesion.

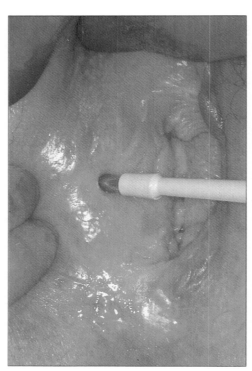

1.2 Use of Punch biopsy.

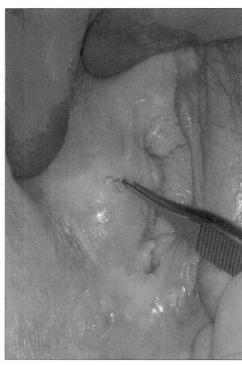

1.3 Tissue disk elevated for removal.

Step 5

Alternatively, a vulvar biopsy can be performed using Adson tissue forceps to elevate the skin (*Fig. 1.6*) followed by excision with small scissors (*Fig. 1.4*). This technique is particularly useful in biopsy of raised lesions.

Alternative procedures to vulvar biopsy are listed in *Fig. 1.7*.

COMPLICATIONS

Complications from vulvar biopsy are exceedingly rare. Bleeding is the most common of these. If the bleeding occurs after the patient has left the office, direct pressure applied by the patient for several minutes is usually sufficient to stop the flow of blood. If bleeding persists, suturing may be necessary.

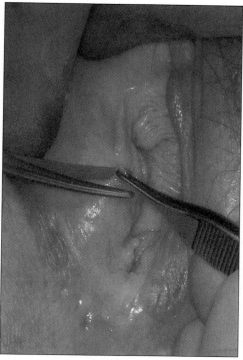

1.4 Removal of abnormal tissue using scissors.

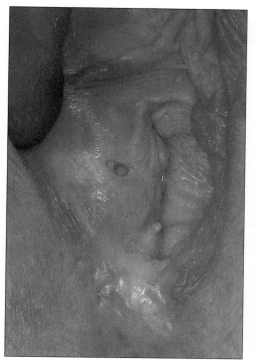

1.5 Hemostasis of vulvar biopsy site obtained.

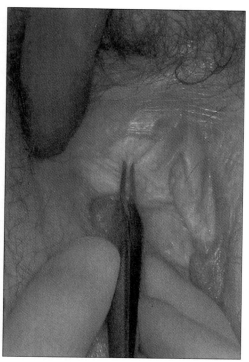

1.6 Elevation of skin with forceps.

Alternatives to Vulvar Biopsy	
Lesion	**Alternative Treatment**
Pruritic area	Empiric trial of antifungal or local steroid application*
Non-healing area	Improved vulvar hygiene*

* Biopsy necessary if prompt improvement does not occur.

1.7 Alternative procedures to vulvar biopsy.

VESTIBULECTOMY

Vestibulectomy, or modified perineoplasty, is the surgical removal of the vestibular skin. This surgical procedure is primarily performed for treatment of vulvar vestibulitis which is unresponsive to conservative management. Vulvar vestibulitis has been defined by the International Society for the Study of Vulvar Disease (ISSVD) as a chronic clinical syndrome characterized by the following criteria: severe pain on vestibular touch; tenderness to pressure localized within the vulvar vestibule; and vestibular erythema as the only physical finding. This definition excludes conditions associated with acute inflammatory processes or immediate postoperative changes.

SURGICAL INDICATION

Surgical treatment of vestibulitis should be reserved for those who meet the above criteria and who fail to respond to more conservative methods discussed below. Some authors have reported a spontaneous resolution of up to 50% of cases over a 6-month period. Although this degree of resolution has been questioned by other investigators, an appropriate trial of non-surgical therapy seems reasonable.

Step 1

The vestibule has been exposed by retraction of the labia majora and minora. Note the extensive erythema (*Fig. 1.8*). Previously in the office, when the patient is not under anesthesia, the areas of localized tenderness on the vestibule are mapped out with a moist Q-tip applicator. An indelible marker is used to outline this same area to be resected (*Fig. 1.9*). This is usually in a horseshoe-shaped area extending from the skin's gland on one side around to the same structure on the other side, incorporating a region, about 1 cm distal and maximal to the hymen. This is to ensure that no area of tenderness inadvertently remains after the procedure has been completed.

Step 2

The vestibular skin is grasped with Allis clamps and a No. 15 scalpel is used to incise the skin of the area to be excised (*Fig. 1.10*).

Step 3

The vestibular skin is dissected free from the underlying connective tissue and removed (*Fig. 1.11*).

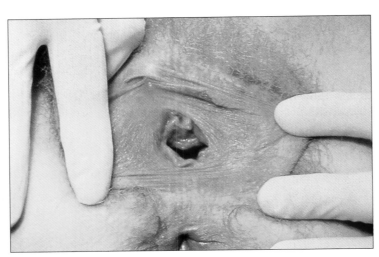

1.8 Vulvar examination.

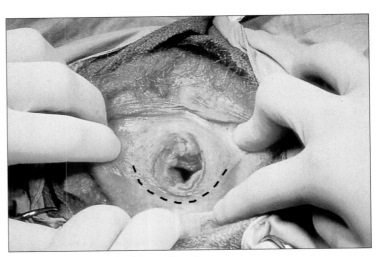

1.9 Area to be excised is outlined.

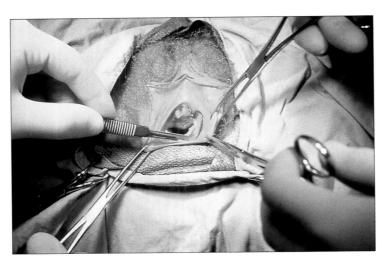

1.10 Skin incision.

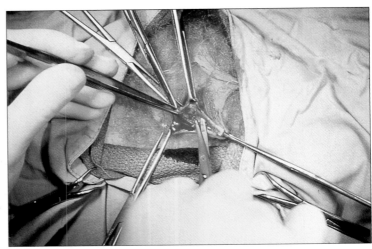

1.11 Dissection of skin from underlying skin.

Step 4

The vaginal skin edge is undermined enough to be advanced so that it can cover the denuded area of the vestibule without tension (*Fig. 1.12*).

Step 5

The vaginal skin edge is reapproximated to the vulvar skin edge using #2-0 or #3-0 synthetic absorbable suture (*Figs 1.13, 1.14*).

ALTERNATIVES TO SURGICAL MANAGEMENT

Treatment guidelines for vulvar vestibulitis have not been established, and no single therapy has been shown to be uniformly successful in treating this condition. *Fig. 1.15* lists alternative therapies that have been successful in some cases. The use of lidocaine jelly has been very helpful in milder cases and in symptomatic therapy in the hope of spontaneous resolution. Amitriptyline in the low dosages used for causalgia (10–75 mg) has proven useful in patients with minimal findings on examination but who continue to complain of constant burning vulvar pain.

COMPLICATIONS

As would be expected from a relatively minor procedure, complications are uncommon. Incision separation is perhaps most frequently found. Small incision breakdowns usually heal without treatment. Sitz bath and routine vulvar hygiene will promote healing of the exposed raw surfaces and provide symptomatic relief from discomfort. To prevent breakdown, approximation of skin edges without tension is essential. In areas where tension cannot be avoided, the use of vertical mattress sutures will decrease breakdown.

Postoperative infection is rare. Routine sitz baths and good vulvar hygiene will prevent most infections. The use of prophylactic antibiotics is not indicated.

Postoperative scarring and stenosis, with resulting worsened dyspareunia, are the most serious, yet uncommon, complications. Avoiding excessive tissue removal and dissection of the deeper connective tissue will help to minimize the possibility of their occurrence, but none the less the patient should be counselled preoperatively about the potential for these complications.

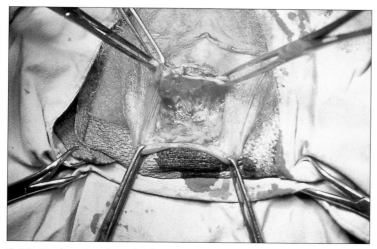

1.12 Undermined vaginal mucosa.

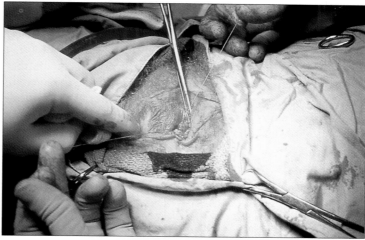

1.13 Reapproximation of vaginal skin edge.

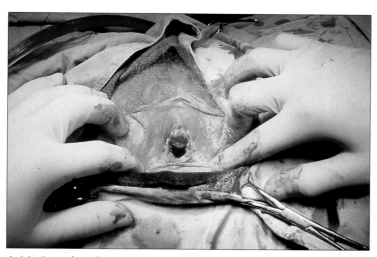

1.14 Completed procedure.

Alternatives to Vestibulectomy
5% lidocaine jelly for symptomatic relief
Interferon injections in presence of human papillomavirus
Topical corticosteriods
Topical antifungals
Low-dose tricyclic antidepressants

1.15 Alternative therapies.

BARTHOLIN GLAND ABSCESS

Infection of the Bartholin gland is a common clinical condition. During acute infection the gland becomes extremely painful and swollen. If abscess formation occurs, the gland becomes fluctuant and often drains spontaneously. If abscess formation does not occur or resolves, the duct frequently becomes scarred and stenotic, with subsequent formation of a chronic mucoid-filled cyst.

Simple incision and drainage of the cyst or abscess is not the optimal treatment for a Bartholin gland abscess. Contraction and scarring of the drainage site frequently results in repeat duct occlusion and cyst recurrence. Placement of a Word catheter, marsupialization, or gland excision is a more appropriate solution.

SURGICAL INDICATIONS

The asymptomatic Bartholin cyst usually requires no therapy. Surgical treatment should be reserved for cysts that are symptomatic or worrisome to the patient. Deep induration or nodularity within an otherwise asymptomatic Bartholin gland cyst, particularly in patients over the age of 40, suggests the possibility of malignancy and requires biopsy or removal of the gland.

The simplicity, high success rate, and minimal complications associated with Word catheter placement make this procedure ideal for initial management of both the acute Bartholin abscess and the chronic symptomatic Bartholin cyst. More extensive procedures are rarely indicated as primary treatment for a Bartholin gland cyst. This is particularly true of the acute Bartholin gland abscess, in which edema and swelling make other extensive procedures very difficult to perform. However, Word catheter placement should not be attempted in the acutely infected Bartholin gland until fluctuance is present.

Marsupialization is usually reserved for the chronic or recurrent Bartholin gland cyst and rarely for initial treatment of an acute Bartholin gland abscess. Marsupialization is a technically less involved procedure than excision, and leads to fewer complications.

Bartholin gland excision is rarely indicated, and should be reserved for patients with repetitive abscess or cyst formation despite more conservative surgery or for patients with suspected malignancy. A summary of indications and suggested procedures is shown in *Fig. 1.16*. Alternatives to surgery are shown in *Fig. 1.17*.

SURGICAL PROCEDURE: WORD CATHETER PLACEMENT
Step 1
A fluctuant right Bartholin gland is shown in *Fig. 1.18*. The surgical approach to the Bartholin gland is through the vulvar vestibule just distal to the hymen. The labia majora and minora are retracted laterally revealing the distended gland (*Fig. 1.19*).

Step 2
A puncture incision with a No. 11 scalpel blade is made over the centre of the bulge (*Fig. 1.20*). Too large an incision will result in the Word catheter falling out of place.

Step 3
In the case of a Bartholin gland abscess, a hemostat can be inserted through the incision into the gland to break up loculi of purulent material. This is frequently not necessary with a chronic cyst. A Word catheter, with the bulb uninflated and inflated, is shown in *Fig. 1.21*.

Indications and Procedures for Lesions of Bartholin Gland	
Condition	**Treatment**
Bartholin gland adenitis	Antibiotics and moist heat
	Surgical therapy not indicated
Bartholin gland abscess	Incision and drainage
	Word catheter placement*
	Marsupialization
Bartholin gland cyst	Incision and drainage
	Word catheter placement*
	Marsupialization
	Excision
Recurrent Bartholin abscess or cyst	Marsupialization*
	Excision
Suspected Bartholin gland carcinoma	Excision*
	* Recommended Procedure

1.16 Surgical treatment options.

Non-Surgical Alternatives for Bartholin Abscess/Cyst	
Non-fluctuant infected gland	Direct heat and broad spectrum antibiotics
	Surgical therapy not indicated
Fluctuant infected gland	Surgical therapy recommended
	Await spontaneous drainage (associated with higher recurrence rate and complications than with intentional drainage)
Asymptomatic cyst	Reassurance only

1.17 Non-surgical therapies.

Step 4

The Word catheter is placed with the help of a hemostat or Kelly clamp (*Fig. 1.22*). After the bulb has been inflated, the catheter should remain in place without assistance (*Fig. 1.23*). If the incision has been made in an appropriate location, the catheter may be directed into the vagina thereby lessening the patient's inconvenience and possible discomfort.

Step 5

The catheter should be allowed to remain in place for a minimum of 2 weeks to allow the tract opening to epithelize.

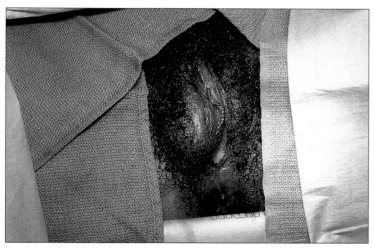

1.18 Bartholin duct cyst.

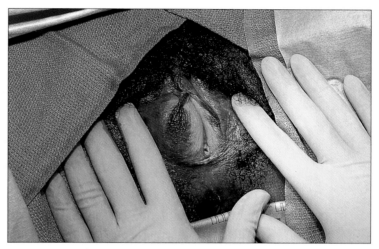

1.19 Area to be incised is identified.

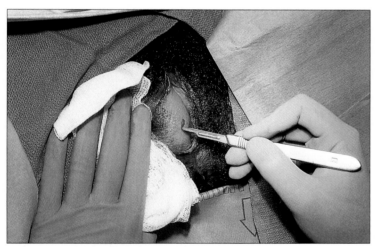

1.20 Incision made in cyst wall.

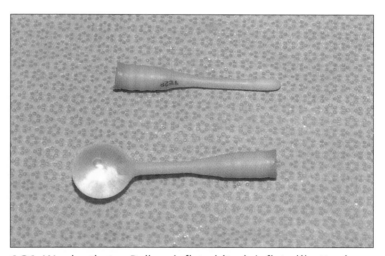

1.21 Word catheter. Bulb uninflated (*top*), inflated(*bottom*).

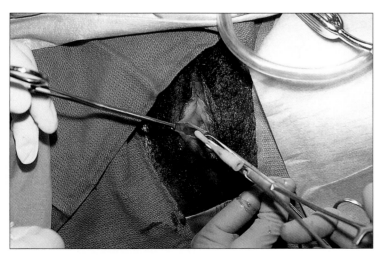

1.22 Placement of Word catheter.

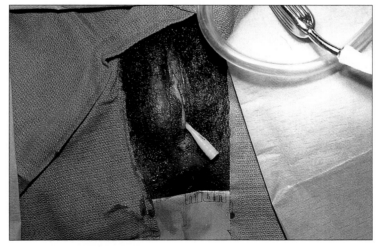

1.23 Completed procedure.

BARTHOLIN GLAND MARSUPIALIZATION
Step 1

The approach for marsupialization of the Bartholin gland is the same as for Word catheter placement, i.e., through the vulvar vestibule. A No.15 scalpel blade is used to remove an elliptical piece of cyst wall about 1 cm in length (*Figs 1.24, 1.25*).

Step 2

The edges of the cyst wall can be grasped with Allis clamps to aid in suture placement (*Fig. 1.26*). In *Fig. 1.26*, mucoid cyst contents can be seen seeping from the opening.

Step 3

The mucosa is now sutured to the edge of the cyst wall with either interrupted or running absorbable suture (*Figs 1.27, 1.28*).

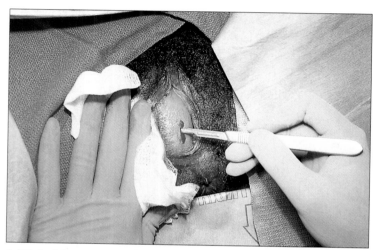

1.24 Incision over Bartholin cyst.

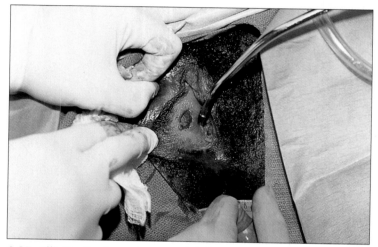

1.25 Elliptically shaped mucosal defect.

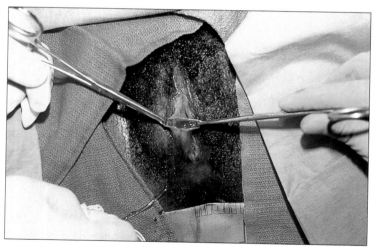

1.26 Mucosa of the cyst wall is grasped with Allis clamps.

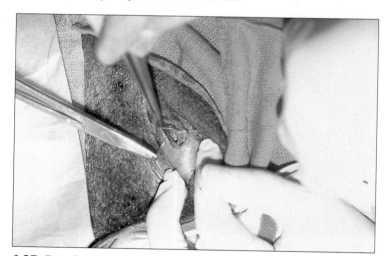

1.27 Exterioration of the cyst lining.

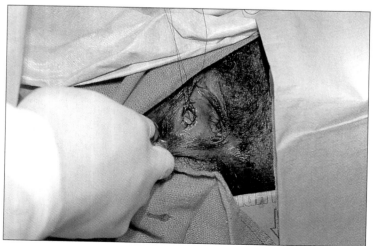

1.28 Completed procedure.

BARTHOLIN GLAND EXCISION

Step 1

An elliptical incision is made in the vaginal mucosa as close as possible to the gland opening (*Fig. 1.29*).

Step 2

The cyst is dissected away from the vaginal wall and cyst bed using sharp dissection (*Fig. 1.30*).

Step 3

Meticulous hemostasis is obtained with needle-point electrocautery (*Fig. 1.31*).

Step 4

The cyst cavity is now obliterated in layers, using fine absorbable suture such as #3-0 chromic (*Fig. 1.32*).

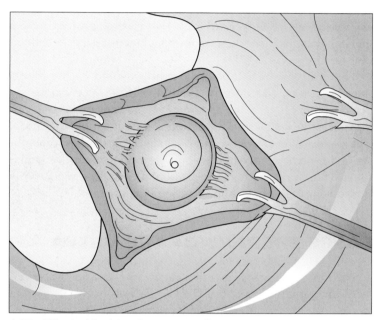

1.29 Elliptical incision into cyst wall.

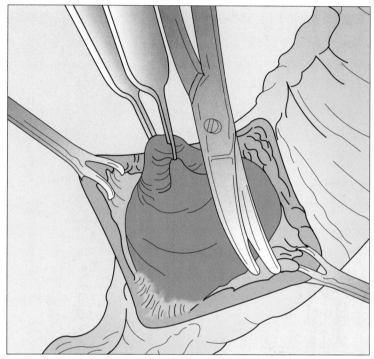

1.30 Sharp dissection of cyst wall.

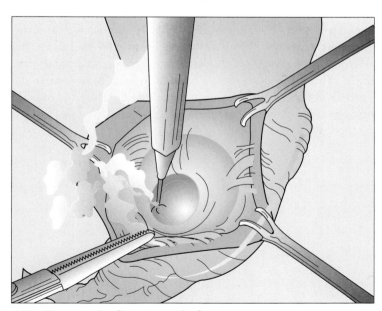

1.31 Hemostasis after removal of cyst.

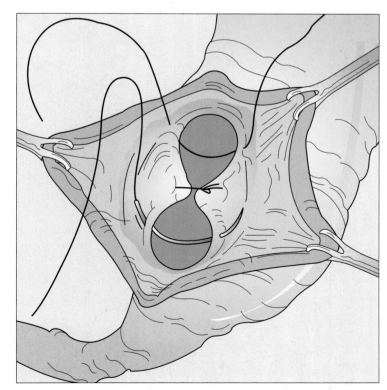

1.32 Layered closure of cyst wall.

Step 5

A closed suction drain is placed into the cyst bed and secured with fine (#5-0) chromic suture (*Fig. 1.33*)

Step 6

The vaginal mucosa is approximated with #0 absorbable suture (*Fig. 1.34*). An ice pack and pressure dressing should be used postoperatively to prevent possible hematoma formation.

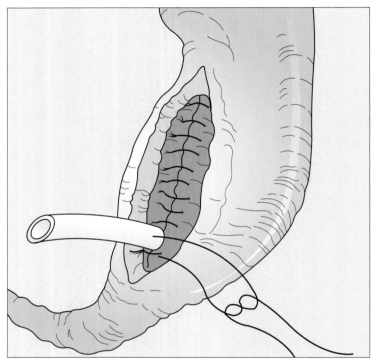

1.33 Closed suction drainage of cyst bed.

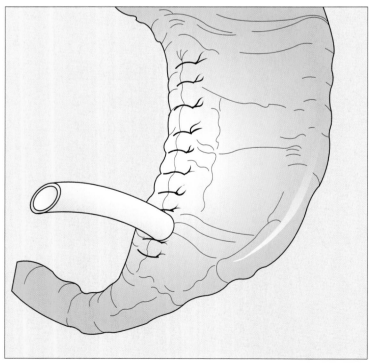

1.34 Completed procedure.

COMPLICATIONS

The most common complication of any of the drainage procedures for a Bartholin cyst or abscess is subsequent recurrence. Although technically the simplest procedure to perform, simple incision and drainage is associated with the highest incidence of recurrence. Therefore Word catheter placement or marsupialization is preferred to incision and drainage whenever possible. Both Word catheter placement and marsupialization allow epithelization of the drainage tract, which reduces the incidence of recurrence. Unfortunately, the extensive edema and swelling associated with acute Bartholin gland abscess often makes marsupialization difficult to perform and increases the likelihood of tract closure.

The close proximity of the Bartholin gland to the highly vascular vestibular bulb may result in vigorous bleeding during gland excision. Despite an apparently hemostatic operative field, postoperative hematoma formation is a frequent complication. The use of sharp dissection and meticulous attention to hemostasis during the procedure will minimize postoperative hematoma. The use of ice packs and pressure dressings postoperatively is also helpful in preventing this complication.

LASER THERAPY OF THE VULVA

The term Laser is an acronym for Light Amplification by Stimulated Emission of Radiation. The CO_2 laser is primarily used in gynecology for vulvar and vaginal procedures. CO_2 laser energy is completely absorbed by water. Since water is the primary component of tissue, CO_2 energy is absorbed by cellular water resulting in vaporization and subsequent disruption of the cell membrane by steam.

Laser surgery of the vagina and vulva is primarily used to treat manifestations of the human papillomavirus such as vulvar intraepithelial neoplasia (VIN) and vaginal intraepithelial neoplasia (VAIN). Since these lesions are confined to the epidermal layer of the skin, the laser beam can be used to selectively remove the epithelium with minimal damage to underlying tissue. As a result, rapid healing without scarring is possible.

SURGICAL INDICATIONS

The primary indications for laser therapy of the vulva or vagina are VIN, VAIN, or condylomata acuminata. In all cases of VIN and VAIN, ruling out the presence of an invasive lesion by biopsy before laser vaporization is a wise precaution. Indications, contra-indications, and alternative treatment options are given in *Fig. 1.35*.

SURGICAL PROCEDURE
Step 1
The anatomy of vulvar skin is illustrated in *Fig. 1.36*. Since both condylomata acuminata and VIN are confined to the epithelial layer, only this layer must be removed.

Criteria for Laser Therapy		
Condition	**Contraindication to Laser**	**Alternatives**
Vulvar condylomata	Invasive carcinoma	Trichloroacetic acid
		Podophyllin
		Cryocautery
		Electro-desiccation
		Interferon injection
Vaginal condylomata	Invasive carcinoma	Trichloroacetic acid
		5-Fluorouracil
		Electro-desiccation
		Interferon injection
VIN	Invasive carcinoma	Local excision
	Hair-bearing area	5-Fluorouracil
		Cryocautery
		Electro-desiccation
VAIN	Invasive carcinoma	5-Fluorouracil

1.35 Criteria for laser therapy.

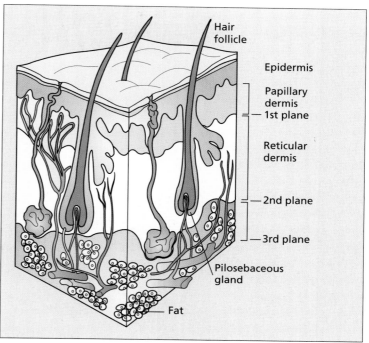

1.36 Anatomy of vulvar skin.

Step 2

The vulva is soaked with 5% acetic acid to highlight the abnormal areas. All procedures should be performed under microscopic guidance to ensure that all abnormal areas are treated *Fig. 1.37*.

Step 3

The abnormal area is outlined with a series of laser dots (*Fig. 1.38*).

Step 4

For vulvar laser surgery, power densities in the range 750–1200 W/cm^2, using a 1–2 mm spot size, are recommended. The laser beam is moved rapidly over the area to be destroyed. When the procedure is performed correctly, bubbles will be seen to form beneath the surface with each pass of the laser beam. This will be accompanied by a characteristic crackling sound. Wiping off the eschar (*Fig. 1.39*) exposes the smooth, intact surface of the papillary dermis (*Fig. 1.40*).

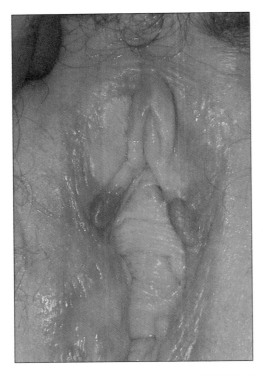

1.37 Acetowhite lesion of the vulva.

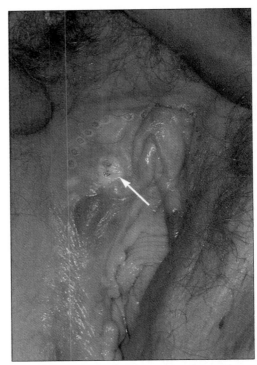

1.38 Lesion to be ablated is arrowed.

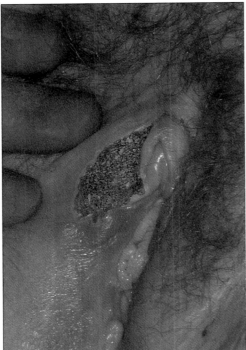

1.39 Completion of ablation.

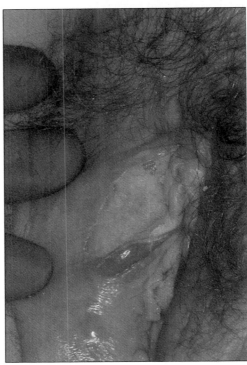

1.40 Papillary dermal layer.

Step 5

For vulvar condylomata, the laser beam is directed into the center of condyloma, allowing it to collapse around the laser beam. Once the condyloma is removed down to the papillary dermis, the power density is reduced to 100–150 W/cm^2, and the area for 2 cm around the condyloma or VIN is 'brushed' to kill latent virus (*Fig. 1.41*).

Step 6

The vaporized area is coated with Silvadene cream (*Fig. 1.42*).

POSTOPERATIVE CARE

Postoperatively, the patient is instructed to use sitz baths three to four times daily and after each bowel movement. The use of sea salt (available at aquarium supply stores) for the sitz bath appears to be soothing and promotes rapid re-epithelization. Silvadene cream is also applied after each sitz bath. Lidocaine jelly 3–5% can be used to supplement oral pain medication during the immediate postoperative period, and in the latter stages of healing is often sufficient alone.

COMPLICATIONS

A common complication of laser surgery is destruction of tissue at a deeper level than intended. Deep tissue destruction will prevent rapid healing and may lead to scarring. This can be avoided by using the appropriate power setting for the surgeon's level of skill and by rapidly moving the laser beam over the target tissue. Frequent removal of escher will allow assessment of the depth of vaporization and prevent inadvertent overpenetration.

A frequent mistake is use of laser vaporization for VIN in hair-bearing areas. Dysplastic epithelium has been shown to extend into the hair shaft. To eliminate these foci of dysplasia, vaporization of the vulva to a depth of 3 mm would be necessary. In many areas of the vulva, this amount of vaporization would produce a full-thickness burn, with slow healing associated with contracture and scar formation. Simple scalpel excision with reapproximation will achieve a more cosmetic result in these cases.

If vaporization is too deep, troublesome bleeding frequently occurs. Defocusing of the laser beam and coagulation of the bleeding vessels usually produces rapid, efficient hemostasis.

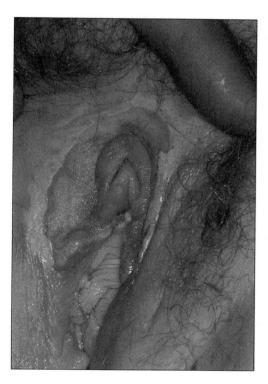

1.41 "Brushing" of surrounding skin.

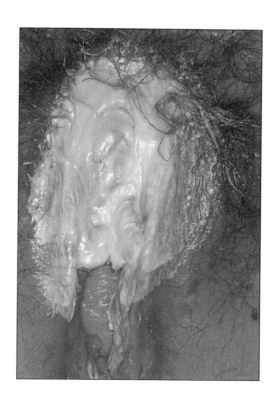

1.42 Application of Silvadene cream.

FURTHER READING

Benedet JL, Murphy KJ. Squamous cell carcinoma of the vulva. *Gynecol Oncol* 1982; 42: 213.

Jacobson P. Marsupialization of vulvovaginal (Bartholin) cysts, *Am J Obstet Gynecol* 1960; 79: 73.

Kaufman RH, Gardner HL, Brown D, Naftalin NJ. Vulvar dystrophies; An evaluation. *Am J Obstet Gynecol* 1974; 120: 363.

Kent HL, Wisniewski PM. Interferon for vulvar vestibulitis. *J Reprod Med* 1990; 35: 1138–40.

McKay M. Dyesthetic (essential) vulvodynia: treatment with amitriptyline. *J Reprod Med* 1993; 38: 9–13.

McKay M, Frankman O, Horowitz B, *et al*. Vulvar vestibulitis and vestibular papillomatosis: Report of the ISSVD on vulvodynia. *J Reprod Med* 1991; 36: 413–16.

Mene A, Buckley CH. Involvement of vulvar skin appendages by intraepithelial neoplasia. *Br J Obstet Gynaecol* 1985; 92: 634.

Reid R. Superficial laser vulvectomy III. A new surgical technique for appendage conserving ablation of refractory condylomas and vulvar intraepithelial neoplasia. *Am J Obstet Gynecol* 1985; 152: 504.

Reid R, Elfont EA, Zirkin RM, *et al*. Superficial laser vulvectomy II. The anatomic and biophysical principles permitting accurate control over the depth of dermal destruction with the carbon dioxide laser. *Am J Obstet Gynecol* 1985; 152: 261.

Word B. New instrument for office treatment of cyst and abscess of Bartholin gland. *JAMA* 1964; 190: 777.

Wright VC, Davies E. Laser surgery for vulvar intraepithelia neoplasia. *Am J Obstet Gynecol* 1987; 156: 374.

2

Surgery of the Bladder and Urethra

Robert L. Summitt, Jr.

Thomas G. Stovall

THE BURCH PROCEDURE

The Burch procedure was first described by Dr John C. Burch in 1961[1] for treatment of stress urinary incontinence. As described in his original report, this technique was devised during a Marshall–Marchetti–Krantz operation in which the sutures continued to pull out of the periosteum of the symphysis pubis. In looking for a more secure point of attachment for the periurethral sutures, the ileopectineal line (Cooper's ligament) was chosen. Subsequently, this operative technique for retropubic urethropexy has been widely used and has undergone a number of modifications. One of the more significant modifications has been described by Tanagho[2]: a wide placement of the periurethral sutures so as to avoid constriction of the urethra. With this procedure well established, extensive postoperative data have demonstrated a high success rate for the cure of stress urinary incontinence, ranging from 85 to 95%[3].

SURGICAL INDICATIONS

The Burch retropubic urethropexy is most commonly used for treatment of primary stress urinary incontinence. However, it is also employed for treatment of recurrent stress incontinence when an anatomic defect is present. There are data to suggest that the failure rate with the Burch procedure is higher in the presence of low urethral closure pressure. More investigation is needed with prospective trials to support this contention. Unless there is a separate gynecologic indication to do so, a hysterectomy is unnecessary at the time of retropubic urethropexy.

The indications for the Burch procedure are as follows:
- Primary stress urinary incontinence.
- Recurrent stress urinary incontinence in the presence of an anatomic urethral support defect.

SURGICAL PROCEDURE
Step 1
The procedure is most easily performed with the patient in the supine lithotomy position. The legs are supported with Allen Universal stirrups, as this allows low placement of the thighs and readily provides access for cystoscopy if this is desired later in the operation (*Fig. 2.1*). The perineum, vagina, and lower abdomen are prepped and a three-way Foley catheter with a 30 ml

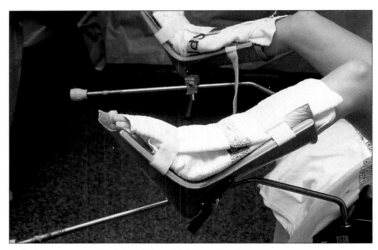

2.1 Legs supported by Allen Universal stirrups.

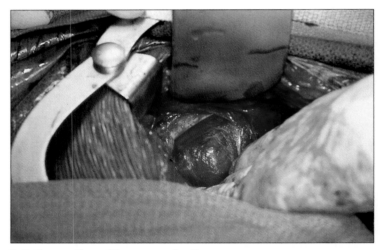

2.2 Separation of loose areolar tissue.

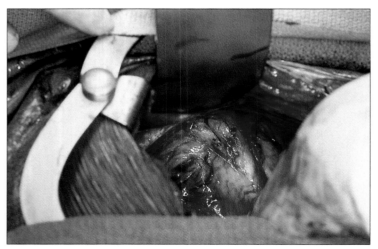

2.3 Deeper dissection to the level of the anterior vaginal wall.

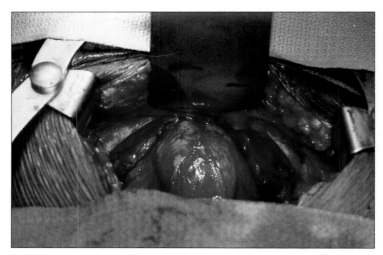

2.4 The large central Foley bulb is a useful reference point for the urethrovesical junction.

balloon is inserted transurethrally. One port of the catheter is attached to cystoscopy tubing and a 1,000 ml bag of sterile water. Drapes are appropriately placed.

Step 2

Through a low Pfannenstiel skin incision, the anterior rectus fascia is entered and the rectus abdominus muscles are bluntly separated from the underlying peritoneum. After a self-retaining retractor is placed beneath the muscles and opened, the retropubic space is entered and exposed. This is initially done by bluntly separating the loose areolar tissue as it extends from the pubic symphysis to the ischial ramus bilaterally (*Fig. 2.2*). The dissection is carried deeper to the level of the anterior vaginal wall, pushing the bladder medially and cephalad (*Fig. 2.3*). Vigorous dissection is avoided in the midline over the delicate urethral structures. Once the urethra, bladder, and vagina have been dropped downward, Cooper's ligament is easily visualized laterally and the large Foley bulb is evident centrally, used as a reference point for the urethrovesical junction (*Fig. 2.4*).

Step 3

The fat overlying the anterior vaginal wall and lateral pelvic sidewall is removed to allow direct contact of tissue surfaces and thus to promote adherence. Removal of fat is aided by pushing the anterior vaginal wall upwards with two fingers in the vagina (*Fig. 2.5*). The fat overlying the urethra is avoided. The inferior margin of the bladder is then pushed upward. This can be facilitated by having the vaginal hand push upwards just lateral to the urethrovesical junction and using a Kitner to dissect against the fingertips (*Fig. 2.6*).

Step 4

Once the fat has been removed and the bladder mobilized upward, placement of sutures can be performed. An O-coated polyester suture on a tapered needle is initially placed at the level of the urethrovesical junction, as far lateral as possible, and almost full thickness through the vaginal wall (*Fig. 2.7*). A figure-of-eight pass is preferred. A similarly placed suture is passed about 1 cm distal to the initial suture (*Fig. 2.8*). The

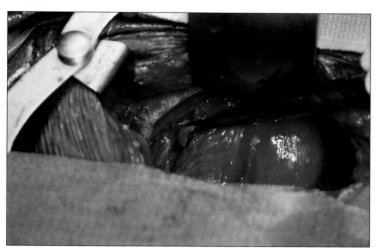

2.5 Removal of fat.

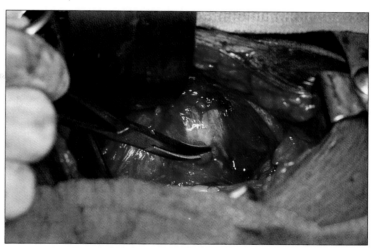

2.6 Application of a Kitner against the fingertips.

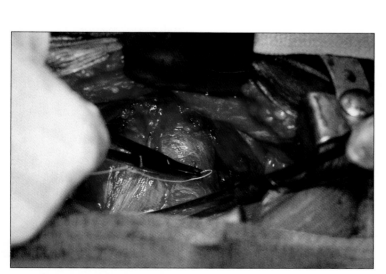

2.7 Placement of a suture at the urethrovesical junction.

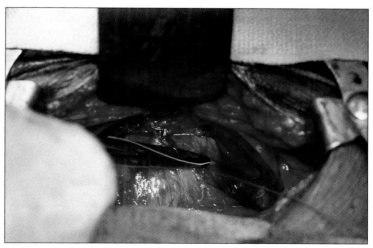

2.8 Second ipsilateral suture placed 1 cm distal.

same procedure is completed on the opposite side (*Fig. 2.9*).

Step 5

After all of the sutures have been placed through the vaginal wall, both ends of each suture are passed through Cooper's ligament. Using a No.6 Mayo needle, the most distal suture is first passed through the ligament at a point almost directly lateral to its origin in the vaginal wall (*Fig. 2.10*). The remaining ends of sutures on the ipsilateral side are successively passed through Cooper's ligament, spacing them by about 0.5–1 cm (*Fig. 2.11*). The same procedure is completed on the contralateral side (*Fig. 2.12*). Care must be taken with the most proximal suture placement, as the external iliac artery and its anastomosis with the inferior epigastric artery are in close proximity.

Step 6

Once all of the suture ends have been placed through Cooper's ligament, the vagina is elevated and the sutures are tied (*Fig. 2.13*). Because no accurate means exists to judge the correct degree of elevation of the vesical neck, the operator's vaginal hand pushes upwards at the level of the urethrovesical junction, simulating a 0° angle from horizontal as if a Q-tip had been passed transurethrally. This is maintained while both distal sutures are initially tied. Both proximal sutures are then tied. The operator can ask the assistant to make adjustments in tension on the sutures before securing the knots by feeling the vesical neck elevation with the vaginal hand. To avoid overelevation, one finger should be able to pass between the urethra and the symphysis pubis. Typically, "banjo strings" of sutures can be seen once the sutures are tied and cut (*Fig. 2.14*).

Step 7

A suprapubic catheter is placed in the bladder after retrograde filling has been completed with about 400 ml of sterile water or saline. We prefer a percutaneous trocar-type catheter with an inflatable balloon on the end (*Figs 2.15, 2.16*). This is simply passed through the abdominal wall, 3–4 cm above the midline of the incision, and is inserted into the bladder (*Fig. 2.17*). After the stylet has been removed and the balloon distended, the retropubic space is irrigated and the abdominal incision closed.

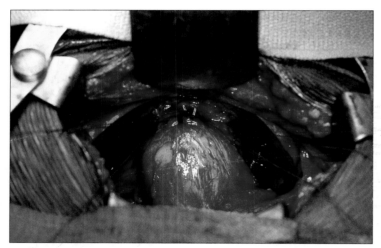

2.9 Same procedure as in **2.8**, completed on opposite side.

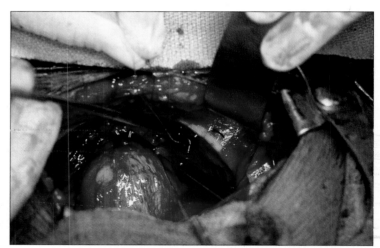

2.10 Passage of most distal suture through Cooper's ligament.

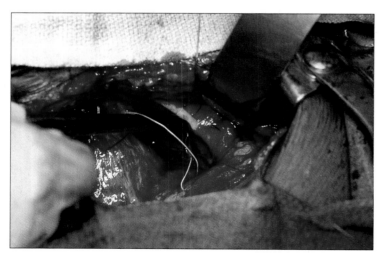

2.11 Remaining ipsilateral sutures are passed though Cooper's ligament.

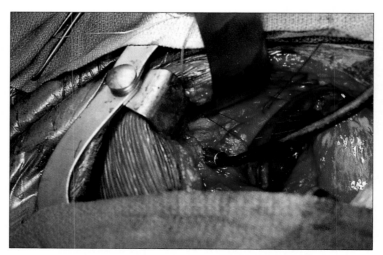

2.12 Same procedure as in **2.10, 2.11**, completed on contralateral side.

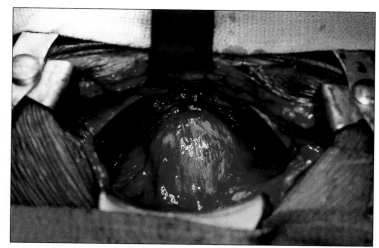

2.13 The sutures are tied when all the ends have been passed through Cooper's ligament.

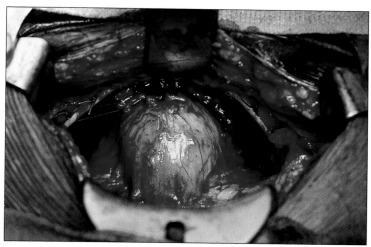

2.14 "Banjo strings" of sutures.

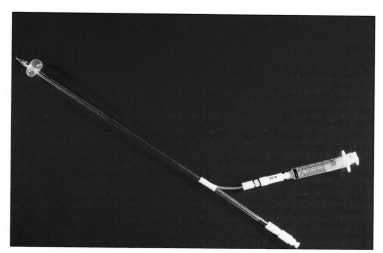

2.15 Percutaneous trocar-type catheter.

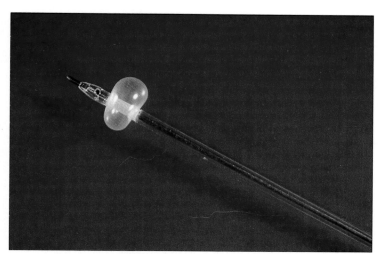

2.16 Inflatable balloon at the end of the catheter shown in **2.15**.

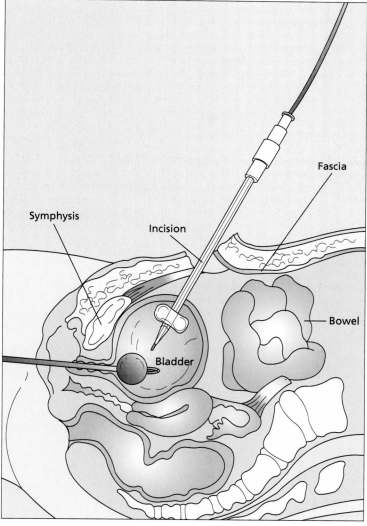

2.17 Insertion of catheter shown in **2.15** into the bladder.

COMPLICATIONS

Complications particular to the Burch procedure can be categorized as those that occur intraoperatively and those that become manifest postoperatively (*Fig. 2.18*).

MODIFIED PEREYRA PROCEDURE

The first needle suspension of the vesical neck for the treatment of stress urinary incontinence was described by Armand Pereyra in 1959[4]. Since that time, many other types of needle suspensions have been described, all variations of Pereyra's original work[5,6]. In general, the cure rates for stress urinary incontinence using the modified Pereyra procedure range from 84 to 97%.

Complications of the Burch Procedure	
A. Intraoperative complications	**B. Postoperative complications**

1. Hemorrhage from
  a. Vaginal venous plexus
  b. Accessory obturator artery
	1. Retropubic hematoma

	2. Infection
	  a. Retropubic abscess
	  b. Osteitis pubis

2. Bladder injury
  a. Laceration or cystotomy
  b. Suture through bladder
	3. Voiding dysfunction
	  secondary to vesical neck
	  elevation

3. Urethral injury
  a. Laceration
  b. Suture through urethra
	4. Ureteral obstruction

	5. Enterocele formation

2.18 Complications particular to the Burch procedure.

SURGICAL INDICATIONS

Utilizing a transvaginal approach, the modified Pereyra procedure is frequently combined with other surgical procedures used to correct genital prolapse. However, needle suspensions are also employed when associated pelvic relaxation is minimal. The indications for the modified Pereyra procedure are:

- Primary stress urinary incontinence.
- Recurrent stress urinary incontinence associated with vesical neck mobility.
- Stress urinary incontinence associated with moderate to severe urogenital prolapse.
- Combination with repair of vault prolapse when manual reduction of the vagina has demonstrated stress incontinence.

SURGICAL PROCEDURE

The operation is performed with the patient in the lithotomy position. Either general or regional anesthesia can be used. The lower abdomen, vagina, and perineum are prepped and draped; an adhesive barrier drape is valuable to cover the lower abdomen and perineum. A Foley catheter is inserted.

Step 1

An inverted-T shaped anterior vaginal wall incision is made. After the transverse portion of this incision has been made with a scalpel, the anterior vaginal wall is undermined to create a vertical midline incision, extending to within 1.5 cm of the external urethral meatus (*Fig. 2.19*).

Step 2

Using sharp and blunt dissection techniques, the underlying vesical, perivesical, and periurethral fasciae are gently separated from the vaginal mucosa. This dissection is carried to the ischial rami (*Fig. 2.20*).

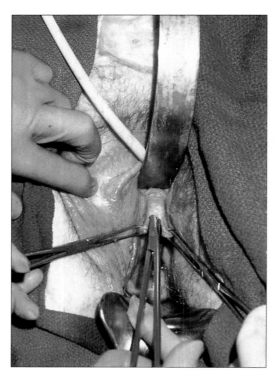

2.19 An inverted-T shaped incision into the anterior vaginal wall.

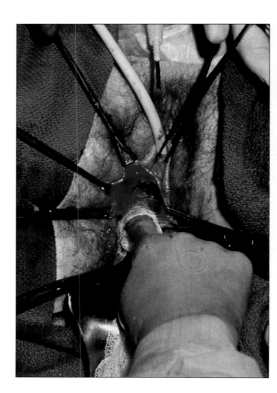

2.20 Separation of the vesical, perivesical, and periurethral fasciae from the vaginal mucosa.

Step 3

Directing the index finger anterolaterally, the urogenital diaphragm is gently penetrated, maintaining contact with the inner aspect of the ischial ramus (*Figs 2.21, 2.22*). This step is completed on each side of the urethra, gaining access to the retropubic space.

Step 4

The band of endopelvic fascia created along the urethra is identified and grasped (*Fig. 2.23*). The bulb of the Foley catheter is palpated to locate the urethrovesical junction. A helical suture of O-prolene is run through the periurethral fascia from the urethrovesical junction to the posterior pubourethral ligament (*Fig. 2.24*). This step is repeated on the opposite side, and the ends are secured with hemostats.

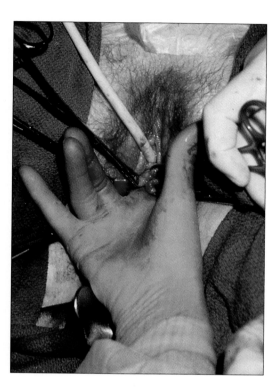

2.21 Penetration of the urogenital diaphragm by anterolaterally directed index finger.

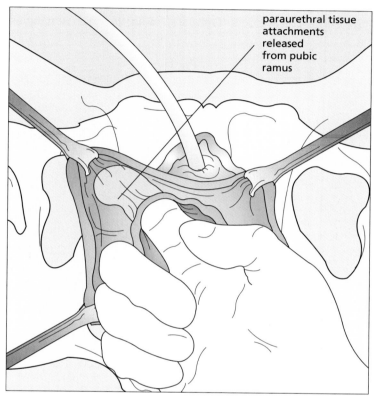

paraurethral tissue attachments released from pubic ramus

2.22 The index finger maintains contact with the inner aspect of the ischial ramus, gaining access to the retropubic space.

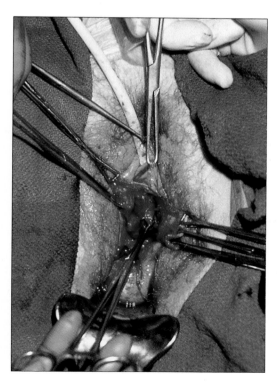

2.23 The band of endopelvic fascia is grasped.

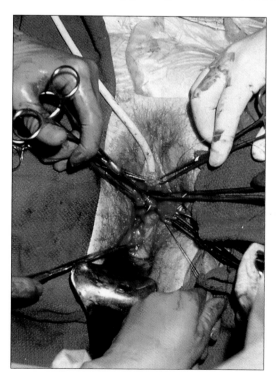

2.24 A suture is placed from the urethrovesical junction to the pubourethral ligament.

Step 5

A 3 cm transverse abdominal incision is made just above the pubic symphysis (*Fig. 2.25*). The incision is taken through the subcutaneous tissue to the level of the rectus fascia.

Step 6

A 0–15° Stamey needle is placed at one corner of the abdominal incision. The index finger of the other hand is in inserted through the vaginal incision on the same side and into the retropubic space. With the vaginal finger, the tip of the needle is contacted through the rectus fascia (*Fig. 2.26*). With the finger serving as a guide, the needle penetrates the fascia adjacent to the ischial ramus and is led through the retropubic space, constantly in contact with the finger. When the needle enters the vaginal field, the ends of the permanent suture from the same side are passed through the hole in the needle tip (*Fig. 2.27*).

Step 7

Once the carrier needle has been passed into the vagina on each side of the urethra, the ends of the prolene sutures are pulled back up into the abdominal field. The ends of the sutures are secured with hemostats (*Fig. 2.28*).

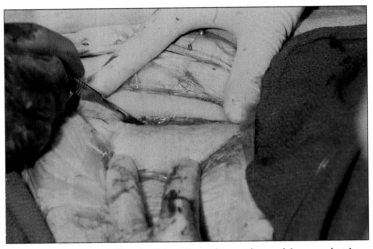

2.25 Transverse abdominal incision above the pubic symphysis.

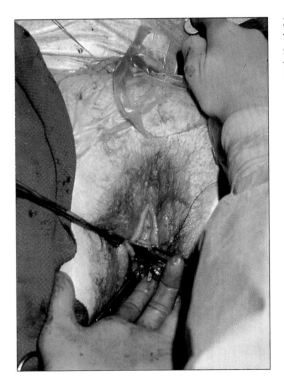

2.27 The ends of the permanent suture are passed through the hole in the needle tip.

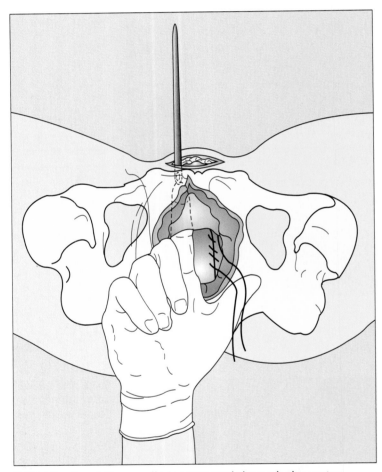

2.26 The tip of the needle is contacted through the rectus fascia with the vaginal finger.

Step 8

After the periurethral sutures have been pulled into the abdominal field, the Foley catheter is removed and cystoscopy is performed to rule out passage of suture or needles through the bladder and urethra. With the bladder full and the cystoscope in place, a percutaneous suprapubic catheter is inserted under direct visualization (*Fig. 2.29*).

Step 9

Before tension on the periurethral sutures is adjusted, the anterior vaginal mucosa is closed with an interrupted #2-0 polyglycolic acid suture (*Fig. 2.30*).

Step 10

Adjustment of the periurethral sutures is performed under urethroscopic guidance. With a 0-15° cystoscopic lens, the tip of the scope is placed just distal to the urethrovesical junction. An assistant then elevates the sutures (*Fig. 2.31*) until the anterior and posterior urethral mucosa will coapt. Tension is maintained while one end of the suture of each side is passed through the rectus fascia with a Mayo-type needle. The sutures on each side are then tied and cut. The skin is closed in a subcuticular fashion. The placement of a vaginal pack completes the operation.

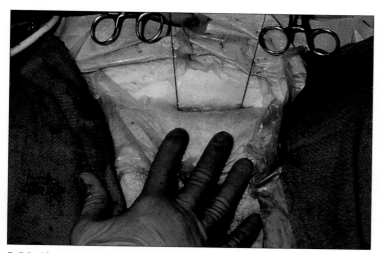

2.28 The ends of the sutures are secured with hemostats.

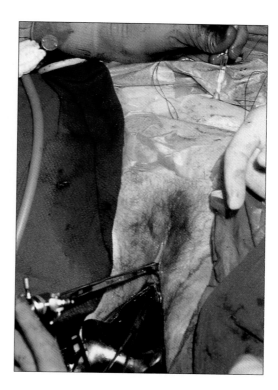

2.29 Insertion of a percutaneous suprapubic catheter under direct visualization.

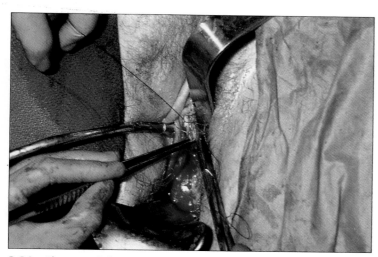

2.30 Closure of the anterior vaginal mucosa.

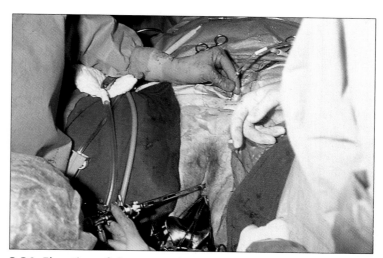

2.31 Elevation of the sutures by an assistant.

PARAVAGINAL REPAIR

Correction of a cystocele with the paravaginal repair is based on the premise that the cystocele results from separation of the pubocervical fascia of the paracolpium from its lateral attachment to the pelvic sidewall. This site of lateral attachment is the arcus tendoneous fascia pelvis (white line). When genuine stress incontinence accompanies a defect resulting from this lateral detachment, the paravaginal repair has been reported to provide success rates of 95% in correcting involuntary urine loss. By reattaching the lateral sulcus of the vagina to the white line, normal anatomy is said to be re-established, thereby restoring continence.

SURGICAL INDICATIONS

Paravaginal repair is indicated both for cystocele resulting from a paravaginal defect and for stress urinary incontinence accompanying a paravaginal defect[7,8].

ANATOMICAL CONSIDERATIONS

A thorough understanding of the anatomic relationships is necessary if the surgeon is to achieve a successful repair. *Fig. 2.32* demonstrates how the bladder lies superior to and is supported by the pubocervical fascia, which attaches to the lateral pelvic sidewalls. This fascial plane encircles the vagina, which is attached laterally to the tendinous arch of the pelvic fascia (white line). The tendinous arch of the pubocervical fascia (white line) is anatomically the tendinous aponeurosis of the obturator internus and levator ani muscles.

SURGICAL PROCEDURE

Step 1

Before selecting the operation for correction of stress urinary incontinence, documentation of a paravaginal defect is necessary. By use of a Sims-type speculum, a cystocele can be demonstrated (*Fig. 2.33*). A paravaginal defect is present if the cystocele is reduced by elevation of the lateral sulci (*Fig. 2.34*).

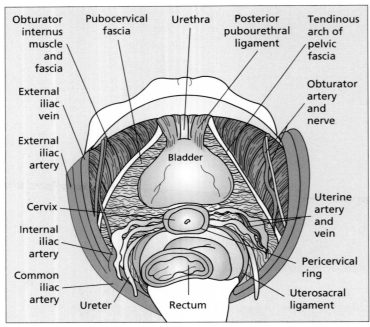

2.32 Position of bladder relative to pubocervical fascia.

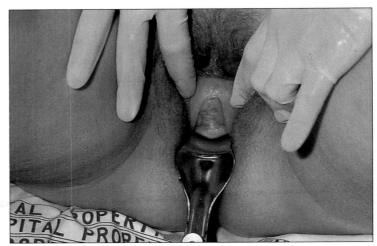

2.33 Demonstration of a cystocele with the use of a Sims-type speculum.

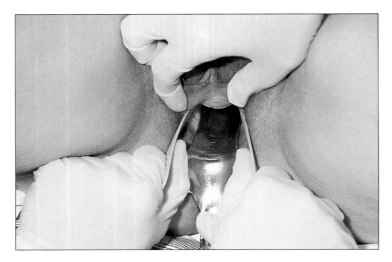

2.34 Reduction of the cystocele by elevation of the lateral sulci indicates a paravaginal defect.

Step 2

The patient is placed in the supine lithotomy position. We prefer to support the legs with Allen Universal stirrups, as this allows low placement of the thighs and provides easy access for cystoscopy if this becomes necessary later in the operation (*Fig. 2.35*). The perineum, vagina, and lower abdomen are prepped, and a three-way transurethral Foley catheter with a 20 ml balloon is inserted transurethrally. Drapes are appropriately placed.

Step 3

Through a Pfannenstiel skin incision, the anterior fascia is entered and the rectus muscles are separated from the underlying peritoneum (the procedure illustrated in this chapter followed an abdominal hysterectomy). After placement of a self-retaining retractor, the retropubic space is entered by bluntly separating the transversalis fascia and loose areolar tissue from the pubis and ischial rami (*Fig. 2.36*). The space is further exposed by

placement of a hand into the vagina for elevation and then pushing the bladder medially and cephalad (*Fig. 2.37*).

Step 4

The fat in the retropubic space is removed from the underlying vagina and lateral pelvic sidewalls, taking care to avoid the urethra. This exposes the lateral sulcus of the vagina and its separation from the sidewall. In many cases, the arcus tendoneus fascia pelvis is not well visualized. However, its location runs from the inferior aspect of the pubic symphysis to the ischial spine (*Fig. 2.38*).

Step 5

On each side of the vagina, the first stitch will determine placement of the remaining sutures. With a hand placed in the vagina, the lateral sulcus of the vagina is elevated at the level of the vesical neck and a suture of 2-0 coated polyester is placed full-thickness

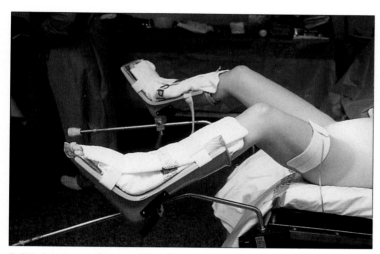

2.35 Support of legs with Allen Universal stirrups.

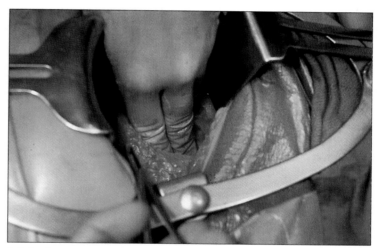

2.36 Blunt separation of the transversalis fascia and loose areolar tissue from the pubis and ischial rami.

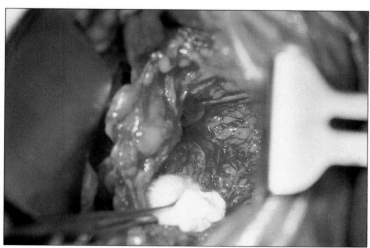

2.37 Further exposure of the space.

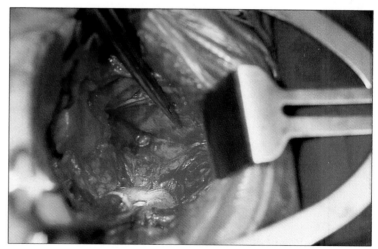

2.38 Location of arcus tendoneus fascia pelvis.

through the lateral sulcus (*Fig. 2.39*). With the needle still held by the needle holder, traction is directed back and toward the arcus tendoneus fascia pelvis until the external urethral meatus is felt to be drawn beneath the pubic symphysis. This is the point at which the suture is placed through the white line (*Fig. 2.40*). The suture is held and not tied.

Step 6

With the intial stich complete, additional sutures are similarly placed, full-thickness through the lateral vaginal sulcus and then to the fascia of the pelvic sidewall (*Fig. 2.41*). Sutures are spaced about 1 cm apart, both dorsally and ventrally. The final stitches are placed 1 cm from the pubic symphysis and 1 cm from the ischial spine (*Fig. 2.42*).

Step 7

Similar rows of sutures are placed along both lateral sulci of the vagina (*Fig. 2.43*). Once these are completed, all sutures are tied and cut, reattaching the lateral sulcus of each side of the vagina to the pelvic sidewall (*Fig. 2.44*). Before the abdomen is closed, a suprapubic catheter can be placed.

COMPLICATIONS

Obvious complications include bladder injury and the potential for infection. One must be cautious not to place sutures too cephalad on the tendinous arch. *Fig. 2.32* shows the relationship of the ureter in this area as it courses to the bladder. Because of this close approximation, ureteral injury is possible.

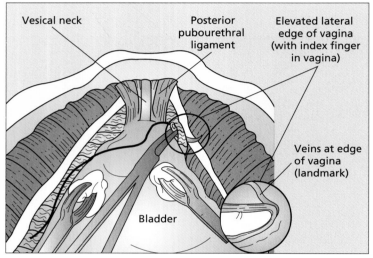

2.39 Placement of suture through the lateral sulcus.

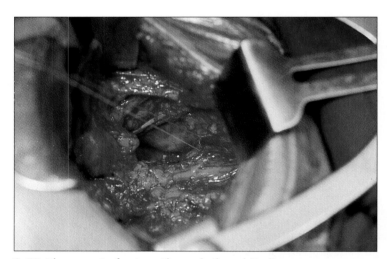

2.40 Placement of suture through the white line.

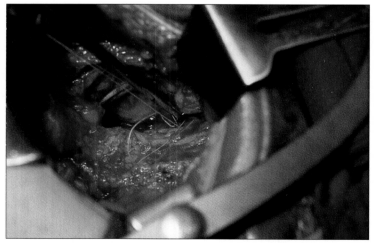

2.41 Placement of additional sutures through the lateral vaginal sulcus to the fascia of the pelvic sidewall.

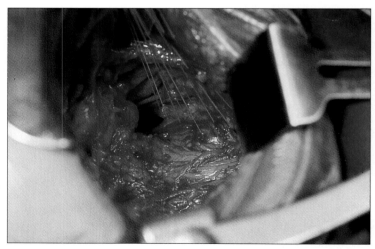

2.42 Placement of final sutures.

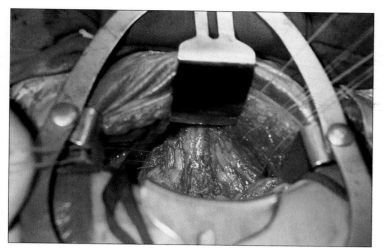

2.43 Placement of rows of sutures along both lateral sulci of the vagina.

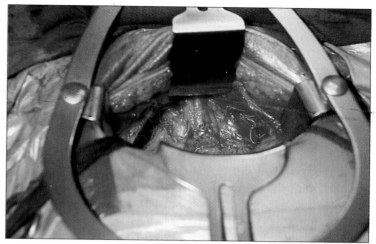

2.44 Reattachment of each lateral sulcus of the vagina to the pelvic sidewall.

SPENCE PROCEDURE

Surgical excision is the principal operative treatment for urethral diverticula[9]. Although success rates are usually good, the operation may require extensive dissection and occasionally results in significant blood loss. In addition, the postoperative development of urethrovaginal fistulae has been reported, with frequencies ranging from 1 to 4%[10].

In 1970, Spence and Duckett[9] described a simplified surgical approach to the treatment of select urethral diverticula in which dissection of the diverticulum is avoided.

SURGICAL INDICATIONS
To avoid complications such as postoperative stress incontinence, candidates for the Spence procedure should be properly selected[11]. The indication for this procedure is a single urethral diverticulum in the distal third of the urethra.

SURGICAL PROCEDURE
The patient is placed in the supine lithotomy position. General, regional, or local anesthesia can be used. The vagina and perineum are prepped and draped, and the bladder is emptied. An indwelling catheter is not used as this would obstruct surgery and the patient can usually void postoperatively.

Step 1
The diverticulum is examined to determine its full anatomic extent (*Figs 2.45, 2.46*).

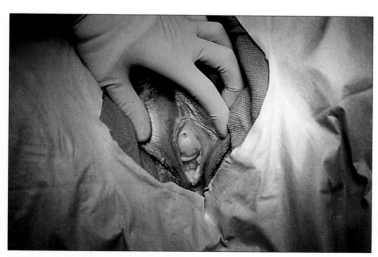

2.45 Examination of the diverticulum.

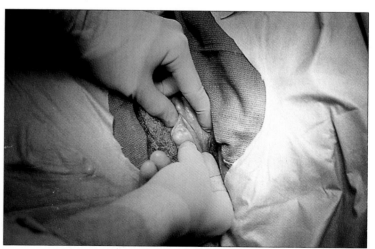

2.46 Examination of the diverticulum.

Step 2

After the diverticulum has been stabilized, a division of the floor of the urethra, between the external meatus and the diverticular orifice, is made by creating a midline incision of the diverticulum and the underlying vaginal wall. This is simply done by placing one blade of Metzenbaum scissors inside the urethra to the diverticular orifice and incising cleanly (*Figs 2.47, 2.48*).

Step 3

Once the incision has been made and any contents evacuated, coaptation of the epithelial margins of the diverticulum to the vaginal mucosa is performed, "saucerizing" the base of the diverticulum. This is performed by using #3-0 polyglactin suture in an interrupted fashion (*Fig. 2.49*). A running suture can also be used.

Step 4

Once all sutures have been placed and tied, the area should be inspected for hemostasis (*Fig. 2.50*). Again, no catheterization of the bladder is needed.

ALTERNATIVE PROCEDURES

Non-surgical procedures include observation if the patient is asymptomatic, and antibiotic therapy. The surgical procedure of choice is excision of the urethral diverticulum.

COMPLICATIONS

The incidence of complications is low with the Spence procedure. The following are complications that are particular to this operation:

- Postoperative stress incontinence. This results from an over-aggressive incision into the urethra in which the urethral sphincter is bisected. This can be avoided by proper selection of surgical candidates (e.g., diverticulum in distal third of the urethra) and by cutting no farther than the ostium of the diverticulum.
- Voiding dysfunction (spraying or stream deviation). This results from an inadequate incision in which the diverticulum is not completely saucerized and a pouch is created. An incision to the ostium avoids this complication.

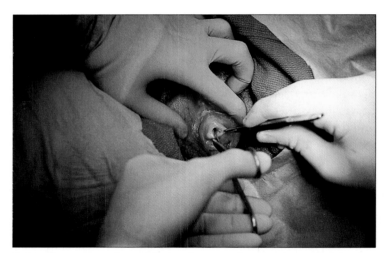

2.47 Placement of one blade of Metsenbaum scissors inside the urethra to the diverticulum orifice.

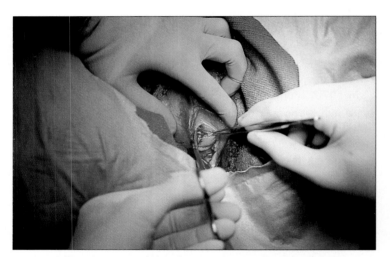

2.48 Midline incision of the diverticulum and vaginal wall.

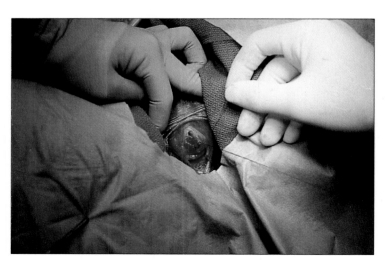

2.49 Coaptation of the epithelial margins of the diverticulum to the vaginal mucosa.

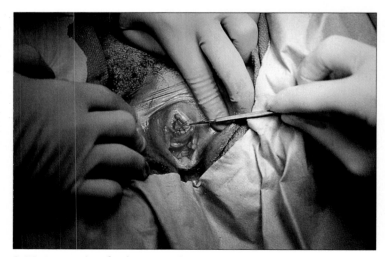

2.50 Inspection for hemostasis.

FASCIAL SUBURETHRAL SLING

In cases of complex urinary stress incontinence, such as those associated with recurrent surgical failures or intrinsic urethral sphincter deficiency, standard abdominal retropubic urethropexies and endoscopic needle suspensions may not provide acceptable cure rates. For these more difficult disorders, the suburethral sling may provide cure rates in excess of 85–90%.

Goebel, in 1910, was one of the first surgeons to utilize a sling, fashioned from pyramidalis muscle, beneath the urethra to treat stress incontinence[12]. Since that time, many modifications of sling procedures have been reported[13,14]. Both autologous (e.g., fascia, muscle, dura) and artificial (e.g., Marlex, Mersilene, Goretex, Silastic) materials have been used to create the sling.

The suburethral sling functions to restore continence by providing adequate support for the urethra within the abdominal sphere when the surrounding tissues are too weak or scarred to give such support. The sling also provides a stable base beneath the urethra, which causes compression of the lumen when abdominal pressure rises. In some cases the sling performs an obstructive function, maintaining continence by means of high urethral resistance. Because of its physiologic properties in restoring continence, complications related to obstruction and excessive pressure on the urethra may result.

SURGICAL INDICATIONS
These include:
- Recurrent urinary stress incontinence.
- Stress incontinence associated with intrinsic sphincter deficiency and the presence of urethral hypermobility.
- Stress incontinence associated with neurologic disorders such as myelodysplasia.

SURGICAL PROCEDURE
The patient is placed in the dorsal lithotomy position with the legs well supported and the lower abdomen exposed widely enough for a low transverse incision to be made. The vagina, perineum, and lower abdomen are prepped and then draped using an adhesive barrier. A transurethral Foley catheter is inserted for bladder drainage and to locate the urethrovesical junction.

Step 1
The first step of the procedure is to harvest the fascial strip that will be used for the sling. A wide Pfannenstiel skin incision is made and the subcutaneous tissue is then bluntly removed from the underlying rectus fascia. Two parallel transverse incisions in the anterior rectus fascia are made, about 2 cm apart and 20 cm in length (*Fig. 2.51*). Before the fascial strip is severed from the rectus sheath, mattress sutures of monofilament O-polypropylene are passed through each end. The strip is then placed in a saline basin until later in the procedure (*Fig. 2.52*). The remaining rectus fascial incision is then closed (*Fig. 2.53*).

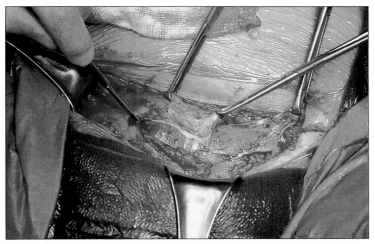

2.51 Parallel transverse incisions in the anterior rectus fascia, to harvest a fascial strip.

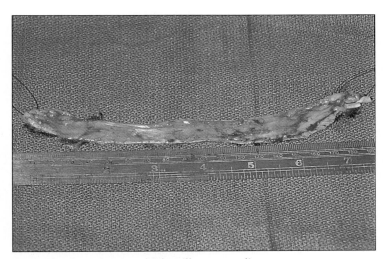

2.52 The fascial strip which will act as a sling.

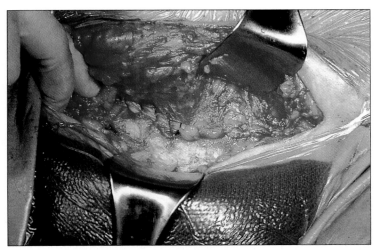

2.53 Closure of remaining rectus fascial incision.

Step 2

The vaginal operating field is now developed. After a weighted speculum has been placed into the vagina, a midline anterior vaginal wall incision is made using an undermining technique. After the bladder and connective tissue have been dissected from the anterior vaginal mucosa, the bladder base, urethrovesical junction, and proximal urethra are exposed (*Fig. 2.54*). Using blunt dissection, the retropubic space is then entered on each side of the urethra by perforating the endopelvic fascia (as in the modified Pereyra procedure) at its attachment to the pubic ramus (*Fig. 2.55*). An opening of 3–4 cm must be created on each side.

Step 3

The sling material is secured in place over the urethrovesical junction before elevating the arms of the sling. The urethrovesical junction is located by palpating the Foley catheter balloon. The fascial sling is then attached at its midportion to this point of the urethra so that it equally covers the proximal and distal portion of the junction. It is secured at four points over the urethrovesical junction with interrupted #2-0 polyglycolic acid sutures (*Figs 2.56, 2.57*).

Step 4

The arms of the sling are now elevated into the abdominal incision. First, two 1 cm incisions are made in the rectus fascia just superior to the pubic rami on each side of the midline. Long reverse-curved DeBakey clamps (*Fig. 2.58*) are then passed down through these incisions, guided with an index finger placed through the vagina, until the tips reach the vaginal field (*Fig. 2.59*). The polypropylene sutures attached to the ends of the sling are grasped by the appropriate clamp and are drawn upward into the abdominal field (*Figs 2.60, 2.61*). Cystoscopy is then performed to exclude injury to the bladder or urethra. A suprapubic catheter is also inserted at this point, using the cystoscope for guidance (*Fig. 2.62*).

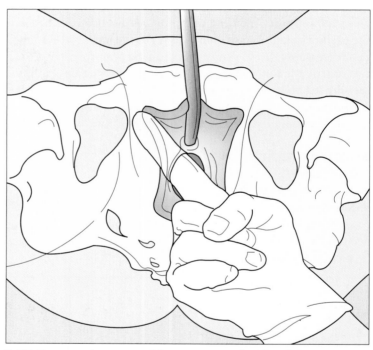

2.55 Entry to the retropubic space on each side of the urethra.

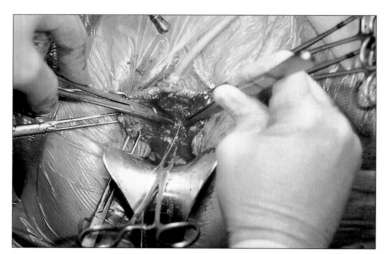

2.54 Exposure of the bladder base, urethrovesical junction, and proximal urethra.

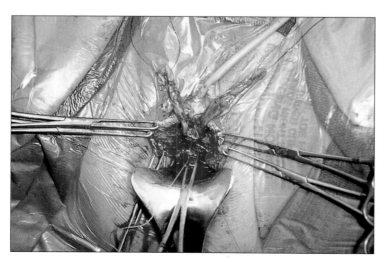

2.56 Attachment of the fascial sling to the urethra.

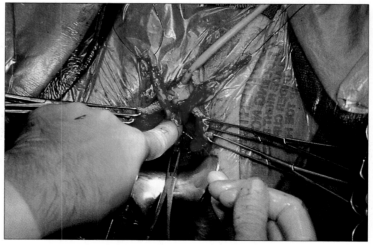

2.57 Fascial sling secured at four points over the urethrovesical junction.

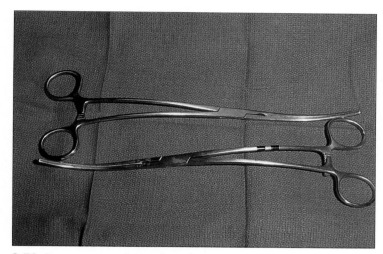

2.58 Reverse-curved DeBakey clamps.

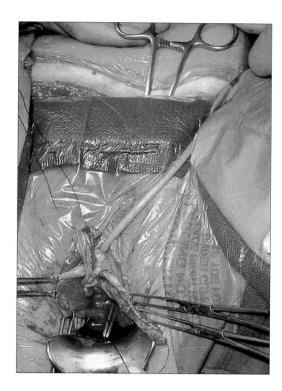

2.59 The clamps are passed down through the incisions until the tips reach the vaginal field.

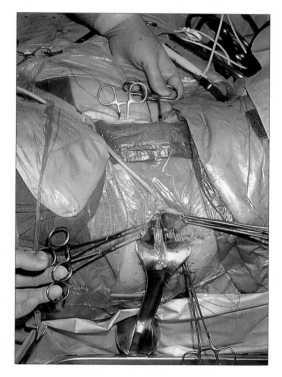

2.60 The sutures attached to the ends of the sling are drawn upward into the abdominal field.

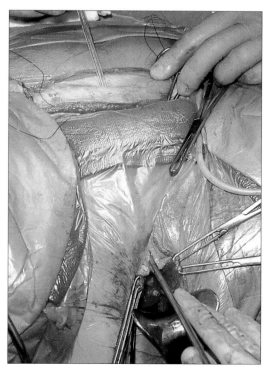

2.62 Insertion of suprapubic catheter.

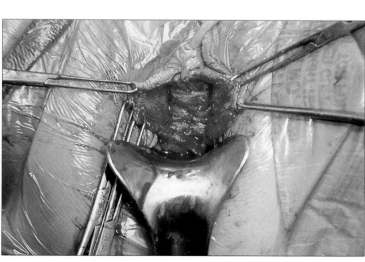

2.61 Sling in place over urethra with ends of sling drawn to the abdominal field.

Step 5

Before the sling is secured in place, the anterior vaginal wall is closed (*Fig. 2.63*). Then, using the polypropylene sutures and a No. 6 Mayo needle, the ends of the sling are sutured to the rectus fascia (*Fig. 2.64*) taking care to avoid placing any tension on the sling. The abdominal incision is closed and the vagina is packed for 24 hours.

ALTERNATIVE PROCEDURES

- Fascial lata suburethral sling: after the fascia lata strip has been harvested, the procedure followed is identical to the one previously described.
- Artificial suburethral sling using Marlex, Mersiline, Goretex, or Silastic: the advantages include easy accessibility of the material and shorter operating time. However, foreign material reactions may take place.
- Artificial urethral sphincter.

COMPLICATIONS

- Urethral obstruction: this complication is avoided by placing no tension on the sling. However, if it occurs, it can be treated with intermittent self-catheterization until voiding resumes. In rare instances, release of the sling may be necessary.
- Detrusor instability: this postoperative complication may occur in 10–30% of patients. It is usually the result of relative urethral obstruction. In most cases it can be treated with anticholinergic medications and/or bladder retraining drills.
- Urethral or vaginal erosion: this usually results from excessive sling tension and is most common with artificial sling materials. It may require loosening or removal of the sling combined with a reconstructive procedure.
- Recurrent urinary tract infection: this usually results from incomplete voiding in the postoperative period. Routine antibiotic therapy will suffice in most cases.

ANTERIOR COLPORRHAPHY

Howard Kelly first reported a repair of stress urinary incontinence and anterior vaginal wall prolapse in 1913, describing the use of vertical mattress sutures beneath the urethra and bladder[15]. Since that time, many modifications of the procedure have been described, primarily focusing on management of the urethra and the use of different suture materials.

Although anterior colporrhaphy has proven successful for the long-term correction of cystocele, it has been replaced in many hands by retropubic urethropexies for the treatment of stress urinary incontinence. However, reports by Beck and by Nichols still show good success rates for the treatment of stress incontinence when steps are added to elevate the urethrovesical junction to a high retropubic position[16,17].

SURGICAL INDICATIONS

Among the surgical indications for anterior colporrhaphy are anterior vaginal wall prolapse (cystocele) and mild urinary stress incontinence.

SURGICAL PROCEDURE

The following description is of our own method for anterior colporrhaphy. The reader should review other techniques to obtain a broad overview of this old and common operation.

The patient is placed in the supine lithotomy position with the feet well elevated. The perineum and vagina are prepped and draped and the bladder is emptied. An indwelling catheter is not used during surgery.

Step 1

After thorough examination under anesthesia, a weighted speculum is placed into the vagina, exposing the anterior vaginal wall and cystocele (*Fig. 2.65*). The vaginal apex is grasped with two Allis clamps and drawn forward. A transverse incision of the

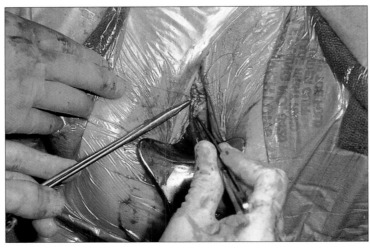

2.63 Closure of the anterior vaginal wall.

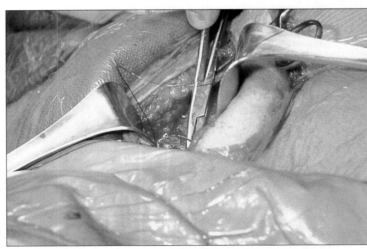

2.64 Attachment of the ends of the sling to the rectus fascia.

vaginal mucosa is made between the Allis clamps, taking care to avoid the underlying bladder (*Fig. 2.66*). Using Metzenbaum scissors, the full thickness of the vaginal epithelium is undermined along the midline of the anterior vaginal wall, maintaining the dissection in the vesicovaginal space (*Fig. 2.67*). As the dissection proceeds toward the urethral meatus, a midline incision is made through the exposed space (*Fig. 2.68*). The incision is continued to within 1–1.5 cm of the external urethral meatus, maintaining

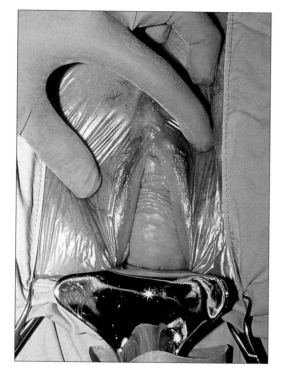

2.65 Insertion of weighted speculum into the vagina.

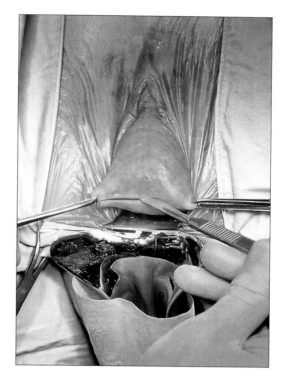

2.66 Transverse incision of the vaginal mucosa.

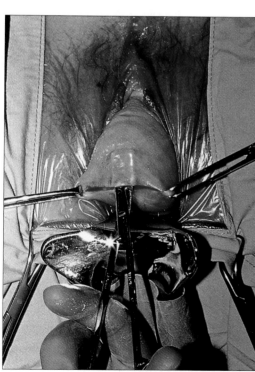

2.67 Dissection into the vesicovaginal space with Metzenbaum scissors.

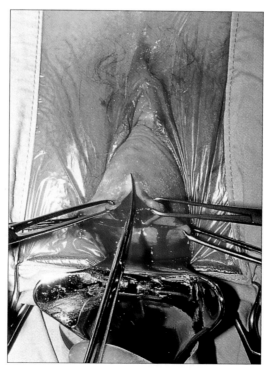

2.68 Midline incision through the exposed space.

attachment of the fibromuscular connective tissue to the vaginal mucosa (*Fig. 2.69*).

Step 2

We prefer to detach the fibromuscular connective tissue from the underside of the vaginal mucosa so that it can be plicated over the bladder herniation, effectively narrowing the prolapse and creating a fibrous shelf beneath the bladder. The fibrous tissue is dissected away from the vaginal mucosa with Metzenbaum scissors, keeping the operator's index finger on the other side of

the mucosa to prevent inadvertent perforation. The tip of the scissors can be slipped beneath the connective tissue attachments, freeing the tissue along the entire length of the anterior vaginal incision (*Fig. 2.70*). Once the dissection has achieved a cleavage plane on each side of the vaginal wall, the fibrous tissue can be pushed off and forward with an open gauze sponge placed over the index finger (*Fig. 2.71*). The tissue is pushed off from the apex of the vagina to the pubic ramus, freeing the underlying bladder from the vaginal walls (*Fig. 2.72*).

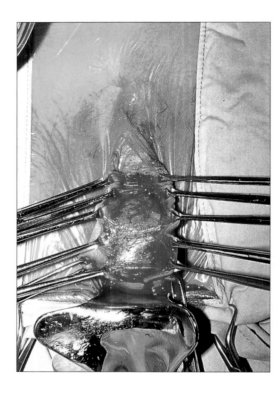

2.69 Incision continued to within 1–1.5 cm of the external urethral meatus.

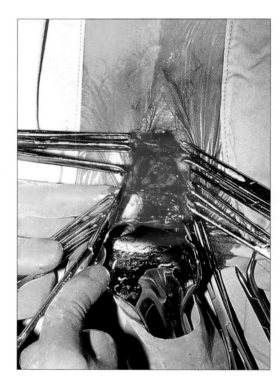

2.70 Use of tip of scissors to free the connective tissue along the length of the anterior vaginal incision.

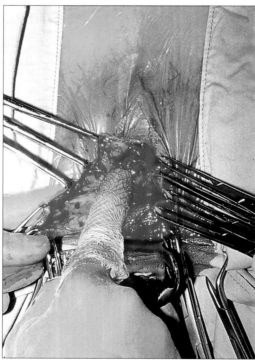

2.71 Open gauze sponge over index finger used to move the fibrous tissue.

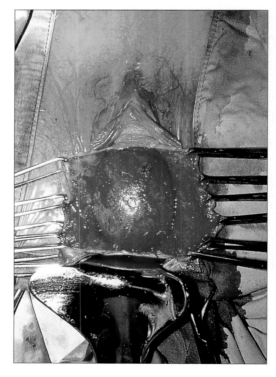

2.72 Underlying bladder freed from the vaginal walls.

Step 3

Plication of the fibrous tissue overlying the bladder is performed using vertical mattress sutures of a delayed absorbable material such as 2-0 polyglycolic acid. Beginning inferiorly, the curved needle of the suture is passed vertically through the fibrous tissue as far lateral as possible on the bladder (*Fig. 2.73*). The suture is then passed through the connective tissue on the other side of the bladder and tied (*Figs 2.74, 2.75*). This plication technique is carried superiorly towards the urethrovesical junction, serially narrowing the cystocele. If a second outer row of imbricating sutures can be placed, this is performed at this point of the operation (*Fig. 2.76*).

Step 4

Although this particular procedure was not performed for stress incontinence, a step to elevate the vesical neck is performed at this time if stress urinary incontinence is noted preoperatively. We prefer to plicate the pubourethral ligaments beneath the urethrovesical

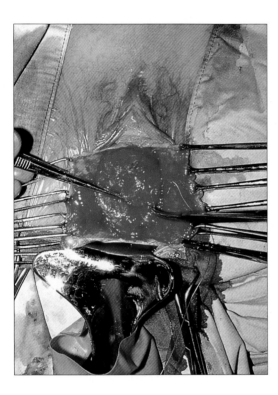

2.73 The curved needle of the suture passed vertically through the fibrous tissue.

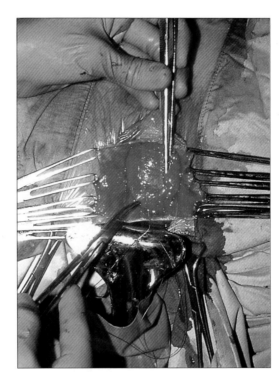

2.74 The suture passed through other side of the bladder.

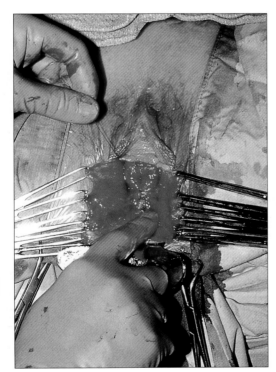

2.75 Suture tied.

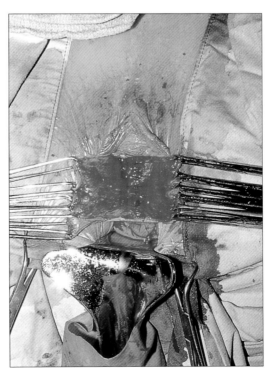

2.76 Placement of an outer row of imbricating sutures.

junction. The ligaments are grasped on each side of the urethra with Kocher clamps and then approximated with a mattress stitch of #2-0 polyglycolic acid suture, effectively elevating the urethrovesical junction to a high retropubic position (*Fig. 2.77*). Some surgeons prefer using a permanent suture material such as Goretex.

Step 5

Once all plicating sutures have been placed and tied, the vaginal mucosa can be closed. Excess mucosa is first removed from each side of the incision with scissors (*Fig. 2.78*). The vagina can be closed with either a running or an interrupted suture technique (*Figs 2.79, 2.80*). At the completion of the procedure, an indwelling bladder catheter is inserted and the vagina is packed for 24 hours.

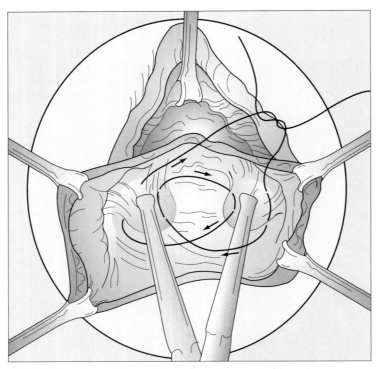

2.77 High retropubic position of urethrovesical junction.

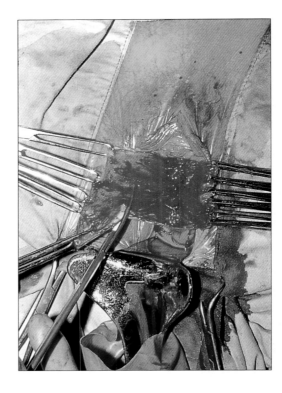

2.78 Removal of excess mucosa.

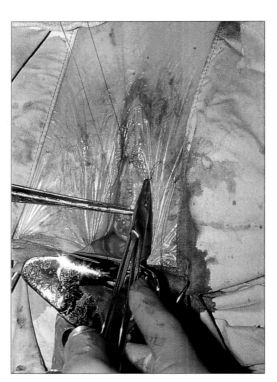

2.79 Closure of vagina.

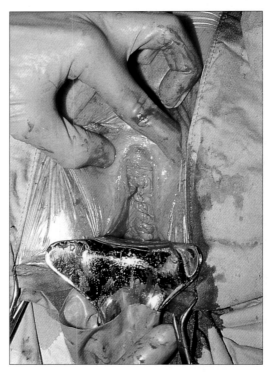

2.80 Closure of vagina.

ALTERNATIVE PROCEDURES

Non-surgical:

- Pessary: preferred pessaries include ring, doughnut, and Gelhorn types.

Surgical:

- Paravaginal fascial repair.
- Burch retropubic urethropexy.
- Endoscopic needle urethropexy.

COMPLICATIONS

The following is a list of complications particularly associated with anterior colporrhaphy:

- Cystotomy: this complication results from incorrect (too deep) development of the proper plane beneath the vaginal mucosa when the midline incision is created. Care must be taken to be superficial and to reach the relatively avascular vesicovaginal space.
- Ureteral obstruction: this complication may occur during repair of a very severe cystocele in which the ureters descend out of the bony pelvis. Care must be taken either to identify the ureters intraoperatively or to avoid extreme lateral and high placement of sutures.
- Postoperative voiding dysfunction: although delayed voiding is common after anterior colporrhaphy, obstruction of the urethra may occur as the result of overaggressive plication of the pubourethral ligaments. This complication is rare, and the surgeon's experience is important in avoiding this problem. In most cases, time allows resolution. However, a surgical takedown procedure may be necessary for prolonged voiding dysfunction beyond 6–8 weeks.

REFERENCES

1. Burch JC. Urethrovaginal fixation to Cooper's ligament for correction of stress incontinence, cystocele and prolapse. *Am J Obstet Gynecol* 1961;**81**:281–90.

2. Tanagho EA. Colopocystourethropexy: the way we do it. *J Urol* 1976;**116**:751–3.

3. Stanton SL, Williams JE, Ritchie D. The colposuspension operation for urinary incontinence. *Br J Obstet Gynaecol* 1976;**83**:890–5.

4. Pereyra AJ. A simplified surgical procedure for the correction of stress urinary incontinence in women. *West J Surg Obstet Gynecol* 1959;**67**:223–6.

5. Cornella JL, Ostergard DR. Needle suspension procedures for urinary stress incontinence: a review and historical perspective. *Obstet Gynecol Surv* 1990;**45**:805–16.

6. Karram MM, Bhatia NN. Transvaginal needle bladder neck procedures for stress urinary incontinence: a comprehensive review. *Obstet Gynecol* 1989;**73**:906–14.

7. Richardson AC, Lyon JB, Williams NL. A new look at pelvic relaxation. *Am J Obstet Gynecol* 1976;**126**:568–73.

8. Richardson AC, Edmonds PB, Williams NL. Treatment of urinary incontinence due to paravaginal fascial defect. *Obstet Gynecol* 1981;**57**:357–62.

9. Spence HM, Duckett JW. Diverticulum of the female urethra: clinical aspects and presentation of a simple operative technique for cure. *J Urol* 1970;**104**:432–7.

10. Davis BL, Robinson DG. Diverticula of the female urethra: assay of 120 cases. *J Urol* 1970;**104**:850–3.

11. Summitt RL, Stovall TG. Urethral diverticulum: evaluation by urethral pressure profilometry, cystourethroscopy, and the voiding cystourethrogram. *Obstet Gynecol* 1992;**80**:695–9.

12. Goebel R. Zur operativen Beseitigung der Angelborenen Incontinenz vesicae. *Zeitschr Gynek Urol* 1910;**2**:187.

13. Blaivas JG, Jacobs BZ. Pubovaginal fascial sling for the treatment of complicated stress urinary incontinence. *J Urol* 1991;**145**:1214–18.

14. Summitt RL, Bent AE, Ostergard DR, Harris TA. Suburethral sling procedure for genuine stress incontinence and low urethral closure pressure: a continued experience. *Int Urogynecol J* 1992;**3**:18–21.

15. Kelly HA. Incontinence of urine in women. *Urol Cutane Rev* 1913;**17**:291–3.

16. Beck RP, McCormick S. Treatment of urinary stress incontinence with anterior colporrhaphy. *Obstet Gynecol* 1982;**59**:269–74.

17. Nichols DH, Milley PS. Identification of pubourethral ligaments and their role in transvaginal surgical correction of stress incontinence. *Am J Obstet Gynecol* 1973;**115**:123–8.

3

Pelvic Support Defects: Surgical Correction

Robert L. Summitt, Jr.

Thomas G. Stovall

SACROSPINOUS LIGAMENT SUSPENSION OF THE VAGINAL VAULT INCLUDING VAGINAL REPAIR OF AN ENTEROCELE

Restoration of vaginal vault prolapse can be accomplished via both the abdominal and vaginal routes. Suspension of the vault through the vagina has the advantages of allowing simultaneous repair of various degrees of accompanying pelvic relaxation and decreased perioperative morbidity.

Sederl[1], in 1958, was the first to describe use of the sacrospinous ligament for fixation of the prolapsed vaginal vault. The procedure was further developed by Richter[2], in Germany, and Randall[3,4], in the United States. The sacrospinous ligament fixation places the vaginal axis in a normal horizontal anatomic position. Although the vagina will deviate slightly to one side after completion of the repair, its position reduces the risk of recurrent prolapse while maintaining the potential for adequate sexual function.

SURGICAL INDICATIONS

In recent years, sacrospinous ligament fixation of the vaginal vault has been proposed as a prophylactic procedure to be performed at the time of vaginal hysterectomy in the presence of moderate to severe uterine prolapse. Although its use with total procidentia is widely accepted, adequate objective data for performing sacrospinous fixation of the vault with first or second degree uterine descensus are lacking. Accepted indications for sacrospinous ligament fixation of the vaginal vault include:

- Post-hysterectomy vaginal vault prolapse of adequate depth.
- Post-hysterectomy vaginal vault prolapse accompanied by cystocele and/or rectocele.
- Total procidentia.

SURGICAL PROCEDURE

This operation is performed with the patient in the lithotomy position. General or regional anesthesia may be used. Prophylactic intravenous antibiotics are typically administered preoperatively. The vagina and perineum are prepped and draped, and the bladder is then drained.

Step 1

The apex of the vagina is grasped with Allis clamps and drawn outward (*Fig. 3.1*). The eventual point of attachment of the vaginal vault to the sacrospinous ligament is marked with the Allis clamp.

Step 2

Two more Allis clamps are placed at the posterior aspect of the hymen. A transverse incision is made between the clamps. The posterior vaginal mucosa is undermined and a vertical midline incision is made toward the middle of the vaginal apex (*Fig. 3.2*).

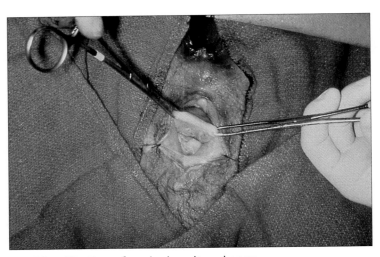

3.1 Identification of vaginal vault and apex.

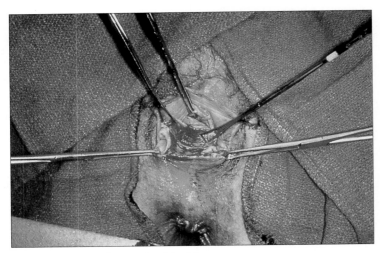

3.2 Initial posterior vaginal incision.

Step 3

The vertical incision is extended to within 1–2 cm of the apex and marked with the Allis clamp. The underlying rectum and its connective tissue are dissected away from the vaginal mucosa (*Fig. 3.3*).

Step 4

In most cases, an enterocele will be encountered during this initial portion of the operation (*Fig. 3.4*). The enterocele should be fully isolated by dissecting away the overlying bladder, the underlying rectum, and the lateral attachments of the vaginal mucosa.

Step 5

Once fully isolated, the enterocele is opened and its contents gently pushed upward. The enterocele is closed by initially placing a purse-string suture (#2-0 permanent suture) as high in the defect as possible (*Fig. 3.5*). A second purse-string suture is placed just distal to the first. The excess enterocele sac is cut away and the ties are allowed to retract (*Fig. 3.6*).

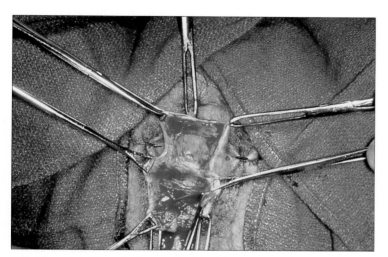

3.3 Completed posterior vaginal incision.

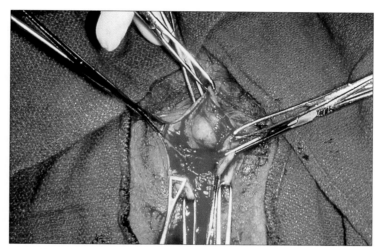

3.4 Identification of enterocele.

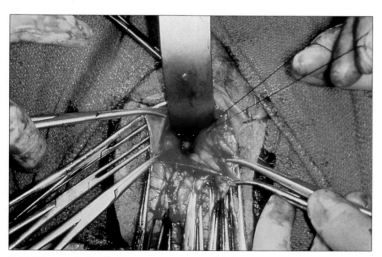

3.5 Placement of permanent suture high in enterocele.

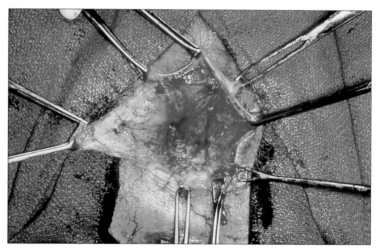

3.6 Completed enterocele closure.

Step 6

Dissection of the sacrospinous ligament is now performed. Alternatively, this step can be performed prior to tying the enterocele sutures in order to avoid disrupting the peritoneal closure. The index and middle fingers of the right hand bluntly separate the loose areolar tissues of the right pararectal space, penetrating the rectal pillar and enter the right pararectal space. A schematic view of this is shown in *Fig. 3.7*.

Step 7

Exposure of the right sacrospinous ligament is obtained by placing a right-angled retractor inferiorly, the tip of the retractor at the ligament. Two Breisky-Navratil retractors are then placed

superiorly and medially (*Fig. 3.8*). The sacrospinous ligament can be grasped with a Babcock clamp for easier identification. This also aids in isolating the ligament from underlying vessels and nerves. The pudendal artery, vein, and nerve pass beneath the sacrospinous ligament, adjacent to the ischial spine (*Fig. 3.9*).

Step 8

Using a Deschamps ligature carrier, Miya hook, or Shutt punch system, a suture of O-polypropylene is passed through the sacrospinous ligament, one and a half to two finger breadths medial to the ischial spine (*Fig. 3.10*). The suture loop that has penetrated the ligament is grasped with a nerve hook (*Fig. 3.11*). The ligature carrier is rotated back through the sacrospinous

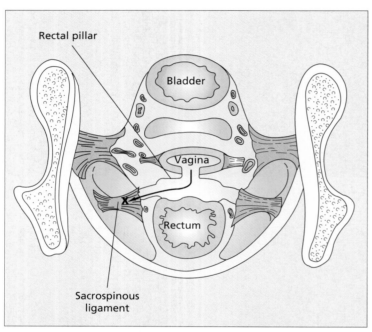

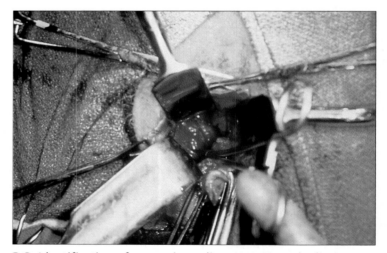

3.8 Identification of sacrospinous ligament. Note the ligament grasped with a Babcock clamp.

3.7 Schematic view of dissection of sacrospinous ligament.

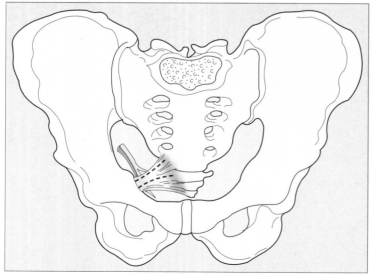

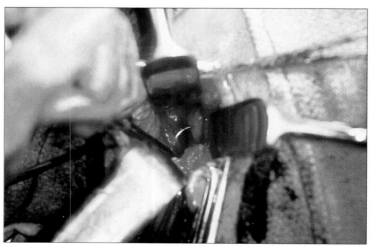

3.9 Relationship of pudendal nerve and vessels to the ischial spine and sacrospinous ligament.

3.10 Placement of initial suture through sacrospinous ligament.

ligament and the nerve hook pulls one end of the suture through the upper aspect of the ligament. The ends of the suture are held. A second suture is then similarly placed 0.5–1 cm medial to the first.

Step 9

The superior end of each suture is sewn through the undersurface of the vagina and tied at the level of the apex (*Fig. 3.12*).

Step 10

Prior to pulling the vaginal vault to the sacrospinous ligament, the vaginal incision closure is started with a running suture of 2-0-polyglycolic acid. When the incision is approximately half closed, the inferior ends of the polypropylene sutures are pulled, approximating the vaginal apex to the ligament (*Fig. 3.13*). After the sutures have been tied and cut, the running closure of the vaginal incision is completed. (Note: excess vaginal mucosa may need to be removed prior to incisional closure. A posterior colporrhaphy is often performed just prior to this closure.)

Step 11

Once the vagina is closed, a slight deviation to the right is seen (*Fig. 3.14*). The procedure is completed by placing a vaginal pack and inserting an indwelling bladder catheter.

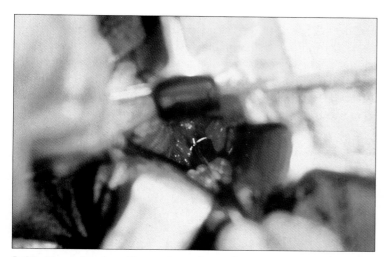

3.11 Nerve hook pulling suture through sacrospinous ligament.

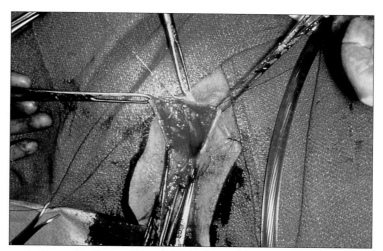

3.12 Placement of sutures through undersurface of vaginal mucosa.

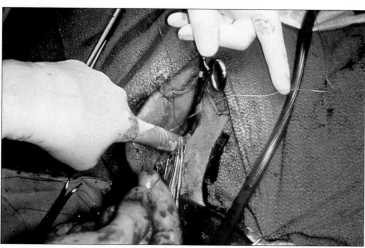

3.13 Securing vaginal apex to sacrospinous ligament after pulling inferior end of polypropylene sutures.

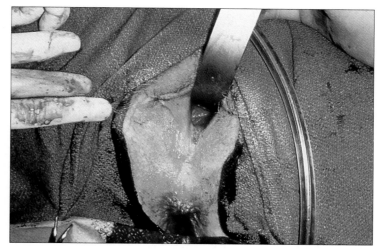

3.14 Completed vaginal vault suspension.

ABDOMINAL SACRAL COLPOPEXY

Surgical correction of vaginal vault prolapse or complete proci-dentia can be repaired either vaginally or abdominally. The abdo-minal approach to the correction of this problem offers potential advantages[5-12]. It is important when considering any operation for correction of genital prolapse that the procedure be associated with correction of the problem, low risk of recurrence, preser-vation of sexual functioning when desired, and low risk of predisposition to the development of other genital defects such as enterocele and stress urinary incontinence.

SURGICAL INDICATION

The indications for the use of an abdominal approach to correc-tion of vaginal vault or genital prolapse are similar to the indi-cations for the vaginal approach. Obviously, vaginal or genital prolapse must be present. Sacrocolpopexy should not be done as a prophylactic procedure. If intra-abdominal pathology exists, an abdominal approach may be preferable. Generally, the decision to proceed vaginally or abdominally is based on the operator's preference.

SURGICAL PROCEDURE

Step 1

The patient is placed in the dorsal lithotomy position with the legs supported in Allen Universal stirrups. This position allows for adequate access to the abdomen, vagina, and perineum while at the same time providing excellent support to the lower limbs. A Foley catheter is placed in the vagina and left in place throughout the procedure.

Step 2

A Pfannenstiel incision is made and a self-retaining retractor is placed. The bowel is packed into the upper abdomen with moist packs so that the pelvis is well visualized (*Fig. 3.15*).

Step 3

An instrument is placed in the vagina to distend and identify the vaginal apex along with the location of the sigmoid colon and bladder (*Fig. 3.16*). Several methods for accomplishing vaginal identification/distension include using an assistant's fingers, or a sponge stick. The use of an EEA sizer is preferable as it provides complete vaginal distension, and cannot be entrapped by sutures as they are placed in the vaginal apex. Use of the fingers can lead to inadvertent needle injury and is not necessary.

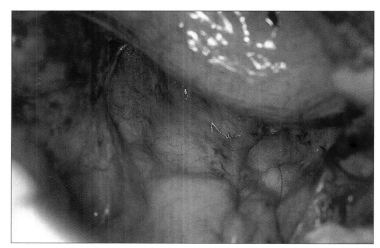

3.15 Visualization of deep cul-de-sac.

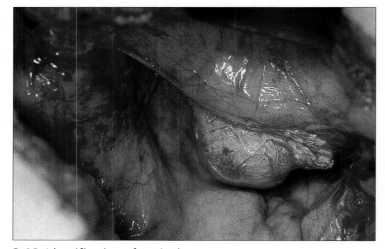

3.16 Identification of vaginal apex.

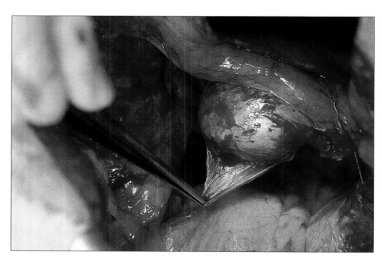

3.17 Dissection of peritoneum from apex of vagina.

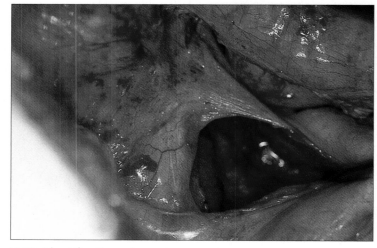

3.18 Identification of sacral promontory.

Step 4

In some patients, a peritoneal covering overlying the vagina can be dissected away from the vagina. This dissection creates a peritoneal covering which can be sutured over the graft material after it has been attached to the vagina (*Fig. 3.17*).

Step 5

The sacral promontory is then identified in the midline and the peritoneum overlying it is incised taking care to avoid the middle sacral artery. This dissection is carried interiorly along the right pelvic sidewall such that the sigmoid colon is retracted to the left. The incision is made so that the ureter is lateral and superior to the incision (*Fig. 3.18*). This peritoneal incision can be extended the full length of the cul-de-sac, or blunt dissection can be used to create a peritoneal tunnel through which the graft is passed.

Step 6

Several types of graft material have been used. The two most common types of material include:
* Polytetrafluoroethylene (GORE-TEX Soft Tissue Patch; W.L. Gore and Associates, Inc., Medical Products Division, Flagstaff, AZ).
* Marlex mesh (BARD Vascular System Division, CR BARD Inc. Billerica, Mass.).

The graft is attached to the anterior and posterior surfaces of the vagina as well as to the vaginal apex using a series of synthetic permanent sutures (*Fig. 3.19*). By attaching the graft on all vaginal surfaces, the tension on the vagina is evenly distributed.

Step 7

To correct an enterocele which is present and in an effort to prevent future enterocele formation, the posterior cul-de-sac is obliterated (*Fig. 3.20*). This can best be accomplished by either a Halban or Moschcowitz techniques[13,14]. In this patient, the Moschcowitz technique was used. The purse-string suture of 2-0-nonabsorbable suture is begun in the deep cul-de-sac. The peritoneum is grasped with the uterosacral ligament, the peritoneum laterally, the sigmoid colon serosa and the vagina superiorly. Care is taken not to constrict the sigmoid colon or entrap the ureters.

Step 8

The graft is passed through the retroperitoneal tunnel and the proper length of the graft is determined. The graft is placed so that minimal tension is placed on the material. A series of three or four synthetic permanent sutures are placed into the ligamentum flavum at the sacral promontory (*Fig. 3.21*).

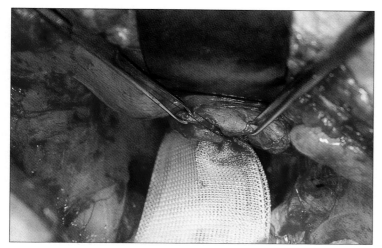

3.19 Attachment of Marlex graft to the vaginal apex.

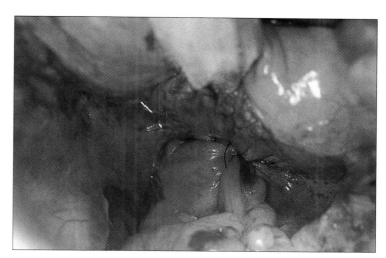

3.20 Completed coldeplasty.

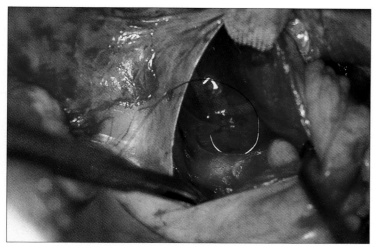

3.21 Passage of suture through sacral promontory.

Step 9

The previously incised peritoneum is closed over the graft material so that the graft is completely retroperitoneal (*Fig. 3.22*). If a retropubic procedure for stress incontinence is required it is performed at this time as is the repair of other pelvic defects.

POTENTIAL COMPLICATIONS

A variety of potential complications can occur as a result of this surgical procedure. Because a synthetic material is used, a foreign body reaction takes place which can lead to erosion of the graft material into the vagina. Hemorrhage can occur from the middle sacral vessels. If this occurs, pressure should be applied to initially control the bleeding. After the bleeding has been controlled, a suture or thumb-tack can be used to occlude the bleeding vessels. Other potential complications include adynamic ileus, wound disruption, and postoperative infection.

ALTERNATIVE SURGICAL PROCEDURES

A variety of surgical procedures and non-surgical techniques such as pessary use have been described. If the patient does not desire to retain her ability to have vaginal intercourse, an obliteration procedure can be performed. Regardless of the operative approach chosen, care must be taken to correct all support defects.

THE ABDOMINAL APPROACH TO ENTEROCELE: THE HALBAN TECHNIQUE

In most cases, a significant enterocele is amenable to treatment from a vaginal approach. Whether or not the enterocele is associated with a vaginal vault prolapse, the sac can be dissected and excised and the remaining peritoneal defect then ligated as high as possible with serial purse-string sutures.

Because the vaginal approach is so accessible and is associated with a lower incidence of morbidity, abdominal repair of an enterocele is less commonly performed. However, if other concomitant disease processes exist that require an abdominal approach (e.g., large uterine leiomyomata), or a procedure that predisposes to enterocele formation such as a retropubic urethropexy is being performed, treatment or prevention of an enterocele is best achieved transabdominally. In the face of a severe enterocele, such as one that accompanies a vaginal vault prolapse, abdominal enterocele repair alone will not support a satisfactory correction. It must be accompanied by some form of transabdominal vaginal vault suspension.

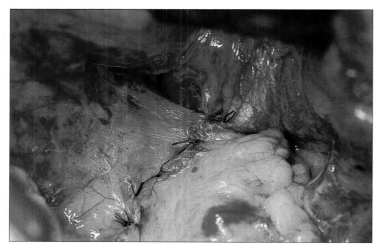

3.22 Completed abdominal sacral colpopexy with reperitonealization.

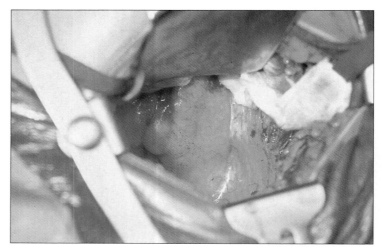

3.23 Full exposure of enterocele.

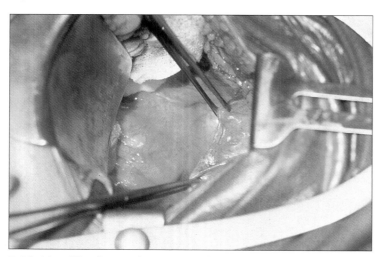

3.24 Identification and grasping of vaginal vault with Allis clamps.

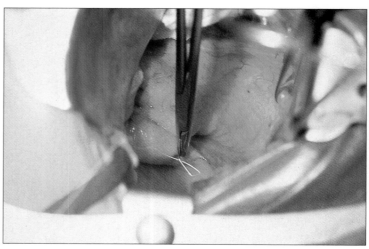

3.25 Placement of permanent suture through peritoneum overlying sacral promontory.

We describe here a simple procedure for prevention and/or treatment of an enterocele. This procedure, the Halban culdeplasty, utilizes sagittally placed serial sutures and has a minimum of complications. If it is performed in conjunction with urethropexy or colpopexy, we perform this procedure first. When performed at the time of a hysterectomy, it is done as a last step.

SURGICAL INDICATIONS

The surgical indications for the Halban culdeplasty include prevention of enterocele, treatment of mild to moderate enterocele when vaginal surgery is otherwise not indicated, and treatment of severe enterocele with simultaneous transabdominal vaginal vault suspension.

SURGICAL PROCEDURE

We prefer to perform this procedure in the dorsal lithotomy position, supporting the legs with Allen Universal stirrups. The culdeplasty shown here was performed before a paravaginal fascial repair.

Step 1

To obtain exposure, a self-retaining retractor should be in place and the intestines must be packed away superiorly (*Fig. 3.23*). With a double-gloved hand, the vagina is pushed upwards from below, demonstrating the apex of the vagina. Allis clamps are then placed on the apical corners of the vagina, taking care to avoid the bladder (*Fig. 3.24*). The vagina is lifted upwards, demonstrating the depth of the cul-de-sac.

Step 2

Suture placement begins laterally, at or just below the sacral promontory (*Fig. 3.25*). Using #2-0 braided polyester suture, the needle is passed beneath the peritoneum in successive bites, running vertically downward to the base of the cul-de-sac (*Fig. 3.26*) and then up the back of the vagina to the apex (*Fig. 3.27*).

Step 3

Successive parallel vertical sutures are then placed in a similar fashion, beginning their spacing by about 1 cm (*Fig. 3.28*). As each suture is completed, the ends are held with hemostats and laid to the side (*Fig. 3.29*).

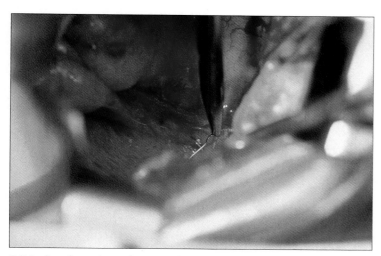

3.26 Continuation of suture shown in **3.25** up posterior aspect of vagina.

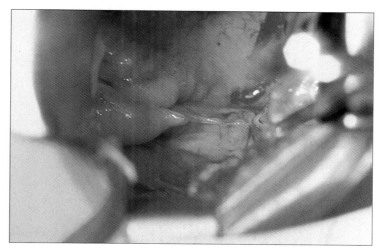

3.27 Completed placement of first suture.

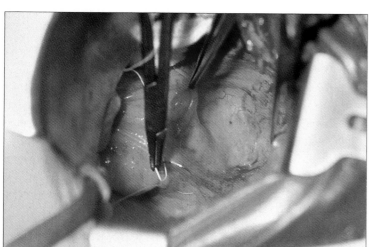

3.28 Placement of second suture 1 cm medial to initial suture.

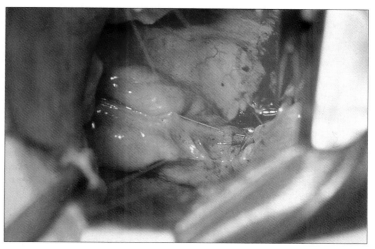

3.29 Completed placement of second parallel suture.

Step 4

Typically, four to six sutures are placed (*Fig. 3.30*). The lateral pelvic peritoneum is undisturbed by these sutures, thereby avoiding medial displacement or obstruction of the ureters. When hemostasis has been achieved and the sidewalls inspected, all sutures are tied and cut. Although small gutters exist on each side of the rectum and vagina, no exposure for enterocele reformation is present and the small bowel cannot be entrapped (*Fig. 3.31*).

ALTERNATIVE PROCEDURES

The Moschcowitz procedure represents an alternative abdominal repair for enterocele. It consists of serial concentric interrupted sutures that begin at the base of the cul-de-sac. Although its success rate is similar to that of the Halban technique, it incorporates the lateral pelvic peritoneum, potentially disturbing the course of the ureters.

Vaginal repair is a further possible approach to correction of enterocele. In some instances, pessary placement can be considered as an alternative.

COMPLICATIONS

Ureteral obstruction

Obstruction of one or both ureters may occur secondary to initial placement of the sutures too widely at the sacral promontory, kinking the ureter as it passes over the pelvic brim.

Hemorrhage or hematoma

The retroperitoneum is highly vascular. However, hematoma formation is usually self-limited. If bleeding continues from suture placement sites, tying the sutures at the end of the procedure usually resolves the problem.

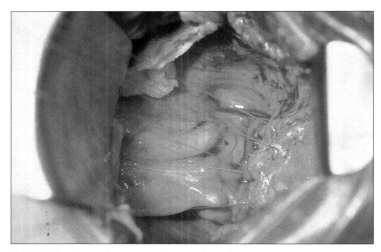

3.30 All sutures have now been placed.

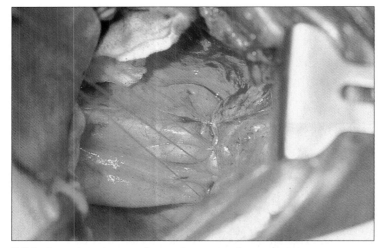

3.31 Completed procedure prior to cutting sutures.

REFERENCES

1. Sederl J. Zur Operation des Prolapses der blind endigenden Scheide. *Geburts u Frauenh*. 1958;18:824–8.

2. Richter K, Aldrich W. Long-term results following fixation of the vagina on the sacrospinal ligament by the vaginal route (vaginaefixatio sacrospinalis vaginalis). *Am J Obstet Gynecol*. 1981;141:811–16.

3. Randall CL, Nichols DH. Surgical treatment of vaginal eversion. *Obstet Gynecol*. 1971;38:327–32.

4. Nichols DH, Randall CL. *Vaginal Surgery*. 3rd ed. Baltimore: Williams and Wilkins; 1989:328–57.

5. Snyder TE, Krantz KE. Abdominal-retroperitoneal sacral colpopexy for the correction of vaginal prolapse. *Obstet Gynecol* 1991;77:944.

6. Timmons MC, Addison WA, Addison SB, Cavenar MG. Abdominal sacral colpopexy in 163 women with posthysterectomy vaginal vault prolapse and enterocele: Evolution of operative techniques. *J Repro Med* 1992;37:323.

7. Ridley JH. A composite vaginal vault suspension using fascia lata. *Am J Obstet Gynecol* 1975;126:590.

8. Addison WA, Timmons MC, Wall LL, et al. Failed abdominal sacral colpopexy: Observations and recommendations. *Obstet Gynecol* 1989;74:480.

9. Sutton GP, Addison WA, Livengood CH III, *et al*. Life-threatening hemorrhage complicating sacral colpopexy. *Am J Obstet Gynecol* 1981;140:836.

10. Cowan W, Morgan HR. Abdominal sacral colpopexy. *Am J Obstet Gynecol* 1980;138:348.

11. Birnbaum SJ. Rational therapy for the prolapsed vagina. *Am J Obstet Gynecol* 1973;115:411.

12. Falk HC. Uterine prolapse and prolapse of the vaginal vault treated by sacropexy. *Obstet Gynecol* 1961;18:113.

13. Moschcowitz AV. The pathogenesis, anatomy, and cure of prolapse of the rectum. *Surg Gynecol Obstet* 1912;15:7–21.

14. Nichols DH. Enterocele. In: *Gynecologic and Obstetric Surgery*. St. Louis: Mosby, 1993:420–30.

4

Surgery of the Cervix

Marian L. McCord

Thomas G. Stovall

CERVICAL BIOPSY

Cervical biopsy is an accurate screening method in the evaluation of abnormal cervical cytosmears. The procedure should be performed under colposcopic direction unless a gross cervical lesion is visible without the aid of the colposcope.

Punch biopsy may fail to reveal the correct diagnosis; under these circumstances conization is required (*Fig. 4.1*).

INDICATIONS

Colposcopically directed biopsies are performed as part of the evaluation of the abnormal cervical cytosmear. Cervical biopsy of all grossly abnormal areas of the cervix should be carried out.

Indications for Conization Following Punch Biopsy

Entire transformation zone not colposcopically defined

Entire lesion not visible/unable to biopsy

Dysplasia on cytology 2° greater than biopsy

Colposcopic impression/cytology suggestive of invasive cancer

Positive endocervical curettage

4.1 Indications for conization following punch biopsy.

CONTRAINDICATIONS

Although there are no absolute contraindications to cervical biopsy, the cervix markedly increases in vascularity during pregnancy. Therefore, cervical biopsy during pregnancy should be undertaken with greater caution.

SURGICAL EQUIPMENT
Forceps

Biopsy forceps (*Fig. 4.2*) are designed to obtain cervical biopsies adequate for histologic diagnosis. The basket can be oval or rectangular in shape; the size of the basket varies among types of forceps and determines the biopsy specimen size. Anchoring teeth are present on some models to help prevent slippage. The teeth may be single or multiple, and may be present on the lower jaw or on both jaws.

Forceps must be kept sharp to decrease their crushing effects at the time of biopsy. Disposable cutting tips are available with some models.

The shaft of the forceps may be straight or angled. Newer designs include a 360° rotating shaft, eliminating awkward positioning of the arm when the biopsy is being obtained.

Hooks

Hooks (*Fig. 4.3*) can be used to manipulate the cervix, providing traction and positioning of tissue to facilitate visualization and biopsy.

(a)

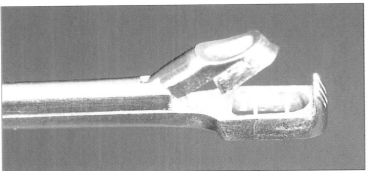

(b)

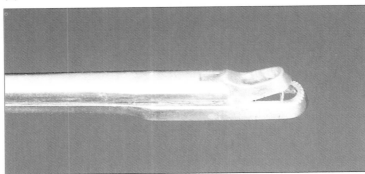

(c)

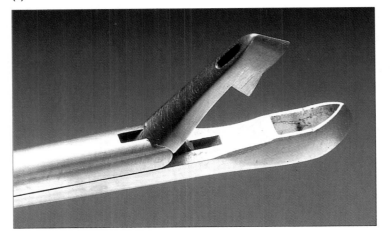

(d)

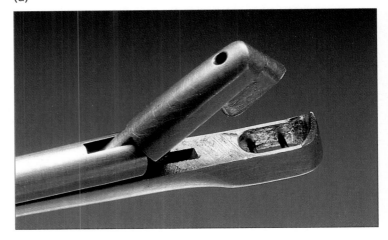

4.2 Types of forceps: (a) Kervormian (b) mini-Tischler (c) Burke (d) Tischler–Morgan

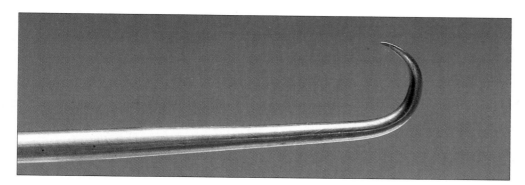

4.3 Hook used to manipulate the cervix.

SURGICAL PROCEDURE

Step 1

Expose the cervix, using as large a speculum as possible. Be careful not to abrade the surface epithelium. The cervix can be cleansed with saline to remove mucus and cell debris.

Step 2

Gross lesions do not require special techniques for identification. For evaluation of abnormal cytology, biopsies should be directed by colposcopy.

Step 3

The biopsy should be cut at right angles to the surface (*Fig. 4.4*). A biopsy depth of 2 mm should be sufficient to obtain stromal cells. The examiner should observe the sampling through the colposcope to ensure that the biopsy has resulted in removal of the abnormal areas.

Step 4

Biopsy specimens can be placed in a cassette on paper, Styrofoam, or cucumber to ensure proper orientation. The surface of the epithelium should be oriented to allow histologic sectioning at a 90° angle.

Each specimen should be individually labeled as to cervical location and placed in a 10% formalin solution. Specimens should never be placed in saline, which can destroy surface epithelium.

Step 5

A number of methods are available to achieve hemostasis.

Monsel's solution (ferric subsulfate)

Monsel's solution should have a thick consistency. It is applied directly into the biopsy groove with a small cotton swab.

AgNO$_3$ sticks

Silver nitrate is applied directly to the bleeding site. However, this agent may leave silver deposits that will interfere with future colposcopy.

Sutures

Non-permanent sutres can be placed if more conservative methods fail to achieve hemostasis.

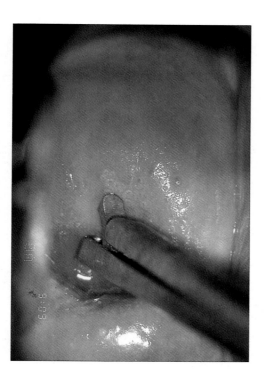

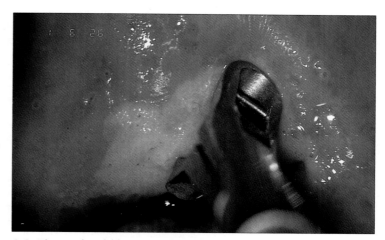

4.4 Biopsy should be cut at right angles to the surface.

CRYOSURGERY

Cryotherapy was introduced during the 1960s as a less destructive alternative to cervical conization. Multiple studies have shown cryotherapy to be efficacious in the treatment of cervical intraepithelial neoplasia, with cure rates of 90%.

INDICATIONS

Cryotherapy is indicated for the treatment of CIN I and unifocal CIN II–III lesions. It is less successful in treatment of multifocal CIN II and CIN III lesions. Other indications for cryotherapy include persistent cervicitis and cervical condyloma.

CONTRAINDICATIONS

Fig. 4.5 shows guidelines that should be used to exclude invasive cancer before cryotherapy. *Fig. 4.6* presents contraindications to cervical cryotherapy.

EQUIPMENT

Cryosurgery equipment does not require sterilization.

It is important to have a cryosurgical unit with a pressure gauge. Pressures must be in the "green zone" during the proce-

dure. Inadequate (low) pressures cause frost but do not freeze. The model pictured (*Fig. 4.7*) has a "gun type" unit with freeze and defrost buttons conveniently located. Cryotips are available in a variety of shapes and sizes (Fig. 4.8). Flat cryotips are preferable for nulliparous patients. Parous patients require a cryotip shape that best approximates the shape of the cervix.

Refrigerants most commonly used for cryosurgery include CO_2 (freezing temperature $-60°C$) and NO_2 (freezing temperature $-90°C$). Nitrous oxide is preferred because of its lower freezing temperature.

SURGICAL PROCEDURE

Cryotherapy is performed in an outpatient setting. Anesthesia is not required, as patient discomfort is minimal.

The ideal timing for cryotherapy is 1 week after the menstrual period because at this time the cervix is less vascular, a possible early intrauterine pregnancy can be ruled out, and problems secondary to menstrual outflow obstruction resulting from transient cervical edema or stenosis can be avoided.

Step 1

The patient is placed on a standard examination table with feet in stirrups and buttocks at the edge of the table.

Step 2

A speculum is selected for size and shape and placed in the vagina allowing complete visualization of the cervix.

Guidelines for the Exclusion of Invasive Cancer
Entire transformation zone and squamocolumnar junction are visible
Entire lesion is visible and can be biopsied
Satisfactory biopsy of most atypical area(s) by colposcopic examination
Endocervical curettage (ECC) negative
Colposcopic impression, cytology, and histology all correlate within one degree
No evidence of cancer on colposcopic impression, cytology, ECC, or biopsy histology

4.5 Guidelines used to exclude invasive cancer before cryotherapy.

Contraindications to Cryotherapy
Invasive cancer not ruled out
Pregnancy
Deep cervical lacerations (e.g., obstetric trauma) that would interfere with adequacy of freeze
Prenatal DES exposure (increased risk of cervical stenosis, infertility, neoplasia)

4.6 Contraindications to cryotherapy.

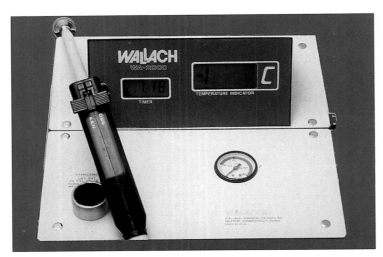

4.7 A cryosurgical unit.

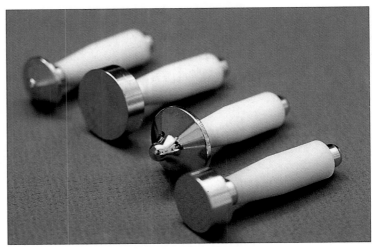

4.8 Cryotips vary in shape and size.

Step 3

The abnormal cervical lesion is identified. Schiller's solution or 3% acetic acid can be applied to the cervix to determine the extent and location of the lesion. The entire lesion must be treated for cryotherapy to be effective.

Step 4

The size of the cryotip selected is dependent on the size of the lesion. The cryotip should cover the entire lesion. If the cryotip does not cover the entire lesion, the lesion must be treated in two or three sections.

Step 5

A thin layer of water-soluble gel (e.g., KY jelly) is applied to the cryotip to ensure even transfer of the freeze to the cervix.

Step 6

The cryoprobe is held flush against the cervix, covering the lesion (*Fig. 4.9*). The cryoprobe is activated and observed for formation of an "ice ball" around the cryotip. The pressure gauge on the tank must show that pressure is in the green zone. The size of the "ice ball" is more important than the actual freeze time. The "ice ball" should extend 5 mm beyond the cryotip. This takes about 3–5 minutes (*Fig. 4.10*).

The cryoprobe is defrosted and then removed by gentle twisting. If gentle twisting does not break the seal, 10 ml of warm tapwater can be placed in the vagina to break the seal.

Clinical studies demonstrate an improved success rate when a "double freeze" is used. The cervix is allowed to thaw for 3–5 minutes and is then re-frozen until a 5 mm ice ball is again formed around the cryotip.

Step 7

The patient is given an instruction sheet which includes post-operative instructions and possible signs of complications (*Fig. 4.11*).

COMPLICATIONS

Potential complications of cryosurgery are presented in *Fig. 4.12*.

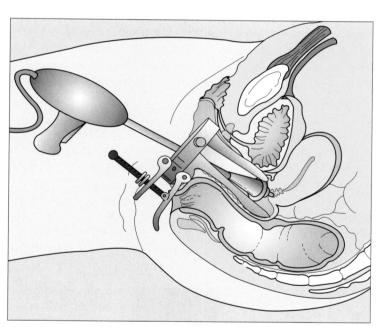

4.9 The cryoprobe held flush against the cervix.

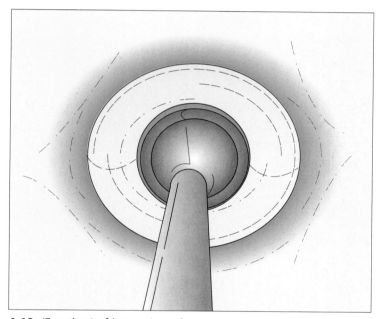

4.10 'Frosting' of inner ring of cervix.

Patient Instructions following Cryosurgery

Mild cramping occurs during the procedure and for 1–2 days afterwards

A clear watery discharge occurs for 2–4 weeks, a result of sloughing of necrotic tissue

The site may become secondarily infected. The patient should call if she develops fever/chills, increasing abdominal pain, or purulent, malodorous discharge. Treatment includes debridement and antibiotics

Avoid intercourse, tampons, and douching for 1 month to prevent contact bleeding and decrease risk of infection

4.11 Post-op patient instructions following cryosurgery.

Complications of Cryosurgery

Early	Late
Cervical infection	Cervical stenosis
Hematometra – rare	Unsatisfactory colposcopic examination (squamocolumnar junction may recede into the cervical canal)
Pyometra – rare	

4.12 Complications of cryosurgery.

SCALPEL CONIZATION OF THE CERVIX

Cervical conization is indicated for diagnostic and therapeutic purposes (*Fig. 4.13*).

The cervical cone should be tailored to the location of the cervical lesion. The base of the cone should be wide enough to encompass the ectocervical lesion. A 4–6 mm margin of normal tissue should be included. Deep conization is required for positive endocervical curettage and in cases of unsatisfactory colposcopy, where the lesion and/or the squamocolumnar junction are endocervical in location.

SURGICAL PROCEDURE

Step 1

The patient is placed in the dorsal lithotomy position and the vaginal area is prepped and draped in sterile fashion. The patient's

---

Indications for Conization

Diagnostic

   Positive ECC

   Unsatisfactory colposcopy

   Discrepancy (two-step) between cervical cytology and histology

   Evidence of possible invasive cancer on cytology, histology, or colposcopic examination

Therapeutic

   Multifocal CIN II–III

   Uncertain patient follow-up

4.13 Indications for conization.

---

buttocks should be at the table's edge to allow maximal visualization. The bladder is drained by in-and-out catheterization.

Step 2

The cervix can be visualized by placing a weighted speculum in the vagina, with one or more right-angled retractors being held by an assistant. Alternatively, a widely opened Graves' speculum can be used (*Fig. 4.14*).

Step 3

Schiller's test is performed by staining the cervix with Lugol's solution (aqueous iodine solution). Normal squamous epithelium contains glycogen and will stain mahogany. Neoplastic cells do not contain glycogen and will not take up the stain. Other causes of nonstaining include cervicitis and normal endocervical columnar epithelium. For photographic purposes, a 3% acetic acid solution has been used to define the cervical lesion.

Step 4

Hemostatic agents may be used to decrease intraoperative blood loss. These include neosynephrine, 1:100,000 solution; phenylephrine lidocaine with epinephrine, 1:100,000 solution; and vasopressin (Pitressin), 1.5% solution. Injections are made directly into the cervical stroma circumferentially at periodic intervals on the ectocervix (*Fig. 4.15*). These agents should be avoided in patients with cardiac, cardiovascular, hyperthyroid, or bronchospastic conditions.

Step 5

A tenaculum is placed horizontally on the anterior lip of the cervix to provide traction. Placement should be at a position outside the intended cone margin.

Step 6

Stay sutures of #1 delayed absorbable suture are placed in the cervix. The purpose of these sutures is two-fold: they allow

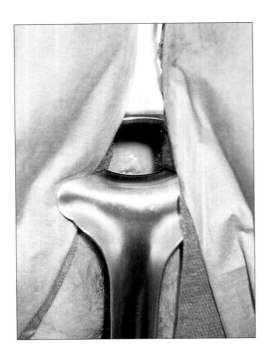

4.14 A weighted Graves' speculum to visualize the cervix.

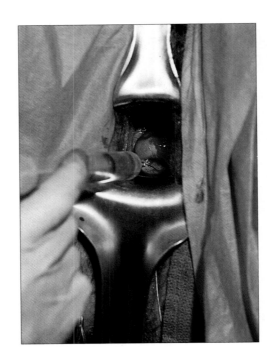

4.15 Anesthetic injections directly into the cervical stroma.

traction on the cervix and they provide hemostasis by ligating the descending cervical branches of the uterine artery.

A figure-of-eight suture is placed at the 3 o'clock and 9 o'clock positions on the cervix (*Fig. 4.16*). Placement should be immediately proximal to the junction of the cervix with the vaginal mucosa.

For the right-handed operator, the 9 o'clock suture is easier to place. The needle is directed anterior to posterior, taking a deep bite into the cervical stroma. The second bite is placed adjacent to the first. After the figure-of-eight stitch has been completed, it is tied and the ends are held with a hemostat. The 3 o'clock suture is placed with the needle directed posterior to anterior. A figure-of-eight suture is placed, tied, and held with a hemostat. (For the left-handed surgeon, the opposite is performed: the 3 o'clock suture is easier to place anterior to posterior; the 9 o'clock suture is placed posterior to anterior.)

Step 7

The endocervical canal is sounded to determine the course and depth of the endocervical canal.

Step 8

A No. 11 or 15 scalpel blade is used to make a continuous incision that encompasses all non-Schiller-staining tissue with a margin of normal tissue of 4–6 mm. The incision should start at the 6 o'clock position so that blood running down from the anterior lip will not subsequently obscure this field (*Figs 4.17, 4.18*). The scalpel blade should be directed towards the canal; the angle will be variable depending on the depth of tissue desired. The apex of the cone can be excised with the scalpel or with curved Mayo scissors (*Fig. 4.19*).

Step 9

The specimen should be obtained in a single piece with as little tissue trauma as possible. A suture is placed at 12 o'clock for pathologic orientation (see *Fig. 4.19*). The pathologist or surgeon then opens the specimen and pins it to a tongue blade before fixation. (The pathologist's preferences as to tissue handling will vary among institutions.)

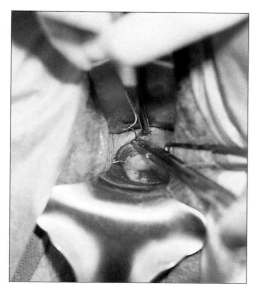

4.16 Figure-of-eight sutures on the cervix.

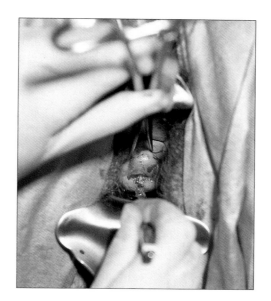

4.17 The incision should start at 6 o'clock so that blood running down the anterior lip will not subsequently obscure this field.

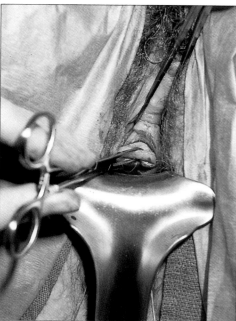

4.18 Allis clamp placed on specimen to be removed.

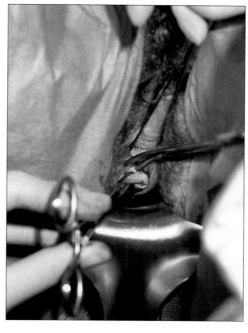

4.19 Excision of the apex of the cone with curved Mayo scissors.

Step 10

The cone bed can be left open or modified Sturmdorf sutures can be inserted, according to the preference of the surgeon. A modification of the Sturmdorf suture provides excellent hemostasis and reconstructs the cervix (*Fig. 4.20*). A #0 or #1 delayed absorbable suture is placed at 2 o'clock about 5 mm from the cone margin. The needle is passed into the endocervix in a shallow outside-to-inside stitch. The needle is then placed at 1 o'clock deep in the cone bed and passed outward. The cone bed is re-entered at 11 o'clock in a deep outside-to-inside stitch. A

shallow inside-to-outside stitch at 10 o'clock completes the anterior suture. A corresponding suture is placed in the posterior lip of the cervix. The anterior and posterior sutures are tied laterally at 3 o'clock and 9 o'clock. The endocervical canal should be checked for patency with a uterine sound or small dilator.

COMPLICATIONS

Potential complications of cervical conization are presented in *Fig. 4.21*.

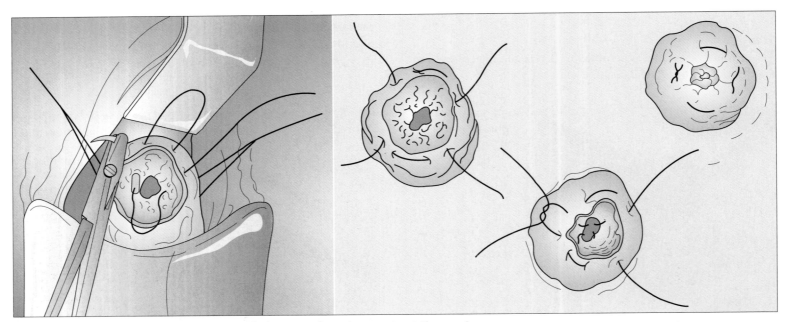

4.20 Modified Sturmdorf sutures to provide hemostasis and reconstruct the cervix.

Complications of Conization

Hemorrhage (immediate or delayed)

Uterine perforation

Cervical stenosis

Incompetent cervix

Infection

Anesthetic risks

4.21 Complications of conization.

CARBON DIOXIDE LASER FOR CERVICAL DISEASE

Carbon dioxide laser can be used for cervical surgery. Conization, ablation, or a combination of these two modalities are used for treatment of cervical disease. Before performing laser surgery, the surgeon must be familiar with laser principles and laser safety.

EQUIPMENT

Many laser delivery systems are available. The surgeon should be familiar with the manufacturer's directions and guidelines for the system used.

Power capability varies among models. In general, power capability of 60–100 watts is desirable for hospital-based systems. Laser energy is delivered through an articulating arm and is aimed at the tissue by a free hand piece or a micromanipulator. The CO_2 laser is in the infrared position of the electromagnetic field, invisible to the naked eye, and thus the laser is aimed at the target by a coincidentally operating helium laser.

The micromanipulator is preferred for cervical surgery, as it provides greater control of the laser. Variable spot size is a desirable feature when the micromanipulator is used; this allows rapid focus/defocus of the beam for cutting and hemostasis.

Colposcope

A colposcope or operating microscope can be coupled to the laser. Colposcopy can be repeated at the time of the procedure to ensure removal of all abnormal tissue with an adequate margin of normal tissue. The laser is coupled to the scope with a microslad. The focal distance of the scope lens and the focus of the laser lens should correspond.

Eye Shields

All personnel in the operating room, including the patient, should have eye protection. For the CO_2 laser, clear safety glasses are required.

Smoke Evacuation

A speculum with a smoke evacuator incorporated into the anterior blade is essential. This can be connected to suction available in the OR.

Operative Instruments

All instruments in the operative field, including the speculum, must be constructed/coated with non-reflective material that is heat- and light-absorbent (*Figs 4.22, 4.23*). Drapes in the operative field should be moistened.

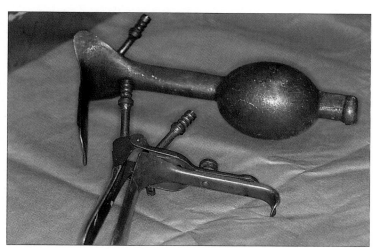
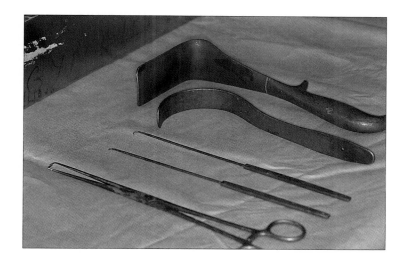

4.22, 4.23 Instruments for carbon dioxide laser treatment.

LASER ABLATION

INDICATIONS

Laser ablation is indicated for treatment of multifocal CIN II–III lesions. It is also indicated for CIN lesions with gland involvement and when deep obstetric lacerations are present, to ensure adequate depth of treatment.

Fig. 4.24 shows the guidelines that should be used to exclude invasive cancer before laser ablation.

SURGICAL PROCEDURE

Step 1
The laser beam should be tested on a moistened wooden tongue blade to determine spot size and depth of penetration at power settings to be used during the procedure (*Fig. 4.25*).

Step 2
The patient is placed in the dorsal lithotomy position. The vaginal area is sterilely prepped and draped. The bladder should be empty; in-and-out catherization can be performed as necessary. Moist towels should be placed over drapes in the operative field (*Fig. 4.26*).

Step 3
The laser speculum is placed in the vagina and positioned to allow complete visualization of the cervix (*Fig. 4.27*).

Step 4
A 3% solution of acetic acid is applied to the cervix. Colposcopy is performed to reconfirm the location and extent of the lesion.

Step 5
The beam is checked for alignment. The focal distance of the colposcope lens and the focus of the laser lens should correspond. If not, the laser beam will be defocused and the spot fuzzy.

Step 6
The peripheral extent of the area to be ablated is outlined with a series of single spots. Five millimeters of normal cervix should be included in the peripheral margin around the abnormal transformation zone (*Fig. 4.28*).

A low-power–density laser beam is used to mark the periphery. The laser is placed on single pulse. A power density of 300–500 W/cm^2 is desired, with spot size of 0.2 mm and power of 15–20 W.

Prerequisites for Laser Ablation

Colposcopy and cervical biopsy have eliminated invasive disease

The entire transformation zone has been colposcopically defined

Any lesion extending into the endocervical canal has been colposcopically defined

Correlation must exist between cytology, colposcopy, and histology, indicating only cervical intraepithelial neoplasia

Negative endocervical curettage

Colposcopist's experience is adequate to rule out an invasive cancer

4.24 Prerequisites for laser ablation.

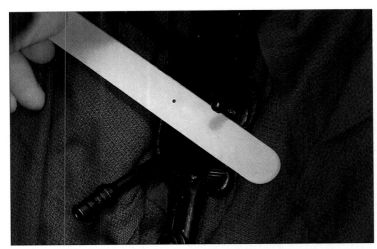

4.25 Testing laser beam on a moistened wooden tongue blade.

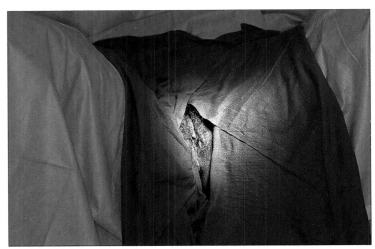

4.26 Moist towels placed over drapes in operative field.

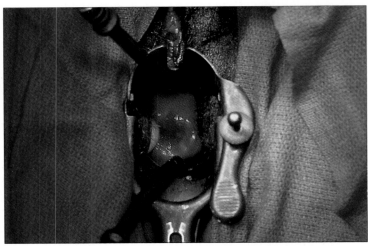

4.27 Laser speculum positioned in vagina to allow complete visualization of the cervix.

Step 7

Laser settings are adjusted for the ablation procedure. Continuous or super pulse modes are employed. A power density of 3,000–3,500 W/cm^2, power of 30–35 W, and a spot size of 0.1 cm^2 are desirable.

Step 8

The spots on the ectocervix are connected with the laser beam, making a circular outline of the transformation zone (*Fig. 4.29*).

Step 9

The area to be ablated is divided into four quadrants. Starting at the posterior lip, vaporization is carried down to a depth of 5–7 mm. The laser beam is moved continuously within each quadrant in a small circular pattern. The purpose of this maneuvre is to create a flat crater devoid of crests and valleys. The depth of the crater can be measured with a millimeter-ruled metal rod or a wooden cotton swab stick scored in millimeters.

The procedure is stopped between quadrants to allow the heat to dissipate. Each quadrant is successively treated (*Figs 4.30, 4.31*).

Step 10

Extending the depth of destruction by 2–3 mm immediately around the endocervical canal creates a "button" of endocervical tissue. The uninvolved endocervical margin must not be destroyed; preservation of this button of endocervix will ensure a visible squamocolumnar junction after healing.

Step 11

Bleeding, if any, can be managed by defocusing the laser beam. Monsel's solution can also be applied.

Step 12

The eschar is washed away with cotton swabs soaked in 3% acetic acid.

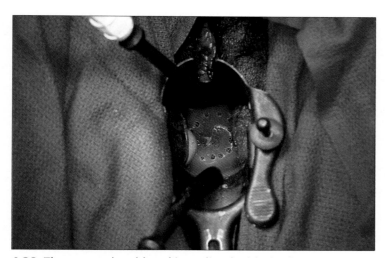

4.28 The area to be ablated is outlined with single spots.

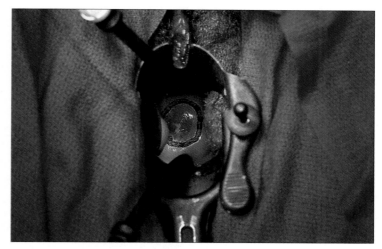

4.29 Spots are connected with the laser beam.

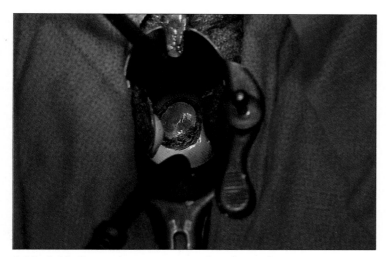

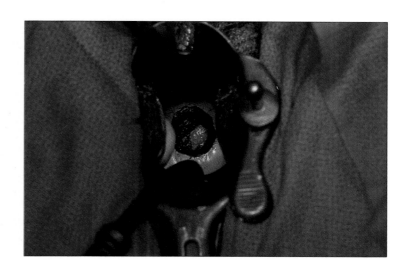

4.30, 4.31 Successive treatment of each quadrant.

Step 13

The patient is given a postoperative instruction sheet (*Fig. 4.32*). *Fig. 4.33* outlines the process of cervical healing after laser ablation.

COMPLICATIONS

Results and complications of laser ablation, as compared with any therapy, are listed in *Fig. 4.34*.

LASER CONIZATION

INDICATIONS

Laser conization is indicated for both diagnostic and therapeutic purposes (*Fig. 4.35*).

Instructions after Laser Surgery

Ibuprofen 400 mg every 6 h to relieve cramping or mild discomfort

Bleeding may occur between 4 and 7 days after laser surgery. The flow may approximate a normal menstrual period and should stop in about 48 h. If bleeding persists or becomes heavy, call your physician

Refrain from sexual intercourse for 2 weeks

Do not douche or place any medications in the vagina for 2 weeks, unless specifically instructed

Return for follow-up examination in 4 weeks

If you develop a fever or abdominal pain, call your physician

Vaginal discharge may be experienced for about 48–72 h

4.32 Postoperative instructions after laser surgery.

Summary Statements: Laser Ablation

The failure rate for CIN treatment increases in direct proportion to the severity of the disease

The recurrence rate after laser vaporization of individual lesions is high; therefore the entire T-zone must be ablated

There is no significant difference in the cure rate between patients with CO_2 laser or cryotherapy

The squamocolumnar junction is visible in 87–100% of patients compared with about 50% of those treated with cryotherapy

Sensations of pain and/or cramping are similar whether patients are treated with laser or cryotherapy

The incidence of significant vaginal discharge is higher when cryotherapy is used

Healing after laser vaporization is more rapid than with cryotherapy

The risk of a significant laser accident is minimal

There is an increased cost of laser treatment compared with cryotherapy

4.34 Summary statements: laser ablation.

Healing after Laser Vaporization

24–48 h	Crater covered with fibrin coagulum
	Bleeds easily on manipulation
	Purulent vaginal discharge
48–96 h	Peak vaginal discharge, appearance similar to 24–48 h cervix
6–7 d	Sharp circumscribed red depression
	Immature epithelium at periphery
	Discharge stops
10 d	Cloudy veil of reserve cells covers depressed wound
14 d	Multi-layered, fragile squamous epithelium
21 d	Wound healed
	Epithelium covers crater completely
	Cervix has rosy hue appearance
28 d	Mature epithelium with complete healing

4.33 Healing after laser vaporization.

Indications for Laser Conization

Diagnostic

Positive ECC

Unsatisfactory colposcopy

Discrepancy (two step) between cervical cytology and histology

Evidence of invasive cancer on cytology, histology, or colposcopic examination

Therapeutic

Multifocal CIN II–III

Uncertain patient follow-up

4.35 Indications for laser conization.

SURGICAL PROCEDURE

Step 1

The patient is placed in the dorsal lithotomy position. The vaginal area is sterilely prepped and draped. The bladder should be empty; in-and-out catheterization can be performed as necessary. Moist towels should be placed over drapes in the operative field.

Step 2

A laser speculum is placed in the vagina and positioned to allow complete visualization of the cervix (*Fig. 4.36*).

Step 3

A 3% solution of acetic acid is applied to the cervix. Colposcopy is performed to determine the location and extent of the lesion.

Step 4

Ten milliliters of 1.5% vasopressin solution (1 ml of vasopressin, 20 units mixed in 29 ml normal saline) is injected via a 25-gauge needle circumferentially into the cervical stroma to induce vascular spasm (i.e., to reduce vessel diameter to less than 1 mm).

Step 5

The peripheral extent of the cone margin is outlined with a series of single spots. Five millimeters of normal cervix should be included within the peripheral margin around the abnormal transformation zone (*Fig. 4.37*). A low-density laser beam is used to mark the periphery. The laser is placed on single pulse. A power density of 300–500 W/cm^2 is desired, with spot size of 0.2 mm and power of 15–20 W.

Step 6

Laser settings are adjusted to provide maximal cutting with minimal thermal artefact. Continuous or super pulse modes are employed. A power density of 3,000–3,500 W/cm^2 with power of 30–35 W and a spot size of 0.1 mm are desirable.

Step 7

The spots on the ectocervix are connected, producing an initial cut 3–5 mm in depth. Increasing depth is achieved by working in quadrants. A fine laser hook is used to provide traction on the specimen, exposing the deepening channel (*Figs 4.38, 4.39*). Once

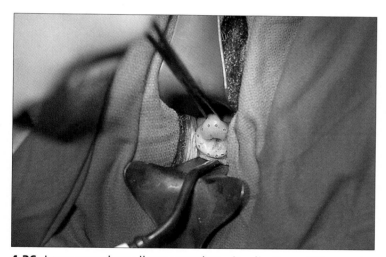

4.36 Laser speculum allows complete visualization of the cervix.

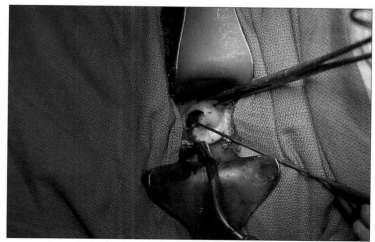

4.37 Five millimeters of normal cervix should be included within the peripheral margin around the abnormal transformation zone.

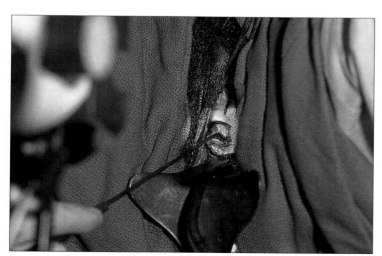

4.38, 4.39 Exposure of deepening channel.

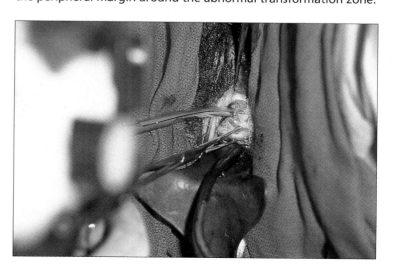

a desirable depth is obtained (1–2 cm), the cone specimen can be removed with the laser beam, a scalpel, or curved Mayo scissors (*Fig. 4.40*).

Step 8
The laser beam is defocused and passed over the conization bed to coagulate small vessels and lymphatics.

Step 9
An endocervical button is created by vaporizing the stroma surrounding the remaining endocervical canal to a depth of 2–3 mm.

Step 10
Management of intraoperative bleeding is outlined in *Fig. 4.41*. Postoperative instructions are the same as for laser ablation (see *Fig. 4.32*).

COMPLICATIONS
Results and complications of laser conization, as compared with cold knife conization, are listed in *Fig. 4.42*.

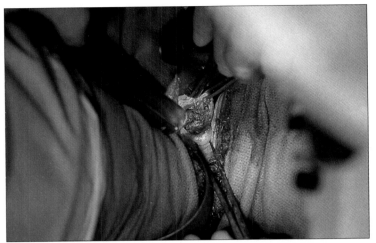

4.40 Removal of cone specimen with curved Mayo scissors.

Management of Intraoperative Bleeding

Maintain same power density: the blood is sucked from the operative site and the blood vessels are simultaneously coagulated

Decrease power density: this can be accomplished by defocusing the laser beam or by decreasing the power

Increase power density: this allows the excessive blood in the field to be vaporized by the laser beam, thus allowing coagulation of the base of the bleeder

Hemostatic sutures

4.41 Management of intraoperative bleeding.

Results and Complications of Laser Conization for CIN

Decreased need for extra hemostatic sutures

Decreased incidence of positive surgical margins

Increased risk of blood loss when the conization is done during menstruation and in the postpartum period

Decreased incidence of late postoperative bleeding

Decreased incidence of postoperative infection

Decreased incidence of cervical stenosis. (More common in menopausal women undergoing conization)

Positive factors must be balanced with the increased cost of the procedure

4.42 Results and complications of laser conization for CIN.

LOOP ELECTROSURGICAL EXCISION PROCEDURE

Diathermy loop excision has been introduced as a method for evaluation and treatment of cervical intraepithelial neoplasia. The European experience indicates that it is effective for such treatment; widespread use in the United States is just beginning.

INDICATIONS

The loop electrosurgical excision procedure (LEEP) is indicated for the evaluation and treatment of cervical intraepithelial neo-plasia and cervical condyloma. American investigators have advocated the following guidelines for use of LEEP: the endo-cervical border of the lesion can be seen in its entirety; there is no colposcopic or cytologic suspicion of cancer; and there is adequate correlation among pap smear, histology, and colpo-scopic impression.

European investigators have been more liberal in their use of LEEP. The LEEP procedure is used in place of cold knife or laser conization for unsatisfactory colposcopy, suspicion of micro-invasive cancer, and discrepancy between cervical cytology and histology.

EQUIPMENT
Electrosurgical generator

Several models are available. The surgeon should be familiar with the manufacturer's guidelines for the model used.

Electrosurgical generators use monopolar outputs. The patient must be properly grounded during the procedure.

Each unit has separate cutting and coagulation modes (*Fig. 4.43*). Cutting modes are used for the LEEP procedure. Cutting modes may be "pure" (cutting only) or "blend" (combining wave forms to provide both cutting power and coagulation). Blend modes are designed for both rapid cutting and hemostasis. The coagulation mode can be used to achieve hemostasis after the procedure is completed. In general, a cutting mode and a coagu-lation mode of 25–45W and 35W of power, respectively are recommended. Power requirements increase with increasing loop size (*Fig. 4.44*). The actual power, and therefore the optimal settings, may vary between units. A surgeon who is unfamiliar with an electrosurgical generator should test it with a pathology specimen or a beef tongue before performing LEEP.

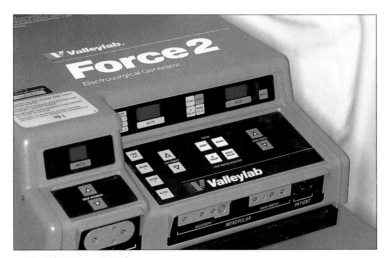

4.43 Electrosurgical generator.

Power Settings for Loop Excision and Fulguration*		
Loop diameter (cm)	**Blend 1** Cutting (W)	**Coagulation** (W)
1.0	25	1
1.5	30–35	1
2.0	35–40	1
2.5	45	1
Ball electrode	35	35

* These power settings were established with the Valley Lab Force 2 generator and may vary with other machines.

4.44 Power settings for loop excision and fulguration.

LEEP electrodes

Loops are made from a thin stainless steel wire attached to an insulated shaft and crossbar (*Fig. 4.45*). A variety of sizes are available. Most commonly used are the 1.5 × 1.5 cm and 2.0 × 1.5 cm loops. Disposable electrodes are available and avoid the problem of carbon build-up associated with resterilized electrodes. Ball tip electrodes are used for hemostasis, if needed, at the end of the procedure (*Fig. 4.46*).

Smoke Evacuator

A smoke evacuator is mandatory for this procedure. Some generators have an evacuator incorporated into the unit. Free-standing smoke evacuators are also available. A vaginal speculum that permits direct connection to the evacuation tubing is preferable.

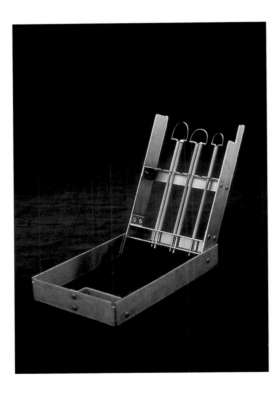

4.45 LEEP electrodes.

SURGICAL PROCEDURE

Step 1

The patient is placed in the dorsal lithotomy position. A disposable grounding pad is placed on the patient's thigh. It is critical to ensure that the patient is properly grounded.

Step 2

An insulated speculum is placed in the vagina. Sidewall retractors can be used to further protect the vaginal wall from inadvertent electrocautery injury.

Step 3

Lugol's solution is applied to the cervix to determine the extent and location of the lesion. Alternatively, 3% acetic acid can be used.

Step 4

Local anesthesia is induced. Paracervical nerve block is performed by injecting 5 ml of 1% lidocaine into each of the uterosacral ligaments. Direct infiltration into the cervical stroma should also be performed. We have found that use of 1% lidocaine with 1:100,000 epinephrine injected directly into the cervical stroma decreases bleeding, thus facilitating the procedure.

Step 5

A loop of sufficient size to allow excision of the lesion in a single pass (if possible) is selected.

Step 6

Cut and coagulation power settings are selected.

Step 7

The loop is positioned 5 mm lateral to the edge of the lesion (*Fig. 4.47*).

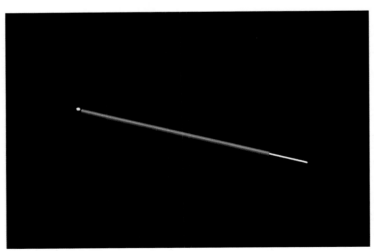

4.46 Ball tip electrodes used for hemostasis at the end of the procedure.

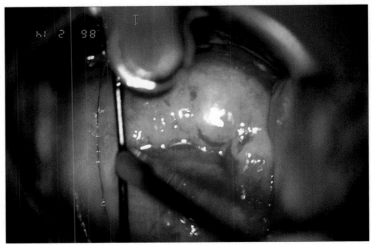

4.47 The loop is positioned 5 mm lateral to the edge of the lesion.

Step 8

The power is activated prior to the loop making contact with the tissue. In a continuous motion, the loop is pushed perpendicular to the surface to a depth of 10 mm, then drawn parallel to the surface to the opposite side, and is then drawn out perpendicular to the surface. (*Fig. 4.48*). Additional passes can be made if the lesion is not completely excised with a single pass (*Fig. 4.49*).

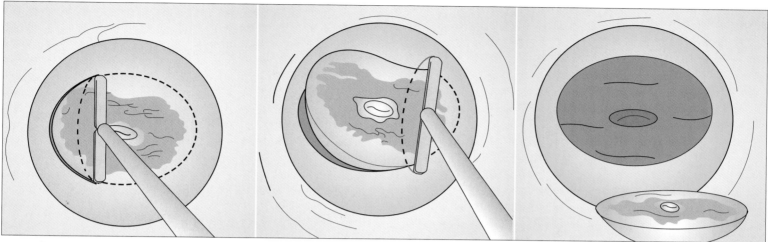

4.48 The loop is drawn out perpendicular to the surface.

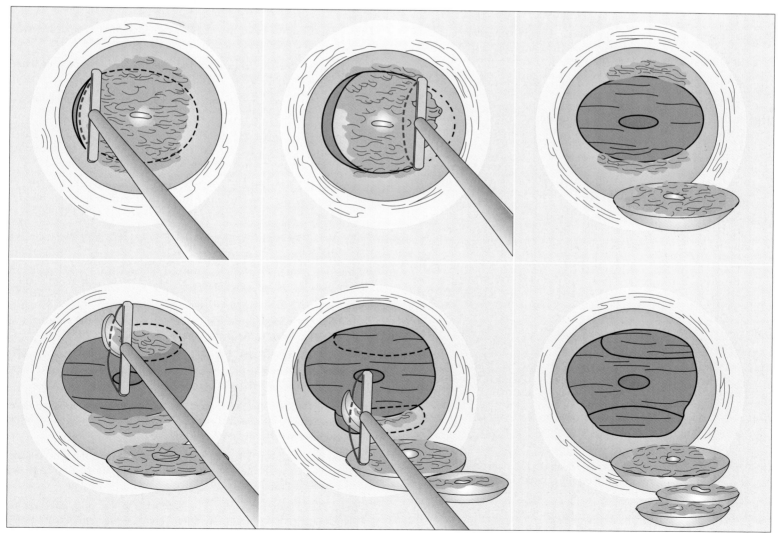

4.49 Additional passes can be made if the lesion is not completely excised with a single pass.

Step 9
Bleeding, if any, can be controlled in several ways. Coagulation can be performed with a ball tip electrode. Monsel's solution is effective for generalized oozing. Rarely, a suture ligature may be necessary.

COMPLICATIONS
Preliminary data indicate that the short- and long-term complications of LEEP procedure are comparable to those of laser conization (*Fig. 4.50*).

Potential Complications of Loop Electrosurgical Excision

Bleeding
  Primary
  Secondary
Infection
Incomplete removal of lesion (positive margins)
Inadvertent burns
  At the active electrode
  Distal burns from inadequate grounding
Cervical incompetence
Cervical stenosis
Inadequate colposcopy post-procedure

4.50 Potential complications of loop electrosurgical excision.

FURTHER READING

Baggish MS. A comparison between laser excisional conization and laser vaporization for the treatment of cervical intraepithelial neoplasia. *Am J Obstet Gynecol* 1986; 155:39.

Baggish MS, Baltoyannis P. Carbon dioxide laser treatment of cervical stenosis. *Fertil Steril* 1987; 24:24.

Baggish MS, Dorsey JH. Carbon dioxide laser for combination excisional–vaporization conization. *Am J Obstet Gynecol* 1985; 151:23.

Bellina JH, Ross LF, Voros JI. Colposcopy and the CO₂ laser for treatment of cervical intraepithelial neoplasia: an analysis of seven years' experience. *J Reprod Med* 1983; 28:147.

Berget A, Andreasson B, Bock JE, *et al*. Outpatient treatment of cervical intraepithelial neoplasia: CO₂ laser versus cryotherapy, a randomized trial. *Acta Obstet Gynecol Scand* 1987; 66:531–6.

Boonstra H, Koudstaal J, Osterhuis JW, Wymnga HA, Amders JA, Jonssens J. Analysis of cryolesions in the uterine cervix: application techniques, extension, and failures. *Obstet Gynecol* 1990; 75:232–9.

Chez RA, Townsend DE. How to do cryosurgery of the cervix. *Contemp Obstet Gynecol* 1979; 13:39–42.

Coney A, Walton LA, Edelmor DA, Loween WC Jr. Cryosurgical treatment of early cervical intraepithelial neoplasia. *Obstet Gynecol* 1983; 62:463–6.

Crapanzano JT. Office diagnosis in patients with abnormal cervico-vaginal cytosmears: correlation of colposcopic biopsy and cytologic findings. *Am J Obstet Gynecol* 1972; 113:967–72.

Creasman WT, Hinshaw WM, Clark-Pearson DL. Cryosurgery in the management of cervical intraepithelial neoplasia. *Obstet Gynecol* 1984; 63:145–8.

Creasman WT, Weed JC, Curry SL, Johnston WW, Parker RT. Efficacy of cryosurgical treatment of severe cervical intraepithelial neoplasia. *Obstet Gynecol* 1973; 41:501–6.

Krebb HB, Helmkamp BF. Assuring successful cone biopsy. *Contemp Obstet Gynecol* 1991; 36:131–49.

Larsson G, Gullberg B, Grundsell H. A comparison of complications of laser and cold knife conization. *Obstet Gynecol* 1983; 62:213.

Mor-Yosef S, Lopes A, Pearson S, Monaghan JM. Loop diathermy cone biopsy. *Obstet Gynecol* 1990; 75:884–6.

Ostergard D. Cryosurgical treatment of cervical intraepithelial neoplasia. *Obstet Gynecol* 1980; 56:231–3.

Partington CK, Turner MJ, Soutter WP, Griffiths M, Krausz T. Laser vaporization versus laser excision conization in the treatment of cervical intraepithelial neoplasia. *Obstet Gynecol* 1989; 73:775.

Richart RM, Townsend DE, Crisp W, *et al*. An analysis of "long term" follow-up results in patients with cervical intraepithelial neoplasia treated by cryotherapy. *Am J Obstet Gynecol* 1980; 137:823–6.

Salim MA, So-Bosita JL, Blair OM, Little BA. Cervical biopsy versus conization. *Obstet Gynecol* 1973; 41:177–82.

Skehan M, Soutter WP, Vim K, Krausz T, Pryse-Davies J. Reliability of colposcopy and directed punch biopsy. *Br J Obstet Gynecol* 1990; 97:811–16.

Stein DS, Ulrich SA, Hasiuk AS. Laser vaporization in the treatment of cervical intraepithelial neoplasia. *J Reprod Med* 1985; 30:179.

Sze EHM, Rosenzweig BA, Birenbaum DL, Silverman RK, Baggish MS. Excisional conization of the cervix uteri: a five part review. *J Gynecol Surg* 1989; 5:235–68, 325–41.

Townsend DE, Richart RM. Cryotherapy and carbon dioxide laser management of cervical intraepithelial neoplasia: a controlled comparison. *Obstet Gynecol* 1983; 61:75.

Whitely PF, Uhah KS. Treatment of cervical intraepithelial neoplasia: experience with the low voltage diathermy loop. *Am J Obstet Gynecol* 1990: 162:1272–7.

Wright TL, Cragnons, Ferenozy A, Richart RM. Excising CIN lesions by loop electrosurgical procedure. *Contemp Obstet Gynecol* 1991; 36:57–74.

5

Tubal and Ovarian Surgery

Peter R. Casson

Thomas G. Stovall

SALPINGECTOMY

The role of salpingectomy in the treatment of tubal disease has changed drastically over the past 20 years. The most frequent reason for performing salpingectomy in the past has been for ectopic pregnancy. However, as more conservative approaches have been shown to be effective, salpingectomy is being done less frequently. However, it is still an important technique with which every gynecologic surgeon should be familiar[1].

SURGICAL INDICATIONS

Indications for salpingectomy are listed in *Fig. 5.1*. Salpingectomy can also be used after a failed tubal occlusive procedure.

SURGICAL PROCEDURE

Step 1

Laparoscopic removal of the fallopian tube is one of the easiest operative surgical techniques to learn and perform. However, once the decision has been made to proceed with laparotomy, the fallopian tube is identified and any adhesive attachments for the ovary are removed (*Fig. 5.2*). This case illustrates the removal of a normal fallopian tube and was done at the time of hysterectomy for another indication.

Step 2

The cornual portion of the tube is clamped with a Kelly or Heaney clamp, and the distal portion of the tube is elevated with tissue forceps. The remainder of the mesosalpinx is clamped with a similar type of clamp so that the tips of both clamps meet (*Fig. 5.3*).

Step 3

Once hemostasis is secured, Metzenbaum scissors are used to cut above the two clamps and the fallopian tube is removed (*Fig. 5.4*).

Step 4

A synthetic absorbable suture material is used to suture the clamped portion of the mesosalpinx. A suture is placed at the tip of the clamp and the tissue ligated (*Fig. 5.5*). This procedure is repeated, and the distal portion of the mesosalpinx is removed (*Fig. 5.6*). If the surgeon desires, a running interlocking suture technique can be used.

Step 5

The abdomen is irrigated and the operative site is inspected for hemostasis. Because the cornual portions of the uterus and the mesosalpinx are extremely vascular, the surgeon should inspect these areas carefully for hemostasis. The laparotomy incision is then closed in a standard fashion.

Indications for Salpingectomy in the Treatment of Tubal Disease
Ectopic pregnancy
Pyosalpinx
Hematosalpinx
Hydrosalpinx
Fallopian tube torsion
Sterilization

5.1 Indications for salpingectomy in the treatment of tubal disease.

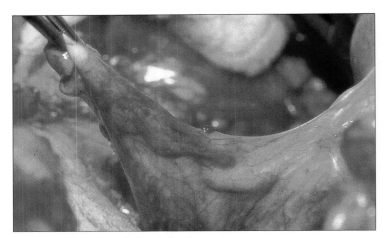

5.2 Identification of the fallopian tube.

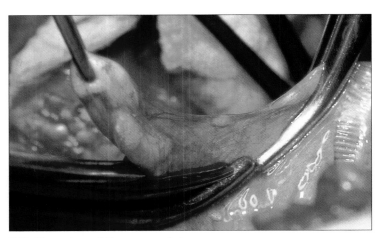

5.3 Clamping of the mesosalpinx.

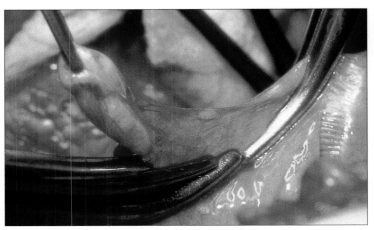

5.4 Removal of the fallopian tube.

ALTERNATIVE PROCEDURES

The decision that the surgeon most often faces when deciding about the treatment of a pathologic tubal process is whether to perform a total salpingectomy or a partial salpingectomy of only the tubal segment involved, or to proceed with a salpingostomy. This decision should be guided by the patient's hemodynamic condition, the degree of tubal pathology present, a history of infertility, and the amount of tubal damage that has occurred.

In the past some authors have advocated the resection of the interstitial portion of the fallopian tube to prevent the possibility of a subsequent interstitial pregnancy. However, this appears to increase the risk of uterine rupture if the patient should become pregnant. In addition, because the subsequent risk of an interstitial pregnancy is small, the procedure is no longer recommended.

COMPLICATIONS

There are no surgical complications specific to salpingectomy. However, the more commonly encountered problems include mesosalpinx bleeding and postoperative adhesion formation. These potential complications can be minimized by using surgical techniques that promote gentle tissue handling, meticulous hemostasis, and use of minimally reactive sutures.

SALPINGO-OOPHORECTOMY/OOPHORECTOMY

Oophorectomy or, more commonly, salpingo-oophorectomy, is the most common concurrent surgical procedure performed at the time of hysterectomy. Until recently, it was suggested that if the ovaries required removal at the time of hysterectomy, the procedure should be approached from an abdominal incision. However, this recommendation was not based on clinical trial experience. Data now available suggest that 95% of ovaries can be removed transvaginally if a hysterectomy is done via this approach. However, if the primary indication for surgery is adnexal disease, it is more appropriate to approach the procedure abdominally. Oophorectomy/salpingo-oophorectomy can also be accomplished via operative laparoscopy. However, the advantages of this approach and the indications for its use have not been clearly defined. Until such time that they are, gynecologic surgeons will continue to use both approaches.

INDICATIONS

Fig. 5.7 outlines the indications for oophorectomy and/or salpingo-oophorectomy. Except for prophylactic ovarian removal, oophorectomy is used when the disease process involves

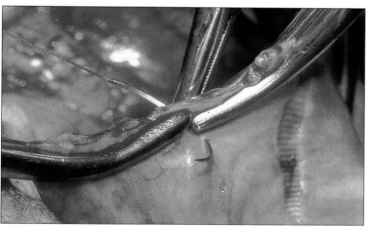

5.5 Ligation of mesosalpinx.

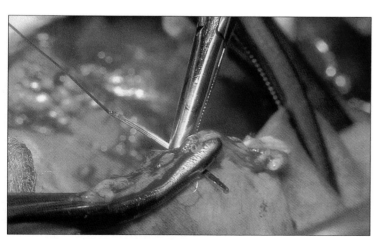

5.6 Removal of distal portion of mesosalpinx.

Indications for Oophorectomy/Salpingo-oophorectomy
Prophylactic Removal–postreproductive age, or patients with a strong familial history of ovarian carcinoma
Persistent Adnexal Mass
Treatment for Estrogen Dependent Disease Process
Ovarian Pregnancy
Tubo-ovarian Abscess Unresponsive to Antibiotic Therapy
Pain
Adnexal Torsion
Note: Many of these indications can be managed by medical therapy or more conservative surgical therapy such as ovarian cystectomy.

5.7 Indications for oophorectomy/salpingo-oophorectomy.

the ovary to such an extent that the ovary cannot be conserved owing to technical difficulties, or in the postreproductive patient when ovarian conservation is usually not necessary. *Fig. 5.8* shows an ovary that has undergone torsion. This mass could be demonstrated on both physical examination and ultrasound (*Fig. 5.9*).

Concurrent removal of the fallopian tube is indicated only when future childbearing is not an issue or when the disease process has enveloped the fallopian tube, such as in the case of pelvic adhesive disease.

SURGICAL PROCEDURE
Step 1
The first step in any pelvic surgical procedure is normalization of the pelvic anatomy. To accomplish this, adhesions should be lysed and the fallopian tube and ovary mobilized from the pelvic sidewall or bowel. This step will help to ensure that all ovarian tissue is removed and that a remnant of tissue is not left behind.

Step 2
The round ligament is ligated near the pelvic sidewall using synthetic absorbable suture material (*Fig. 5.10*). The ligament is also ligated about 1–2 cm from its point of insertion into the uterus and cut so that the posterior leaf of the broad ligament is opened (*Fig. 5.11*).

Step 3
The anterior and posterior leaves of the broad ligament can be separated by sharp and blunt dissection and the ureter identified on the medial surface of the broad ligament (*Fig. 5.12*). This step will help to ensure that the ureter is not injured during clamping of the infundibulopelvic ligament.

Step 4
An opening is then created in the posterior leaf of the broad ligament superior to the ureter (*Fig. 5.13*). The defect can then

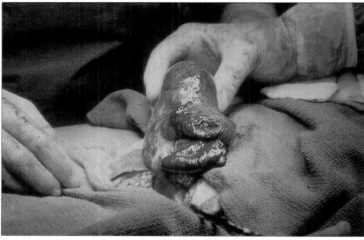

5.8 An ovary that has undergone torsion.

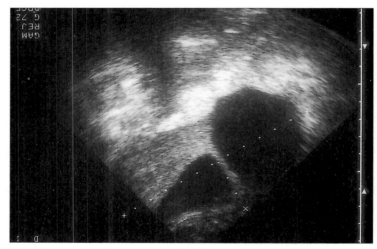

5.9 Ultrasound of ovary seen in **5.8**.

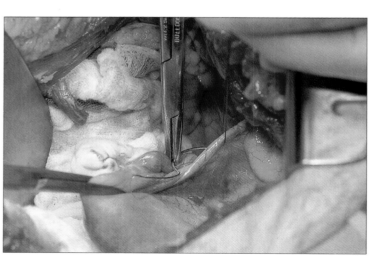

5.10 Ligation of the round ligament.

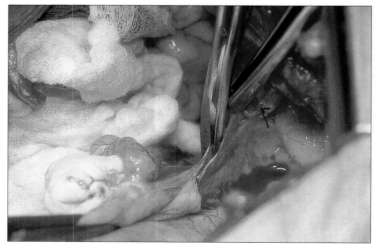

5.11 Incision to open the posterior leaf of the broad ligament.

be extended with Metzenbaum scissors above the ureter toward the uterine artery caudad and cephalad toward the infundibulo-pelvic ligament. This step also mobilizes the ureter out of the operative field and further isolates the ovary and infundibulo-pelvic ligament. It also ensures that the entire ovary is removed, reducing the risk of leaving an ovarian remnant (*Fig. 5.14*).

Step 5

A Haney-type clamp is placed on the proximal portion of the infundibulopelvic ligament (*Fig. 5.15*). Scissors are used to transect the ligament between these two clamps (*Fig. 5.16*). A synthetic absorbable suture tie is placed proximal to the clamp (*Fig. 5.17*). The clamp is "flashed" and a suture ligature is placed

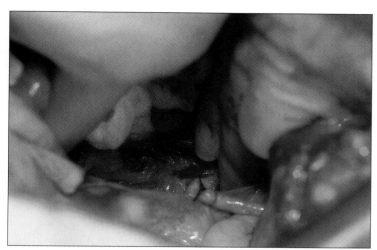

5.12 Identification of the ureter.

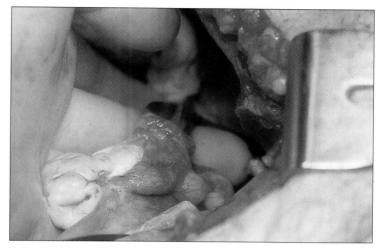

5.13 Creation of an opening in the posterior leaf of the broad ligament.

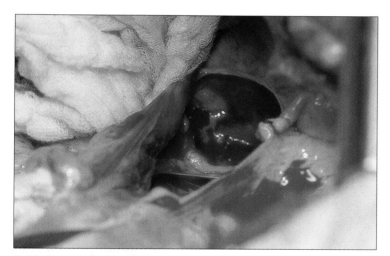

5.14 Removal of entire ovary.

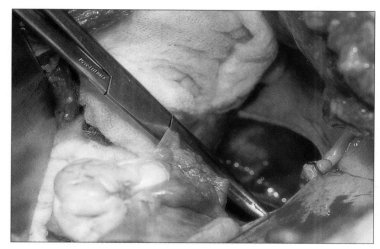

5.15 Clamping of the infundibulopelvic ligament.

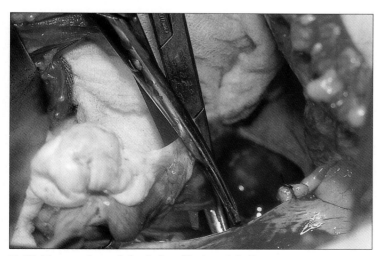

5.16 Transection of the infundibulopelvic ligament.

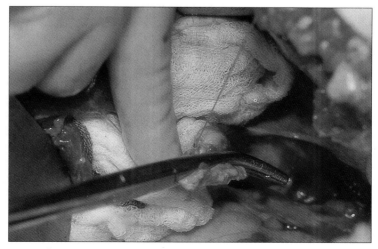

5.17 Placement of suture proximal to the clamp.

distal to this suture ligature (*Fig. 5.18*). By double-ligating this vascular pedicle, excellent hemostasis is obtained.

Step 6

A Haney clamp or similar-type instrument is used to clamp the utero-ovarian attachment (*Fig. 5.19*). Once clamped, the specimen can be removed with scissors and the pedicle ligated with either a suture ligature or suture tie. If the tube is to be salvaged, this clamp should be positioned in such a way that the cornual portion of the tube is not ligated and the fallopian tube blood supply is not compromised.

ALTERNATIVE PROCEDURES

The alternative procedures to oophorectomy are ovarian cystectomy and medical management of the disease process. In selected patients, percutaneous drainage of a tubo-ovarian abscess or vaginal drainage can also be used as an alternative to oophorectomy. In selected patients with ovarian torsion, the ovary can be untwisted and an oophoropexy performed. If this is done, the ovary must be secured to the pelvic sidewall peritoneum in two planes so that it does not undergo torsion again.

COMPLICATIONS

Complications specific to oophorectomy include retroperitoneal hemorrhage and ovarian remnant syndrome. Retroperitoneal hemorrhage can occur secondary to retraction of one or more of the veins, and ovarian remnant syndrome results from incomplete removal of all ovarian tissue. This complication is most commonly encountered in patients with endometriosis, pelvic inflammatory disease or severe pelvic adhesive disease.

TUBOPLASTY/FIMBRIOPLASTY

Tubal fimbrioplasty is defined as deagglutination and reconstruction of damaged fimbriae. Before the availability of *in vitro* fertilization (IVF), it represented the only option for enhancing fertility in patients with this condition. Success rates are generally disappointing, reflecting global tubal damage. Distal fimbrioplasty pregnancy rates vary from 22 to 60%, with increased rates of ectopic pregnancy in the range 5–15%[3]. Good prognostic signs include abscence of hydrosalpinx, easily recognizable fimbriae, no significant peritubal, periovarian, or pelvic adhesions, and healthy intratubal rugae[4]. A tubal diameter of greater than 2.5 cm and a thickened tubal wall portend a poor prognosis[5].

Given the disappointing pregnancy rates and the availability of IVF, distal fimbrioplasty is now more selectively applied to patients with good prognostic indicators and to those who cannot afford advanced reproductive technologies. This surgery may also be an option for younger patients, who have the luxury of deferring IVF without significant impairment of their fertility rate. However, the occurrence of distal tubal damage represents the most visible facet of what is really pan-tubal disease with depletion of steroid receptors and extensive decilliation, conditions unlikely to improve with surgery[3]. This, in conjunction with the fact that IVF clinical pregnancy rates range as high as 30–40% in many programs, indicates that this procedure is now outmoded. Others suggest that given the low pregnancy rates and the significant morbidity associated with exploratory laparotomy, this procedure should be performed laparoscopically[6]. Several large laparoscopic series demonstrate equivalent pregnancy rates, although no direct comparison has been made

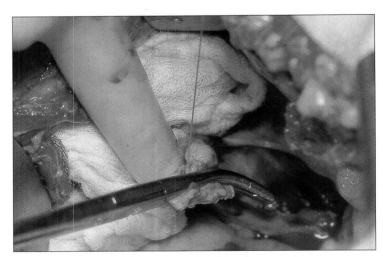

5.18 Placement of suture distal to first suture.

5.19 Clamping of the utero-ovarian attachment.

between laparoscopy and microsurgery[3].

This surgery should be reserved for patients with good prognostic factors as determined by a hysterosalpingogram and laparoscopy. Preoperative semen analysis is of course essential.

It is conventional wisdom that use of the operating microscope enhances results. Adhesion prevention adjuvants are more controversial. At various times, interperitoneal and systemic steroids, antihistamines, low molecular weight dextran (Hyskon), and barrier methods have been used[7]. In the absence of conclusive data, their use is left to the judgment of the individual surgeon.

SURGICAL INDICATIONS

The indications for microsurgical distal fimbrioplasty are shown in *Fig. 5.20*.

SURGICAL PROCEDURE

Step 1

If the condition of the distal tubes is not known, preoperative laparoscopy may be indicated. In this particular patient it had demonstrated some fimbrial preservation. Before the surgical procedure the operating microscope is readied for use. Intraocular widths and eyepiece focus are adjusted by both the surgeon and the assistant, and a 250- or 300-mm objective is placed on the scope. It is then placed in a sterile drape (*Fig. 5.21*) and positioned in the operating room for easy access (*Fig. 5.22*).

Step 2

A Foley catheter is placed in the patient's bladder, and a pediatric Foley (No. 10 or 12) is introduced into the uterine cavity and attached to a closed system to chromopertubate with diluted indigo carmine dye (*Fig. 5.23*). The intrauterine catheter enables the uterus to be manipulated more than with other more rigid chromopertubation systems.

Microsurgical Distal Fimbrioplasty: Surgical Indications and Alternative Procedures	
Indications	**Alternative Procedures**
Partial distal tubal obstruction with fimbrial agglutination	Laparoscopic fimbrioplasty
	In vitro fertilization/embryo transfer

5.20 Microsurgical distal fimbrioplasty: surgical indications and alternative procedures.

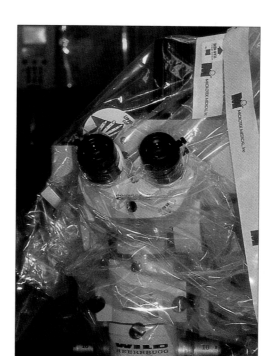

5.21 Sterile drape over the microscope.

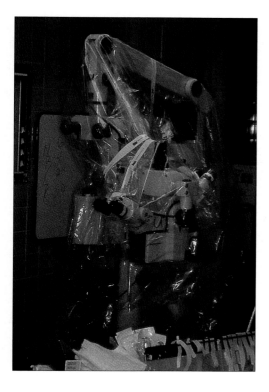

5.22 Positioning of microscope within operating room.

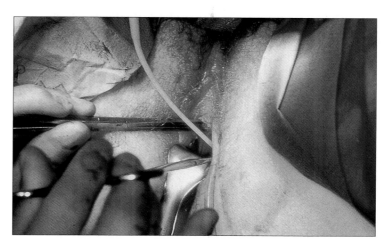

5.23 Cannulation of the uterine cavity.

Step 3

The abdomen is opened in the usual fashion (*Fig. 5.24*, in this case through a previous incision). The surgeons then rinse off the glove talc, and intra-abdominal adhesions, if any, are lysed (*Fig. 5.25*).

Step 4

Once the pelvic cavity has been exposed, an intra-abdominal drape is placed to minimize blood pooling (*Figs 5.26, 5.27*). A retractor (Kirschner or otherwise) is then placed for maximal exposure (*Fig. 5.28*). A gauze roll, fitted into a washed glove, is inserted into the cul-de-sac and elevates the uterus, ovaries, and fallopian tubes (*Figs 5.29, 5.30*). This patient had undergone a previous salpingectomy for ectopic pregnancy and therefore unilateral fimbrioplasty is required. A necrotic paratubal cyst, visible in the cornual region, was later removed.

Step 5

The necessary microsurgical instrumentation is seen in *Fig. 5.31*. A pediatric feeding tube attached to a syringe filled with dilute indigo carmine dye can be used for distal chromopertubation. Glass rods are used for atraumatic manipulation and 50 ml syringes filled with heparinized lactated Ringer's are used for

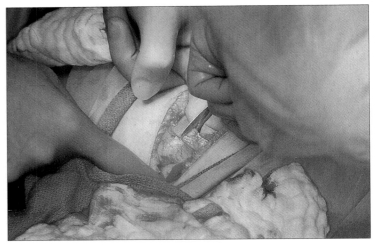

5.24 Opening of the abdomen.

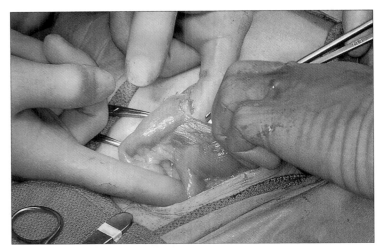

5.25 Lysing of intra-abdominal adhesions.

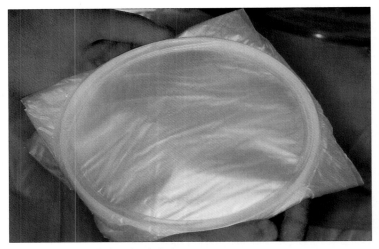

5.26 An intra-abdominal drape.

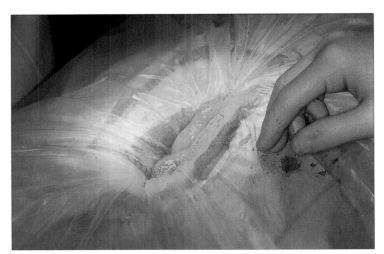

5.27 Placement of intra-abdominal drape to minimize blood pooling.

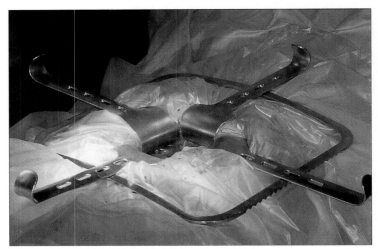

5.28 Placement of retractor.

irrigation. Hemostasis is obtained with a microsurgical unipolar needle tip or bipolar electrocautery. The suture material used is #5-0 and #8-0 or #9-0 polyglactin. After the microscope is brought into the operative field, positioned correctly, and focused, any remaining tubo-ovarian adhesions are lysed with micro-

surgical technique. This process allows maximal mobilization of the distal tube from the ovary (*Fig. 5.32*) and optimal identification of the remnants of the fimbriae. Adhesions are excised completely, with meticulous hemostasis (*Figs 5.33, 5.34*).

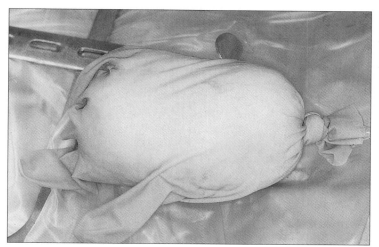

5.29 A gauze roll inside a washed glove.

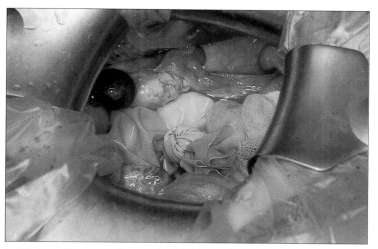

5.30 Insertion of roll seen in **5.29** into the cul-de-sac.

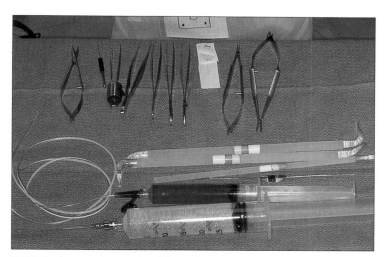

5.31 Instruments required for microsurgery.

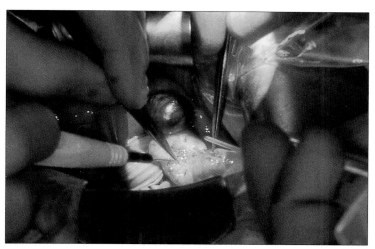

5.32 Mobilization of the distal tube from the ovary.

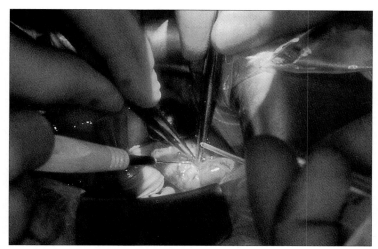

5.33 Excision of adhesions.

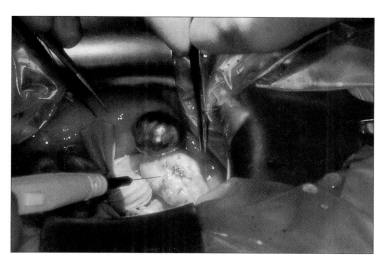

5.34 Excision of adhesions.

Step 6

After full mobilization of the tube, the most distal portion (with fimbrial remnants) is distended with dye and examined closely (*Fig. 5.35*). The tissue is handled atraumatically. The process of tubal agglutination and hydrosalpinx formation occurs as a process of inversion, and therefore a point can be identified in the serosal adhesions at which incision and circumferential peeling of the eschar tissue will release the trapped fimbria (*Fig. 5.36*). This is also demonstrated in *Fig. 5.37*. In most fimbrioplasties, little actual incision of the fallopian tube is necessary to allow full fimbrial eversion. This process, akin to peeling skin off an orange, is assisted by placement of a lacrimal duct probe in the tubal ampulla (*Fig. 5.38*). The process is continued in *Fig. 5.39* with satisfactory eversion of the fimbria (*Fig. 5.40*).

Step 7

Meticulous hemostasis is obtained by the judicious use of unipolar or bipolar needle-tip electrocautery (*Fig. 5.41*). Intratubal adhesions or bipolar agglutinating the fimbria are identified and lysed (*Figs 5.36, 5.42*), normalizing the ampulla.

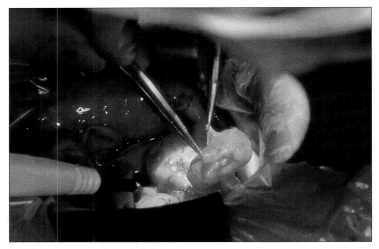

5.35 Exposure of fimbrial remnants.

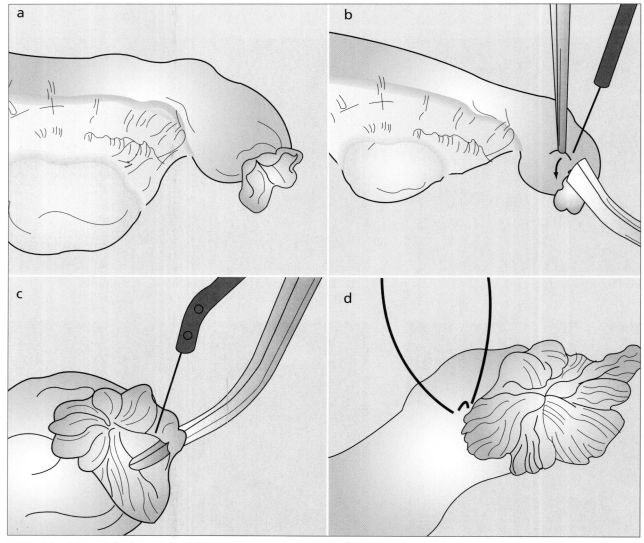

5.36 Principles of fimbrioplasty. The eschar trapping the fimbriae is identified, incised, and peeled away circumferentially (**a, b**). Intratubal adhesions, if any, are lysed (**c**), and the fimbriae are held everted by #8-0 serosal sutures (**d**).

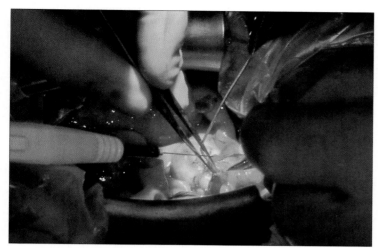

5.37 Release of trapped fimbria.

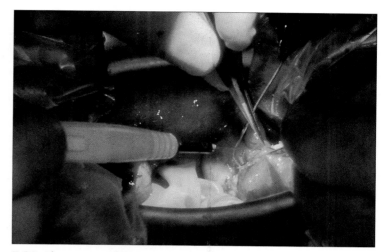

5.38 Placement of lacrimal duct probe in tubal ampulla.

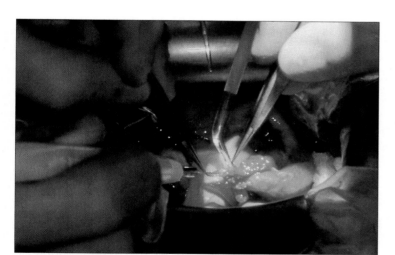

5.39 Continued eversion of fimbria.

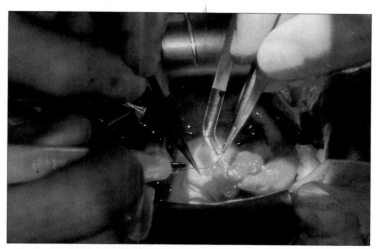

5.40 Satisfactory eversion of the fimbria.

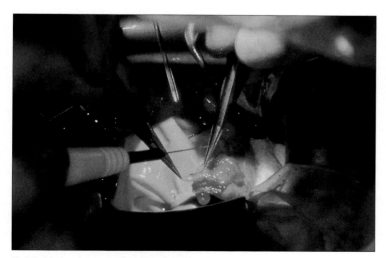

5.41 Unipolar needle-tip electrocautery.

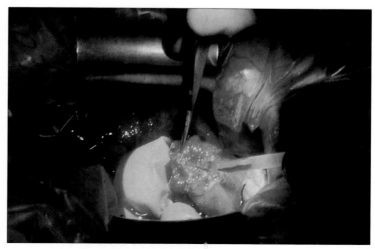

5.42 Identification and lysis of intratubal adhesions.

Step 8

Microsurgical suture (#8-0 or #9-0 polyglactin) is then used to further evert the fimbria. This suture is placed through the serosa of the fallopian tube, then through the serosal aspect of the fimbria (*Figs 5.36, 5.43, 5.44*) to provide such eversion. *Fig. 5.45* illustrates the result of placement of this suture, with good eversion and moderately healthy endosalpinx. Further serosal sutures are placed as required to bring about full eversion (*Fig.*

5.46), and to bring the fimbria into apposition to the ovarian surface (*Fig. 5.47*).

Step 9

In this case, a resorbable anti-adhesion barrier was placed around the reconstructed distal tube, as seen in *Figs 5.48, 5.49*. If these barriers are used, hemostasis must be meticulous, and care is taken to prevent dislodgement when the abdomen is closed.

COMPLICATIONS

The most serious complications are those associated with exploratory laparotomy. Complications specific to distal tubal surgery are listed below.

Ectopic pregnancy

Because of significant pan-tubal functional disease, the risk of ectopic pregnancy is increased. Early recognition of ectopic pregnancy makes possible conservative surgical therapy that permits subsequent functional tubal salvage. Postoperative ectopic pregnancy presages a poor prognosis for future intrauterine pregnancy, and these patients should be treated by IVF.

Adhesion re-formation

Some degree of adhesion re-formation and fimbrial reagglutination can be expected. These complications are thought to be

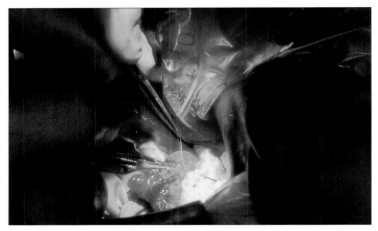

5.43 Placement of suture through the serosa of the fallopian tube.

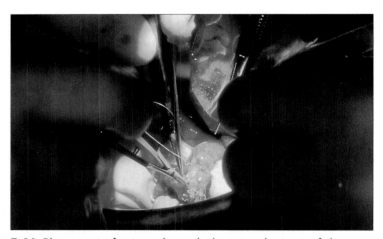

5.44 Placement of suture through the serosal aspect of the fimbria.

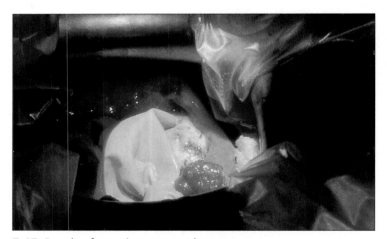

5.45 Result of everting suture placement.

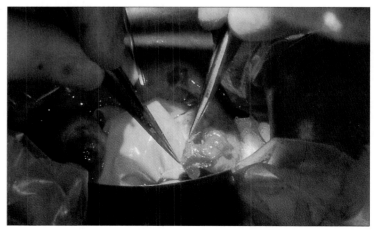

5.46 Placement of further sutures to produce full eversion.

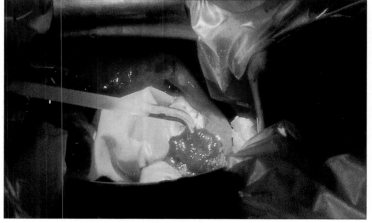

5.47 The fimbria is in apposition to the ovarian surface.

minimized by use of adhesion prevention agents. Their usefulness remains unproven[5]. The best prophylaxis against this complication remains meticulous hemostasis and copious irrigation.

Pelvic and tubal infection

In most cases, the tubal damage necessitating this procedure is caused by *Chlamydia* infection. The surgery may aggravate a latent infection, causing a postoperative salpingitis or, in the worst case, a tubo-ovarian abscess. Prophylactic antibiotic coverage with doxycycline, as well as meticulous surgical technique, should reduce the risk of this complication. The occurrence of a postoperative pelvic infection greatly reduces the possibility of pregnancy and further increases the risk of ectopic pregnancy. An interval postoperative hysterosalpingogram may demonstrate tubal occlusion, indicating a poor prognosis and suggesting treatment by IVF.

Failure

Although these patients often conceive many years after surgery, lack of conception after 1 year, even with open tubes, should indicate a change to IVF. Given the low rates of pregnancy achieved, the patient should be warned of the likelihood of failure before surgery is performed.

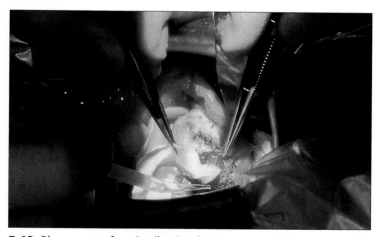

5.48 Placement of anti-adhesion barrier around the reconstructed distal tube.

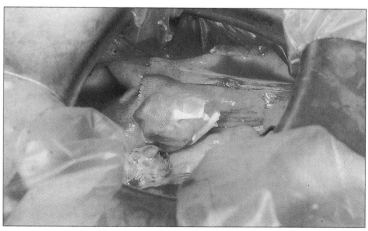

5.49 The anti-adhesion barrier in place.

TUBOPLASTY: MICRORESECTION AND REANASTOMOSIS OF THE FALLOPIAN TUBE

The introduction of microsurgical technique into the field of tubal reconstructive surgery has resulted in an increase in pregnancy rates and a decrease in rates of ectopic gestation[8]. This is especially true with fallopian tube reanastomosis, where intrauterine pregnancy rates range from 60 to 82% and ectopic pregnancy rates are less than 5%[9]. With pregnancy rates proportional to the postoperative tubal length, results are disappointing if the remaining fallopian tube measures less than 4 cm. Another contributing factor to low success rates is the occurrence of proximal and distal segment luminal disparity at the anastomosis site[10].

Most microsurgical tubal reanastomoses are performed for reversal of a previous tubal ligation most often after modified Pomeroy tubal ligations, and unipolar or bipolar tubal cautery. These are usually isthmic–ampullar reanastomoses. Unipolar cautery, because of extensive degrees of adjacent tissue damage, has disappointing results after tubal ligation reversal[11]. Conversely, reversal after a fallope ring or Blier clip application (often isthmic–isthmic anastomoses) is technically easier and associated with higher pregnancy rates.

Other indications for microsurgical resection and reanastomosis of the fallopian tube include proximal cornual obstruction secondary to salpingitis isthmica nodosa (SIN), pelvic inflammatory disease, or endometriosis. These types of proximal block may benefit from an initial attempt at hysteroscopically or fluoroscopically guided tubal cannulation[12].

The preoperative work-up for microsurgical tubal reanastomosis includes a semen analysis, a hysterosalpingogram, review of the operative note of the tubal ligation, and demonstration of ovulatory status.

SURGICAL INDICATIONS

The surgical indications for tubal reamastomosis are shown in *Fig. 5.50*.

Surgical Indications for Microsurgical Resection and Reanastomosis of the Fallopian Tube	
Indication	**Alternative Procedures**
(1) Reversal of tubal ligation	IVF
(2) Proximal tubal block	IVF
Salpingitis isthmica nodosa (SIN) Pelvic infection Endometriosis Medically treated ectopic pregnancy Previous failed tubal ligation reversal	
(3) Previous partial salpingectomy	IVF
Surgical treatment of isthmic ectopic pregnancy	

5.50 Surgical indications for microsurgical resection and reanastomosis of the fallopian tube.

SURGICAL PROCEDURE

Step 1

Most surgeons perform a preliminary laparoscopy (*Fig. 5.51*) to ensure the presence of adequate proximal and distal tubal remnants. In the case of a clip or a fallope ring tubal ligation, laparoscopy can be omitted, but the patient should be informed about the possibility of an unnecessary laparotomy. Diagnostic laparoscopy will also identify concurrent pelvic disease that would preclude fertility. Surprisingly, operative notes from tubal ligation frequently fail to mention significant concurrent pelvic disease.

Step 2

Optimal tubal reanastomosis requires intraoperative chromopertubation of the proximal tubal segments. Therefore, an intrauterine pediatric Foley catheter (as shown in *Figs 5.52–5.54*) or another intrauterine dye injection device is placed in the uterine cavity. The bulbs on these devices should be inflated before insertion, and after placement traction should be applied (see *Fig. 5.54*) to ensure a good seal. A Foley catheter is also placed in the patient's bladder, and after repositioning in the supine position, a 50 ml catheter tip syringe filled with dilute indigo

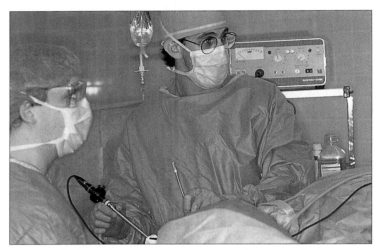

5.51 Preliminary laparoscopy to ensure adequate tubal remnants are present.

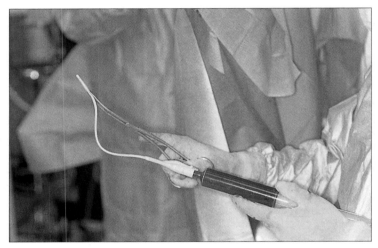

5.52 The intrauterine pediatric Foley catheter.

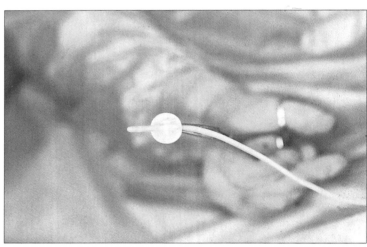

5.53 Close-up view of the Foley catheter.

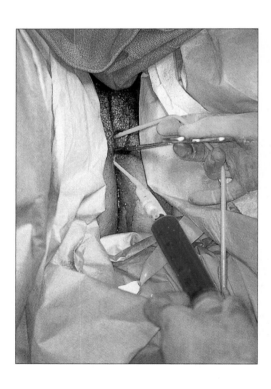

5.54 Insertion of the intrauterine Foley catheter.

carmine dye is taped to the end of the intrauterine Foley catheter and affixed to the patient's thigh (*Fig. 5.55*). It is thus readily accessible through the drapes during the procedure. Others prefer to attach intravenous extension tubing to the catheter and to place the syringe in the operative field.

Step 3

In multiparous women with a good deal of pelvic mobility, this procedure can often be performed through a mini-laparotomy. The uterus can then be elevated on to the rectus muscles, obvia-

ting the need for a retractor. When this cannot be done, a formal exploratory laparotomy is necessary. The patient's abdomen is then opened through a Pfannenstiel or vertical incision (*Fig. 5.56*). Paradoxically, microsurgery requires excellent exposure and therefore a large incision. We use a wound protector to minimize blood seepage into the pelvis (*Fig. 5.57*). On entering the abdominal cavity, the surgeon and assistants wash their gloves thoroughly to remove any talc (*Fig. 5.58*). The bowel is then packed away in the usual fashion (*Fig. 5.57*). A medium gauze roll is then placed in a surgeon's glove, washed, and inserted in

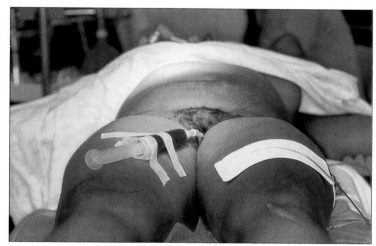

5.55 Syringe of dye, attached to catheter and taped to the patient's thigh.

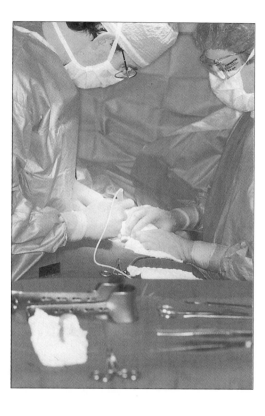

5.56 Opening the patient's abdomen.

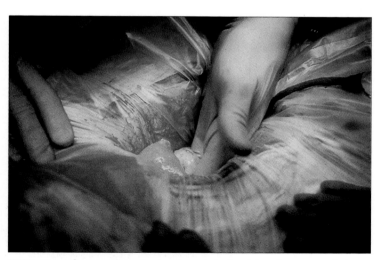

5.57 Use of wound protector to minimize blood seepage into the pelvis.

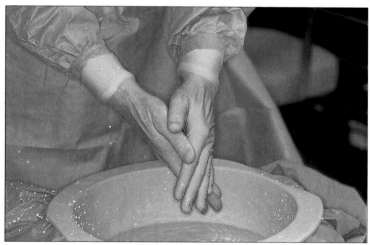

5.58 Gloves are washed to remove any talc.

the cul-de-sac (*Fig. 5.59*) to elevate the uterus and fallopian tubes.

Step 4

When the uterus and adnexa are positioned, the operative microscope is brought into the field (*Fig. 5.60*). Before the procedure, the surgeon and assistant have optimized the width and the focus of each eyepiece and have attached a 250 or 300 mm objective lens to allow unimpeded hand movement below the microscope. Some surgeons prefer to sit, whereas others find it more comfortable to stand; the key is to be comfortable, with minimal back strain, so as not to hurry the surgery. Irrigation is provided with a 50 ml syringe and a 20-gauge intravenous catheter with heparinized lactated Ringer's solution (5,000 units heparin/l). Tissues should be kept moist to minimize adhesion formation.

Optimal performance of this operation is dependent on appropriate microsurgical instrumentation, as illustrated in *Fig. 5.61*. Two pairs each of toothed and non-toothed microsurgical forceps are required, as well as either a locking or nonlocking microsurgical needle driver. Unipolar microneedle-tip cautery is preferred. A pair of iris scissors is useful, as is a separate pair of microsurgical scissors to cut the suture material. Double-armed #8-0 or #9-0 polyglactin suture is used. Atraumatic traction on tissues is achieved using 90° and 45° glass rods. A lacrimal duct probe can be used to cannulate the cornual region, and distal tubal chromopertubation is obtained with a pediatric feeding tube attached to a syringe filled with dilute indigo carmine dye.

Step 5

This patient had a previous postpartum modified Pomeroy tubal ligation, and the operative result is shown in *Fig. 5.62*. The first step is to accurately identify the proximal and distal stumps of the fallopian tube. In this case no mesosalpingeal dissection was required. Usually, however, some degree of dissection is necessary to provide free and mobile proximal and distal stumps, allowing satisfactory approximation.

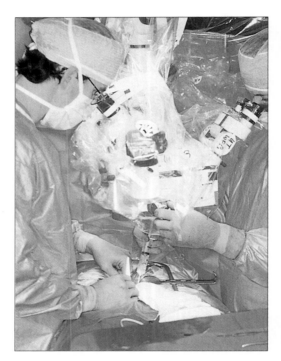

5.60 The operative microscope.

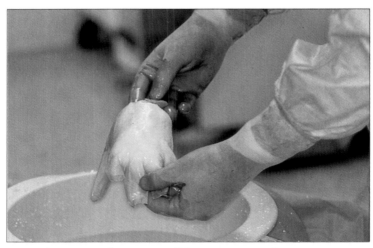

5.59 Placement of a gauze roll in a surgeon's glove.

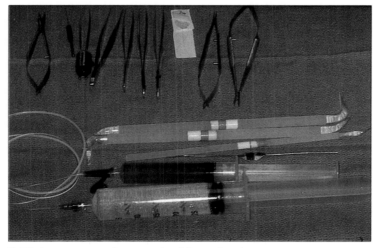

5.61 Instrumentation required for tuboplasty.

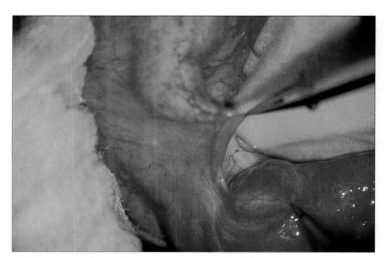

5.62 Result of previous postpartum tubal ligation.

Step 6

After the serosa has been peeled back from the muscularis and mucosa of the proximal stump by dissection and microtip electrocautery, a pair of iris scissors is used to cut a minuscule piece of stump away, until the proximal lumen can be identified with the aid of chromotubation (*Figs 5.63, 5.64*). The meticulous hemostasis needed in the transected area of the proximal stump is achieved by using high magnification and needle-point electrocautery.

Step 7

Identification of the most proximal part of the distal segment of the fallopian tube is a critical step; often it lies buried in the mesosalpinx and requires extensive dissection. This step is assisted by distending the distal fallopian tube with a pediatric feeding tube. This tube is guided into the tubal ampulla and dye is gently injected (*Figs 5.65, 5.66*). This distends the distal stump, making the anatomy of the proximal portion much clearer. After the distal stump has been mobilized, the serosa is gently peeled back and the iris scissors are used to make an extremely small ostium (*Fig. 5.67*). It is critical that the size of this ostium matches that of the

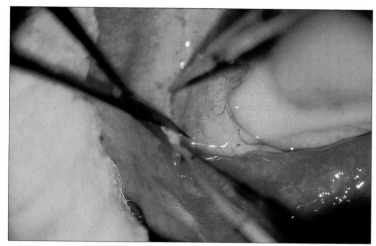

5.63 Use of iris scissors to remove a minuscule piece of proximal stump.

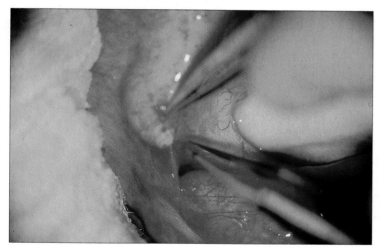

5.64 Chromotubation to identify the proximal lumen.

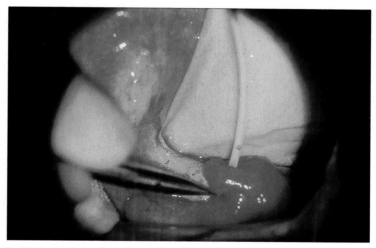

5.65 Insertion of pediatric feeding tube into the tubal ampulla.

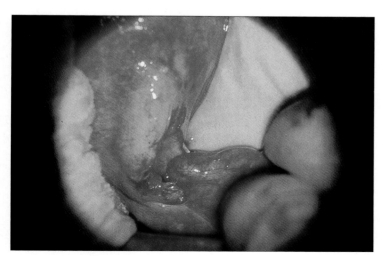

5.66 The distended distal stump.

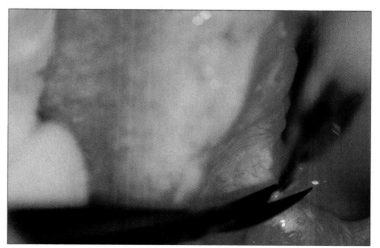

5.67 Use of iris scissors to make a small ostium.

proximal stump. If it is too large, luminal disparity of the anastomosis will exist, the likelihood of pregnancy will be lessened, and the procedure will be complicated by the persistent eversion of the abundant ampullary fimbria into the operative site. This is seen to a degree in *Fig. 5.68*. Although some endosalpingeal eversion into the operative site is inevitable (*Fig. 5.68*), the folds can be gently reduced with a lacrimal duct or glass probe.

Step 8

After the proximal and distal anastomosis sites have been prepared, a #5-0 polyglactin stay suture is placed in the mesosalpinx equidistant and close to the inferior margin of each stump (*Fig. 5.69*). This stitch not only provides the strength of the anastomosis but also ensures mesosalpingeal hemostasis. With the stay suture tied on the lateral aspect of the mesosalpinx (*Fig. 5.70*), the two stumps are brought into close apposition. The microsurgical anastomosis can then be performed with a minimum of tension. The principles of microsurgical tubal reanastomosis are shown in *Fig. 5.71*. Four interrupted sutures of #8-0 or #9-0 polyglactin are passed through the muscularis and submucosa at the 6, 3, 9 and 12 o'clock positions respectively, to reappose the lumina accurately. These sutures are placed under high magnification and are tied individually. The knots should be extraluminal. Particularly on the proximal stump, the suture should not encroach into the lumen, but distally this is less important. Placement of the 6 o'clock stitch is illustrated in *Fig. 5.72*, and the 3 o'clock stitch in *Fig. 5.73*. *Fig. 5.74* shows the appearance after all four sutures have been placed.

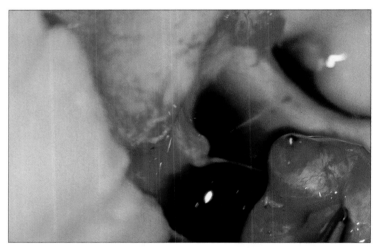

5.68 Slight endosalpingeal eversion of the operative site.

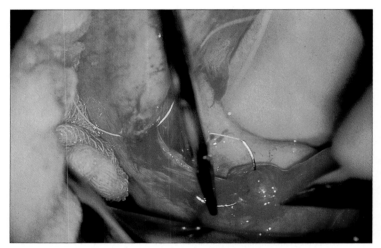

5.69 Placement of the mesosalpingeal stay suture.

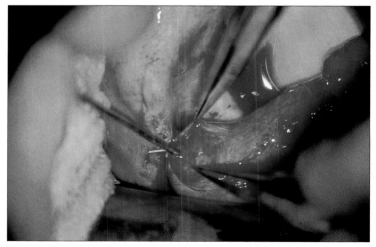

5.70 Stay suture tied on the lateral aspect of the mesosalpinx.

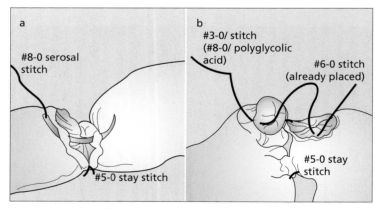

5.71 Principles of microsurgical tubal reanastomosis: placing the muscularis submucosal sutures (**a**); reapposing the serosa (**b**).

Step 9

Serosal stitches are then placed to provide further support for the reanastomosis. Usually, five or six simple interrupted sutures of #8-0 or #9-0 polyglactin acid are used (*Figs 5.71b, 5.75, 5.76*). *Fig. 5.77* demonstrates the completed isthmic–ampullar anastomosis with distal spill of indigo carmine dye. Although a water-

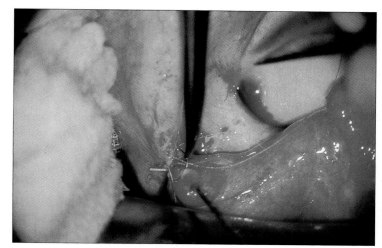

5.72 Placement of the 6 o'clock stitch.

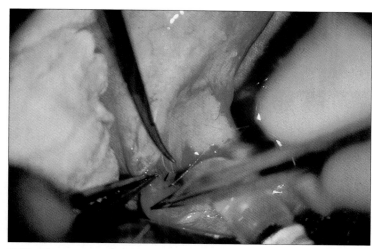

5.73 Placement of the 3 o'clock stitch.

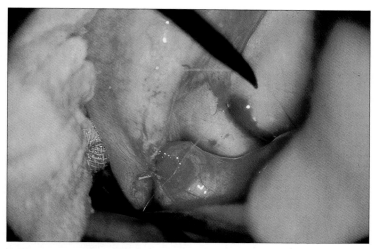

5.74 Appearance after placement of all four sutures.

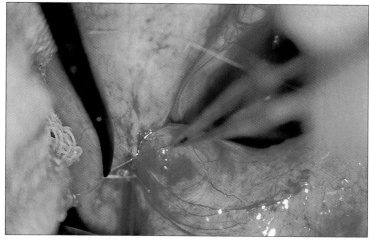

5.75 Placement of a serosal suture.

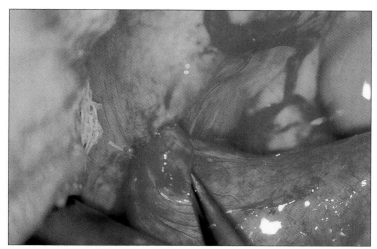

5.76 Placement of a serosal suture.

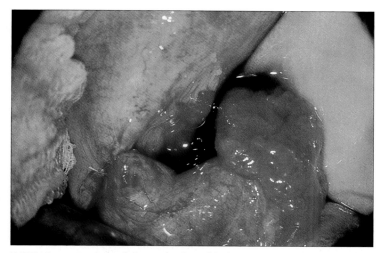

5.77 Appearance of the completed isthmic–ampullar anastomosis with distal spill of indigo carmine dye.

tight anastomosis site is esthetically appealing, there is no evidence that it improves the outcome. *Fig. 5.78* illustrates the approximately 4–5 cm of tube present after reanastomosis.

Step 10

Attention is then turned to the other fallopian tube, and in the same fashion the proximal and distal stumps are prepared (*Figs 5.79, 5.80*). The stay suture is placed in the mesosalpinx (*Fig.*

5.81) and the microsurgical isthmic–ampullar reanastomosis is performed (*Fig. 5.82*). This 39-year-old patient became pregnant 8 months after the surgery.

COMPLICATIONS

Most complications of microsurgical tubal reanastomosis are those associated with laparotomy. They include bleeding, hemorrhage, deep venous thrombosis, anesthetic morbidity, and infection. Complications specific to this procedure are as follows.

Occluded anastomosis sites

This is recognized by failure to obtain pregnancy postoperatively; the diagnosis is made by an interval hysterosalpingogram at 3 or 6 months. If the initial procedure resulted in relatively long tubal remnants, the possibility of repeat anastomoses can be entertained. Occasionally, occluded anastomosis sites can be recannulated with hysterscopically guided fallopian tube catheterization. Despite the availability of these techniques, most authorities agree that occluded anastomosis sites are an indication for IVF.

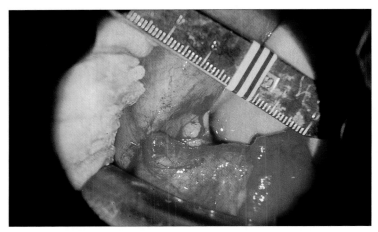

5.78 Length of the tube after reanastomosis.

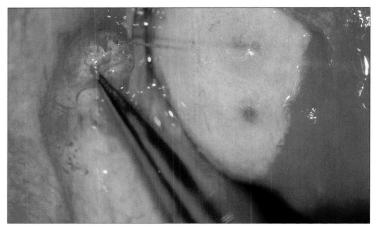

5.79 Preparation of the proximal stump of opposite fallopian tube.

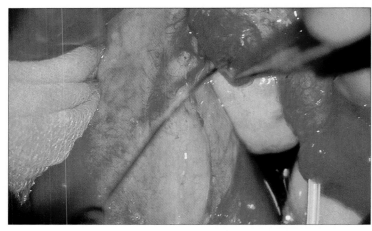

5.80 Preparation of the distal stump of opposite fallopian tube.

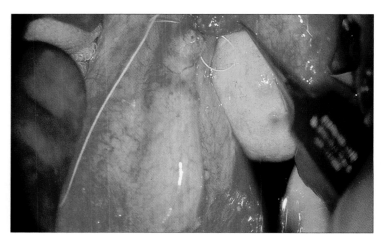

5.81 Placement of stay suture in mesosalpinx.

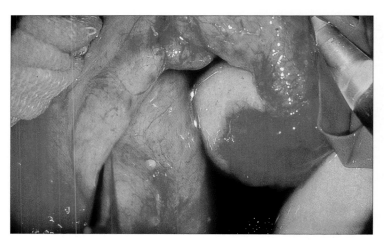

5.82 Appearance of the second isthmic–ampullar reanastomosis.

Failure to achieve pregnancy with patent fallopian tubes on hysterosalpingogram

This is often secondary to inadequate tubal length; this type of patient would best benefit from IVF. If the fallopian tube remnants are sufficiently long, one can entertain either gamete intrafallopian transfer (GIFT) or empiric human menopausal gonadotropin therapy, with or without intrauterine insemination.

Tubal fistula

This complication, delineated on the postoperative hysterosalpingogram, may in theory result in an increase in the incidence of ectopic pregnancy. Although repeat anastomosis can be considered, IVF is probably the most effective route to pregnancy.

Ectopic pregnancy

Ectopic pregnancy rates are slightly increased in patients who have undergone fallopian tube reanastomosis. Surveillance for ectopic pregnancy with early ultrasound, serial serum human chorionic gonadotropin (hCG) levels, and serum progesterone levels is important. Modern surgical and non-surgical treatments for ectopic pregnancy may not preclude salvage of the reconstructed fallopian tube, particularly with timely diagnosis.

OVARIAN CYSTECTOMY

Ovarian cystectomy is the treatment of choice for reproductive-aged patients who have a benign ovarian neoplasm. It is almost always possible to remove the ovarian pathology and preserve normal and functional ovarian tissue. Thus, the advantage of this procedure is that functional ovarian tissue remains. A technique using a laparotomy incision will be presented here, although it is possible to manage many such patients with operative laparoscopic techniques. However, to date, a prospective clinical trial has not been reported comparing these two techniques[13-16].

SURGICAL INDICATION

Surgical removal of an ovarian mass in a reproductive-aged female is indicated when there is persistence of the mass over 6–8 weeks, when it is responsible for pain, if it has undergone torsion, when it is associated with hemorrhage, or if it is larger than 7–8 cm (Fig. 5.83).

SURGICAL PROCEDURE

Step 1

After induction of anesthesia, a thorough examination should be performed to make certain that the ovarian mass is still present. It is possible for the mass to have regressed between the time the patient was scheduled for surgery and the time of surgery. A full bladder or rectum can be confused with an adnexal mass when the pelvic examination is done in an ambulatory setting.

Step 2

In patients of reproductive age, the chance of encountering an ovarian malignancy is low, and therefore a transverse incision is acceptable. In older patients, and especially those who are menopausal or postmenopausal, it is probably more prudent to make a lower midline incision in the event that the incision requires later extension for exploration of the upper abdomen.

Step 3

As soon as the peritoneum is opened, pelvic cytology is obtained. This is easily done using a 50 ml bulb syringe filled with about 25–39 ml of saline. The saline is placed into the pelvis and then removed. Any ascites fluid should also be removed and sent for cytologic analysis (Fig. 5.84).

The pelvis and upper abdomen are explored. The contralateral ovary should be inspected to make certain there is not a bilateral ovarian mass present. The surgeon should take special note of any excrescences on the ovary or studding of the pelvic peritoneum.

Indications for Surgical Removal of an Ovarian Mass

Size >7cm

Persistence over 6–8 weeks

Torsion

Rupture with hemorrhage

Pain

5.83 Indications for surgical removal of an ovarian mass.

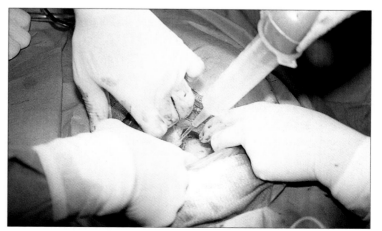

5.84 Use of bulb syringe to obtain a pelvic cytology sample.

Step 4

In this procedure the ovary has been exteriorized and moist packs have been placed around the incision to prevent any material spilling from the cyst in the case of rupture. This technique also allows excellent exposure without requiring the placement of packs inside the abdomen, thus reducing the risk of adhesion formation. The ovarian capsule is incised with a scalpel (*Fig. 5.85*). Because the ovarian cortex is very thin, care should be taken not to rupture the cyst if possible.

Step 5

Traction is applied on the cut edge of the ovarian cortex using either Allis clamps or tissue forceps (*Fig. 5.86*). The remainder of the cyst wall is separated from the ovarian cortex and parenchyma using the back of a knife handle or Metzenbaum scissors (*Fig. 5.87*). The cyst can then be shelled out without rupture in

most instances (*Fig. 5.88*), and submitted for pathologic analysis (*Fig. 5.89*).

Step 6

Hemostasis within the base of the cavity from which the cyst was removed can be obtained with electrocautery or sutures. This space can be sutured with a small gauge synthetic absorbable material using either an interrupted or a continuous purse-string type technique (*Fig. 5.90*). The cortex can be reapproximated with a subcortical running stitch of a fine gauge synthetic absorbable suture (*Fig. 5.91*). Some authors have suggested that leaving the ovary open and not reapproximating the cortex layer will result in decreased adhesion formation. It is not known if this technique reduces the incidence of adhesion formation. If excessive cortical tissue is encountered, this can be removed.

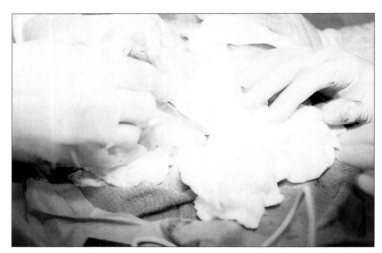

5.85 Incision of the ovarian capsule.

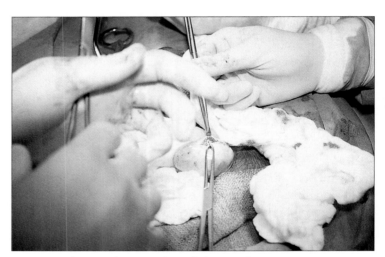

5.86 Traction on the cut edge of the ovarian cortex.

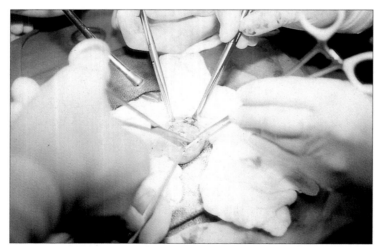

5.87 Separation of cyst wall from the ovary.

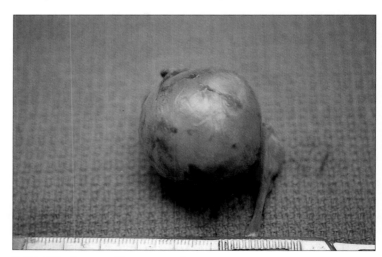

5.88 Whole cyst after removal.

Step 7

The abdomen is irrigated with Ringer's lactate solution and the abdominal incision is closed in a standard fashion (*Fig. 5.92*).

ALTERNATIVE PROCEDURES

Not all ovarian masses require surgical intervention. The majority of functional ovarian cysts will resolve with observation alone. If surgery is required, an alternative approach to laparotomy is operative laparoscopy. However, to date no randomized studies have shown that this approach to the management of an ovarian cyst is better. In fact, because it is a potentially difficult procedure, it might be that the surgeon would perform oophorectomy by laparoscopy when a cystectomy might be possible if the procedure were done with a laparotomy incision.

Oophorectomy rather than cystectomy should be performed in all postmenopausal patients with an adnexal mass, and may be necessary in the older patient of reproductive age or if there is a suspicion of malignancy.

COMPLICATIONS

Complications specific to ovarian cystectomy include cyst rupture and incomplete removal of the cyst. If cyst rupture occurs and the mass is subsequently found to be malignant, most surgeons believe that this does not necessarily worsen the patient's prognosis. If the cyst fluid from a mature teratoma spills, pseudomyxoma peritoni can result. In an effort to prevent this, copious amounts of warm 5% dextrose–water irrigation should be used. Every effort to remove the entire cyst wall should be made. If this is not possible, oophorectomy can be performed or electrocautery can be used to destroy any functional epithelium left behind. This technique is most often used in the face of an endometriotic cyst in which a portion of the capsule cannot be removed.

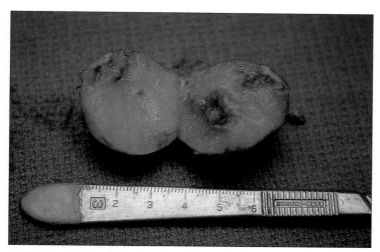

5.89 Dissection of the cyst for pathologic analysis.

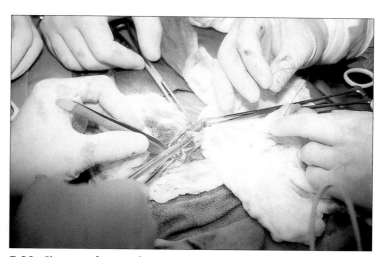

5.90 Closure of space from which cyst was removed.

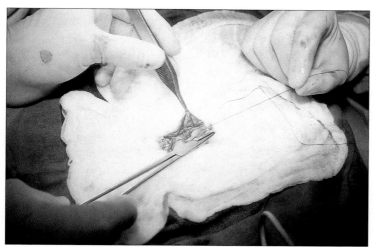

5.91 Reapproximation of the cortex.

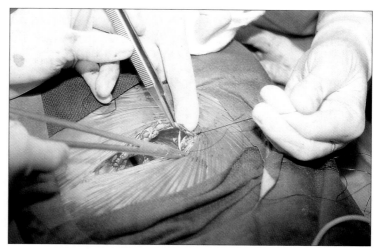

5.92 Closure of the abdomen.

REFERENCES

1. Herbst AL, Mishell DR, Stenchever MA, Droegemueller W, eds. *Comprehensive Gynecology*, 2nd ed. St. Louis: Mosby–Year Book, 1992: 518–21.

2. Stovall TG, Ling FW, eds. *Extrauterine Pregnancy: Clinical Diagnosis and Management*. New York: McGraw–Hill, 1993: 203–17.

3. Bateman BG, Nunley WC, Kitchin JD. Surgical management of distal tubal obstruction–are we making progress? In: Wallach EE, Kempers RD, eds. *Modern Trends in Infertility and Conception Control,* Vol 4. Chicago: Yearbook Medical Publishers, 1988; 305–24.

4. Rock JA, *et al*. Factors influencing the success of salpingostomy techniques for distal tubal obstruction. *Obstet Gynecol* 1978; 52:591.

5. Dohnez J, Casanas-Roux F. Prognostic factors of fimbrial microsurgery. *Fertil Steril* 1986;46:200.

6. Mettler L, *et al*. Treatment of female infertility due to tubal obstruction by operative laparoscopy. *Fertil Steril* 1979;32:384.

7. Schwartz LB, Diamond MP. Formation, reduction, and treatment of adhesive disease. *Semin Reprod Endocrinol* 1991; 9:89–99.

8. Patton GW. Microsurgical reconstruction of the oviduct. In: Behrman SJ, Kistner RW, Patton GW, eds. *Progress in Infertility*, 3rd ed., Boston: Little Brown and Co., 1989:125–54.

9. Siegler AM, Hulka J, Peretz A. Reversibility of female sterilization. In: Wallach EE, Kempers RD, eds. *Modern Trends in Infertility and Conception Control*. Vol. 4. Chicago: Yearbook Medical Publishers, 1988:573–84.

10. Patterson PJ. Factors influencing the success of microsurgical tuboplasty for sterilization reversal. *Clin Reprod Fertil* 1985;3:57.

11. Rock JA. Infertility: surgical aspects. In: Yen SSC, Jaffe RB, eds. *Reproductive Endocrinology,* 3rd ed. Philadelphia: WB Saunders, 1991;710–38.

12. Flood JT, Grow DR. Transcervical tubal cannulation. *Obstet Gynecol Surv* 1993;48:748–755.

13. Steinkampf MP, Hammond KR, Blackwell RE. Hormonal treatment of functional ovarian cysts: a randomized prospective study. *Fertil Steril* 1990;54:775.

14. Oelsner G, Graebe RA, Boyers SP, *et al*. A comparison of three techniques for ovarian reconstruction. *Am J Obstet Gynecol* 1986; 154:569.

15. Marge G, Canis M, Manhes H, *et al*. Laparoscopic management of adnexal cystic masses. *J Gynecol Surg* 1990;6:71.

16. Hurwitz A, Yagel S, Zion I, *et al*. The management of persistent clear pelvic cysts diagnosed by ultrasonography. *Obstet Gynecol* 1988;72:320.

6

Other Procedures

James G. Blythe

Thomas G. Stovall

HYPOGASTRIC ARTERY LIGATION

In 1893, Howard Kelly[1] reported the first bilateral hypogastric artery ligation, which was performed to decrease bleeding during a hysterectomy. Since its first description, much work has been done to determine why this procedure decreases pelvic bleeding. In 1964, Burchell[2] determined that hypogastric artery ligation worked because it decreased the arterial pulse pressure, thus providing the opportunity for a clot to form.

The chief difficulty with using this procedure lies in waiting too long to perform it rather than in its actual execution. Consequently, hypogastric artery ligation is a procedure that should be in the surgical repertoire of any well-trained gynecologic surgeon[3-6].

SURGICAL INDICATIONS

Indications can be divided into obstetric versus gynecologic and prophylactic versus therapeutic. Some surgeons have questioned the value of prophylactic ligation (*Fig. 6.1*).

Indications for Hypogastric Artery Ligation	
Gynecologic	**Obstetric**
Bleeding from vaginal cuff after hysterectomy	Placenta accreta
Bleeding from pelvic carcinomas	Abdominal pregnancy
Fibroids requiring morcellation	Uterine atony
Broad ligament hematomas	Couvelaire uterus
	Ruptured uterus

6.1 Indications for hypogastric artery ligation.

SURGICAL PROCEDURE

Access to the hypogastric artery can be gained through either a transabdominal or an extraperitoneal approach. The transabdominal approach is a familiar gynecologic technique preferred by most gynecologists because it facilitates easy visualization of pelvic pathology, viewing of both hypogastric arteries through one incision, and easy access to both the hypogastric and ovarian vessels.

Step 1

Elevate the round ligaments. Place a hemaclip or suture across the proximal portion and a #3-0 delayed absorbable suture across the distal portion. Elevating the round ligament exposes the lateral pelvic wall peritoneum (*Fig. 6.2*).

Step 2

The round ligament is cut and the incision is extended though the lateral pelvic wall peritoneum parallel to the infundibulo-pelvic ligament to the level of the ovary (*Fig. 6.3*).

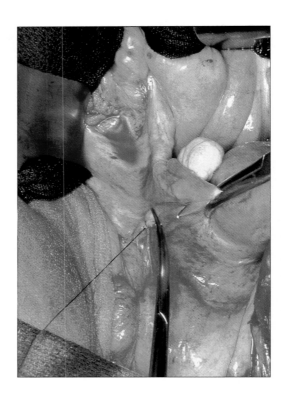

6.2 Cutting of round ligament.

Step 3

The lateral pelvic wall retroperitoneal space is exposed. This space is filled with filmy areolar tissue extending from the medial to lateral pelvic peritoneum (*Fig. 6.4*)

Step 4

This loose, filmy areolar tissue should be removed with sharp dissection. Small blood vessels that may be encountered are easily cauterized. This dissection should be performed down to the level of the external iliac artery (*Fig. 6.5*).

Step 5

Insert the index finger of both hands into this area and sweep them gently, parallel to the external iliac artery down to the level of the hypogastric artery. Sweeping parallel to the pelvic wall should not injure the pelvic vessels (*Fig. 6.6*).

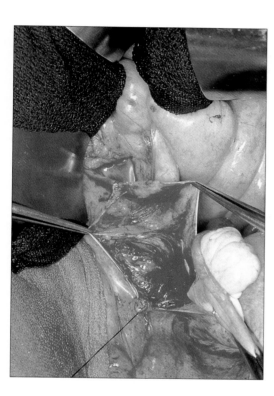

6.3 Exposure of retroperitoneal space.

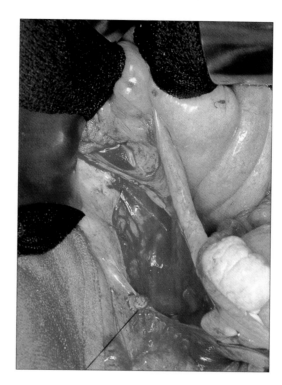

6.4 Dissection of retroperitoneal space.

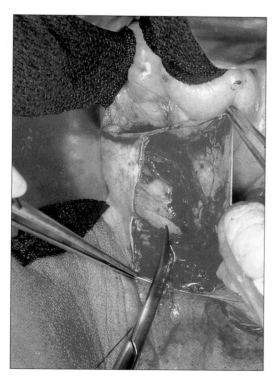

6.5 Removal of loose areolar tissue.

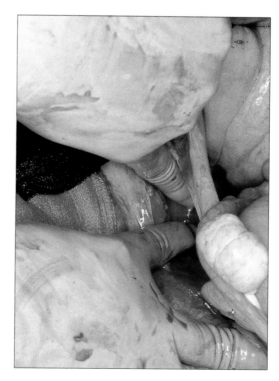

6.6 Use of blunt dissection.

Step 6

The ureter is identified on the medial leaf of the peritoneum. It bisects the bifurcation of the internal and external iliac arteries (*Fig. 6.7*).

Step 7

A thorough knowledge of these anatomic relationships is important to a successful hypogastric artery ligation (*Figs 6.8, 6.9*).

Step 8

The surgeon performing the procedure ligates the artery on the opposite side of the pelvis. This aids in visualization and identification of the hypogastric artery. Before the artery is ligated, both the surgeon and the assistant should agree that the artery to be ligated is the hypogastric artery. With both blunt and sharp dissection, the areolar and surrounding fatty tissues are dissected away from the hypogastric artery. A right-angled clamp is placed beneath the bifurcation of the external iliac and hypogastric

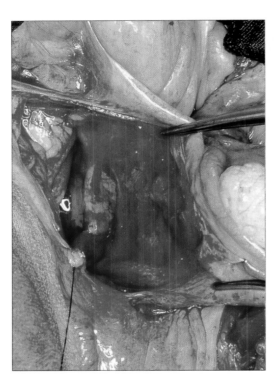

6.7 Ureteral identification.

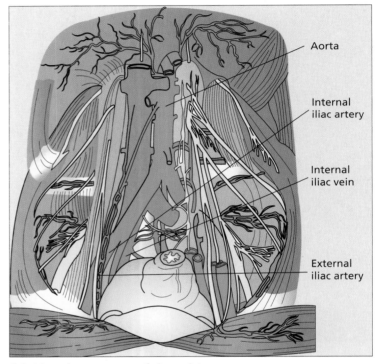

6.8 Vascular anatomy of the pelvis.

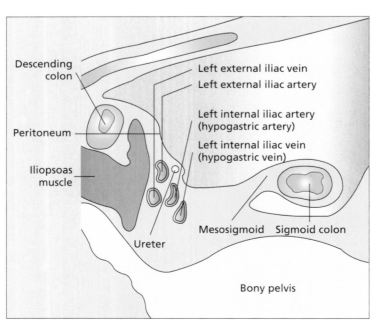

6.9 Cross-sectional anatomy of the pelvis.

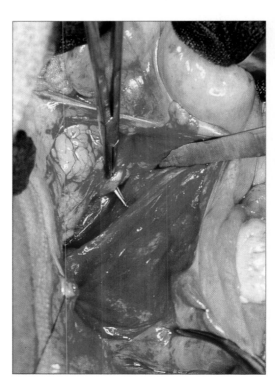

6.10 Placement of right-angled clamp.

arteries. The clamp is placed beneath the hypogastric artery from the lateral side. This decreases the potential damage to the hypogastric vein (*Fig. 6.10*). The correct and incorrect placements of the right-angled clamp are illustrated in *Fig. 6.11*. In position #1, the clamp will puncture the hypogastric artery, while in position #2 the clamp will pass safely between the hypogastric artery and vein. In position #3, the clamp will puncture the hypogastric vein. In *Fig. 6.12* the pelvic sidewall has been completely dissected to illustrate the anatomic relationships. It is neither advisable nor necessary to expose the anatomy to this extent.

Step 9
The right-angled clamp beneath the artery is opened, a suture is passed to this clamp, and the clamp is withdrawn. The suture is tied, thus ligating the hypogastric artery. This procedure is repeated on the opposite side (*Figs 6.13, 6.14*).

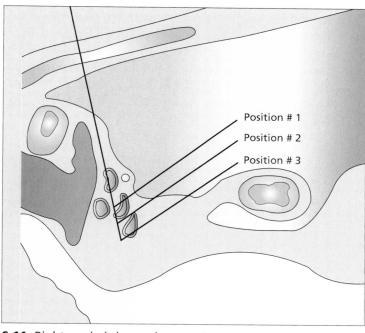

6.11 Right-angled clamp placement.

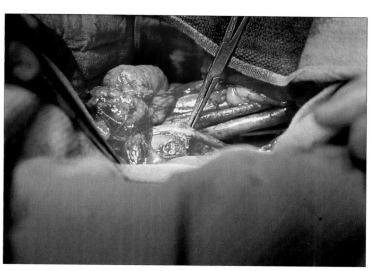

6.12 Lateral pelvic sidewall anatomy.

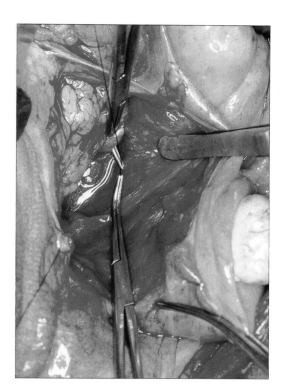

6.13 Placement of the suture beneath artery.

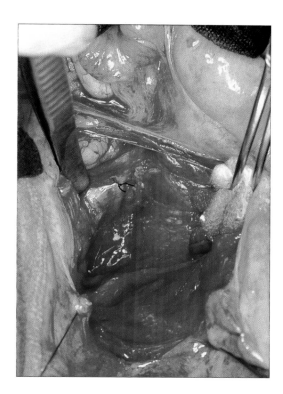

6.14 Completed procedure.

An acceptable alternative procedure after the artery has been exposed (as described in Step 7) is to grasp the artery with a Babcock clamp. Step 9 is now completed (*Fig. 6.15*). Other alternative surgical and non-surgical procedures for hypogastric artery ligation are listed in *Fig. 6.16*.

COMPLICATIONS

- The most common potential complication of this procedure is waiting too long before its performance. The results of this action are obvious.
- It is all too easy to ligate the external iliac artery instead of the hypogastric artery. This is why it is imperative to have the artery identified by both the surgeon and the assistant before it is ligated. After the surgery has been completed, it is wise to palpate the dorsalis pedal pulse. Absence of this pulse, followed in a few hours by cyanosis of the affected limb, indicates an erroneous ligation. Corrective procedures require reopening of the abdomen and removal of the tie.

- Puncture of the hypogastric vein may occur if the surgeon is unfamiliar with the anatomic relationships. The danger to the patient is not due to the injury to the vein but rather to the immediate bleeding that will ensue; this increased bleeding worsens the patient's condition. The vein can be repaired by immediate pressure on it below the level of the injury. This will stop the venous bleeding, after which the venous laceration can be closed either by a Ligaclip or by a #4-0 permanent suture.
- Necrosis of the gluteus maximus muscle has been reported, and is more likely to occur if the ligature is placed above the posterior branches of the hypogastric artery (iliolumbar, lumbosacral, superior gluteal). This may occur because the ligature is placed too close to the bifurcation or because these vessels originate at a lower point than expected. Treatment should include removal of the ligature, provided the artery has not been divided, followed by wound care of the necrotic area.

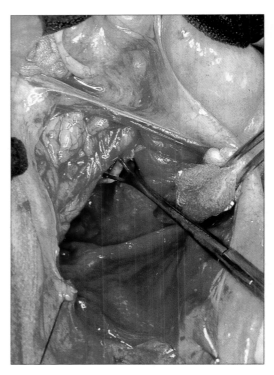

6.15 Alternative procedure.

Alternative Procedures	
Surgical	**Non-surgical**
Uterine artery ligation	Pack
Hysterectomy	Vaginal
Ovarian artery ligation	Pelvic
Hemostatic sutures	Cervical
	MAST suit
	Arterial embolization
	Microfibrillar collagen

6.16 Alternative procedures for hypogastric artery ligation.

APPENDECTOMY

Several surgical techniques for removing the appendix exist today. These include: the time-honored tie, incision technique; the laparoscopic clip technique; and the gastrointestinal stapling technique. Since many gynecologists perform appendectomies incidentally at the time of another procedure, the well-trained gynecologic surgeon should be proficient in all of these techniques.

SURGICAL INDICATIONS

In the majority of gynecologic cases, an appendectomy is an incidental procedure (*Fig. 6.17*)[7–9]. It may also be performed as part of the staging procedure in a gynecologic oncology patient[10].

SURGICAL PROCEDURE

Step 1

The appendix is identified. If it is retrocecal, it should be dissected free and adequately exposed (*Fig. 6.18*).

Step 2

The junction of the appendix and cecum is identified. The appendicular artery in the appendiceal mesentery is visualized (*Figs 6.19, 6.20*).

Incidental Appendectomy Criteria
1. A stable patient
2. Primary operation uncomplicated
3. No contraindication to additional surgery
4. Original incision provides access to appendix

6.17 Incidental appendectomy criteria.

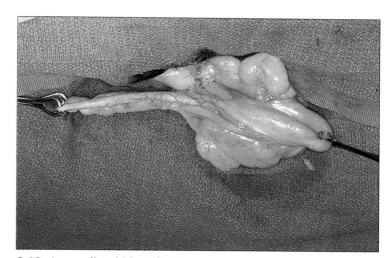

6.18 Appendiceal identification.

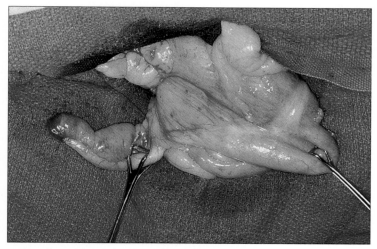

6.19 Identification of the cecal junction.

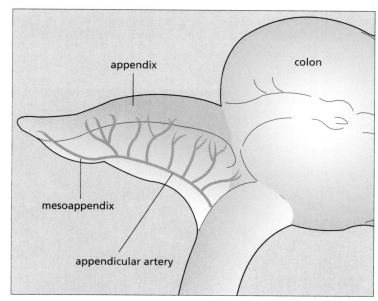

6.20 Anatomy of the appendix.

Step 3

This step involves dividing the appendiceal mesentery. Keeping in mind that the shortest distance between two points is a straight line (*Figs 6.21, 6.22*), the mesentery is incised between points B and C rather than A and B. The starting point can be either point A or point B, whichever is easiest. We prefer to begin by securing the appendicular artery (Point A, *Fig. 6.23*). Either curved or straight hemostats are pushed through the mesentery, one on each side of the artery. The artery is then doubly clamped and incised between the clamps (*Fig, 6.24*).

Step 4

The above procedure is repeated until the mesentery has been divided (*Fig. 6.25*).

Step 5

The appendix is cross-clamped at the appendiceal–cecal junction. A suture is placed in this resulting groove and tied (*Fig. 6.26*).

Step 6

The appendix is clamped and incised 1 cm distal to the tie (*Fig. 6.27*).

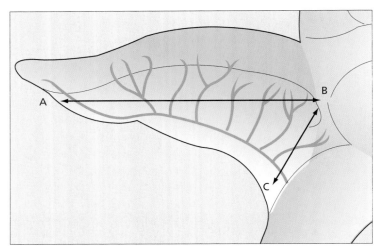

6.21 Illustration of appendicial mesentery.

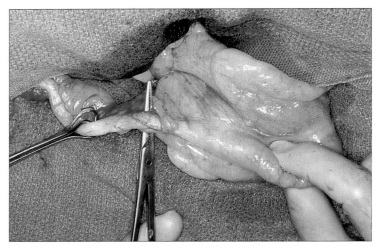

6.22 Appendicial mesentery.

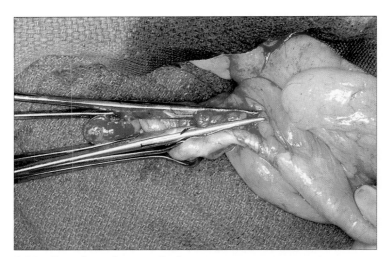

6.23 Clamping of appendicular artery.

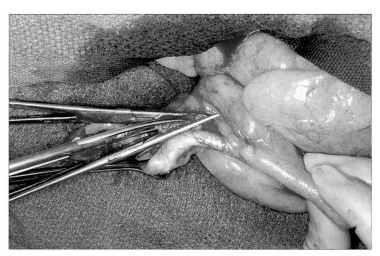

6.24 Incision of artery.

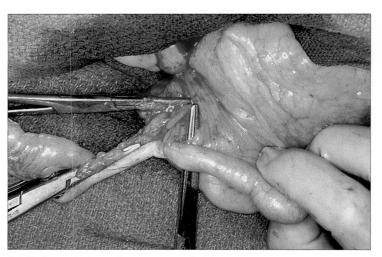

6.25 Completion of mesentery division.

Step 7

Handling of the appendiceal stump is controversial. Several surgeons have demonstrated that no further preparation of this stump is necessary. Traditionally, the appendiceal stump is buried. This, too, is considered optional by many surgeons. If this is done, place a purse-string suture of #2-0 non-absorbable suture about 1 cm from and around the appendiceal stump (*Fig. 6.28*).

Step 8

The appendiceal stump is grasped with a hemostat and indented into the cecum. The #2-0 non-absorbable suture is then tied. All of the appendiceal vessels are ligated with #3-0 delayed absorbable suture *(Fig. 6.29)*.

ALTERNATIVE PROCEDURE

An appendectomy may be performed through either an abdominal incision or the laparoscope. Specifically designed clip applicators are available for appendectomy performed through the laparoscope. If the appendectomy is performed via an abdominal incision, various stapling instruments such as gastrointestinal staples can be used.

COMPLICATIONS

The following intraoperative and postoperative complications can occur and have been listed by various authors:

- The most immediate complication is haemorrhage due to bleeding from one of the mesoappendiceal vessels. If it occurs during the operation, it should be recognized and the vessel immediately secured. If the bleeding occurs postoperatively, it should be diagnosed and treated as any other postoperative haemorrhage.
- The appendiceal stump can leak or perforate, resulting in an abscess and peritonitis. This will require appropriate diagnostic tests, antibiotics, and possibly drainage.
- If intestinal obstruction is reported after an appendectomy, routine treatment for intestinal obstruction should be followed.

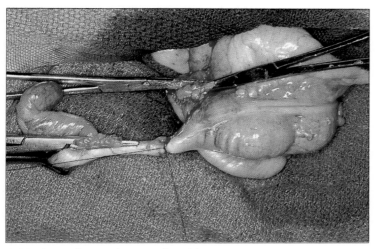

6.26 Cross-clamped appendix with suture.

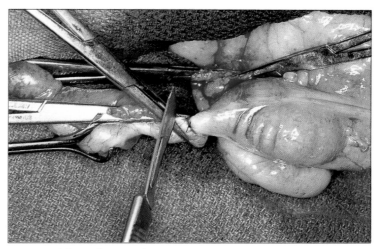

6.27 Excision of appendix.

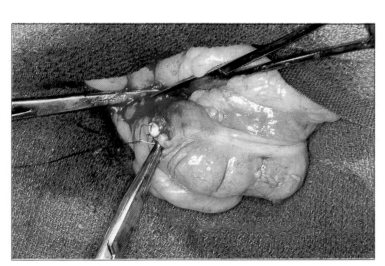

6.28 Placement of purse-string suture.

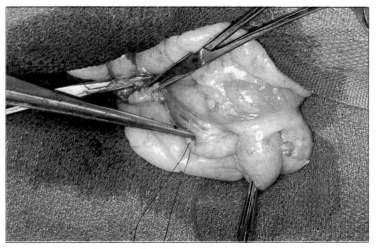

6.29 Burying of appendiceal stump.

BOWEL LACERATION

Laceration of the bowel wall is a fairly common complication faced by the gynecologic surgeon. Krebs[11] reported that 72% of these injuries occurred during uncomplicated gynecologic procedures. The rate of injury to the small intestine is about 75%, and to the large bowel about 25%[12–14]. This is partially due to the multiplicity of surgical procedures that many gynecologic patients undergo. Because of the frequency of lacerations, the gynecologic surgeon should be able to both recognize and repair these complications[15].

SURGICAL INDICATIONS

Areas of bowel and mucosal or muscularis tears require immediate repair, but small serosal lacerations usually require no repair. A classification of bowel injuries can be seen in *Fig. 6.30.*

SURGICAL PROCEDURE

Step 1

When the muscularis and/or mucosa is torn, it must be repaired immediately to prevent peritoneal contamination. The bowel should be dissected free from any structure to which it is adhered. The free injured loop should be isolated by sterile towels or lap pads. If the small bowel has been injured, it should be closed perpendicular to the long axis of the bowel. Traction sutures or noncrushing clamps should be placed at both ends of the laceration. Pulling on either the sutures or the clamps will convert the tear to a transverse laceration (*Fig. 6.31*).

Step 2

Since this laceration penetrates all layers, a two-layer closure is recommended. Using #3-0 absorbable suture on a GI needle, the mucosa is closed with a running stitch that reapproximates the mucosa. The initial stitch of this layer is placed beyond the end of the laceration to ensure that the entire laceration is closed. The end of this stitch is tied and tagged (*Fig. 6.32*) when the opposite end of the laceration is reached, again going one stitch beyond the laceration to ensure that it is closed (*Fig. 6.33*). The end of this suture is tagged for future use (*Fig. 6.34*).

Classification of Bowel Injuries		
Type	**Percentage of Injuries**	**Definition**
Major	31	Muscularis and/or extensive mucosa tears *or* Bowel transection
Minor	69	Localized muscularis and/or mucosa tears
Superficial		Serosal tears

6.30 Classification of bowel injuries.

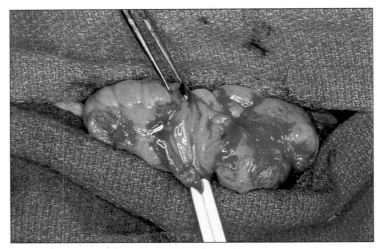

6.31 Placement of non-crushing clamps.

Step 3

The next layers to be closed are the muscularis and serosa. These layers are approximated with #4-0 non-absorbable suture on a GI needle in an interrupted fashion (*Fig. 6.35*). This suture should penetrate only the muscularis and serosa to prevent the needle from passing from a contaminated area (bowel lumen) to a non-contaminated area (*Fig. 6.36*). The first stitch is placed lateral to the tagged non-absorbable suture. This ensures that the initial suture tissue is buried, thus eliminating potential contamination from the absorbable suture that penetrated all layers. The non-

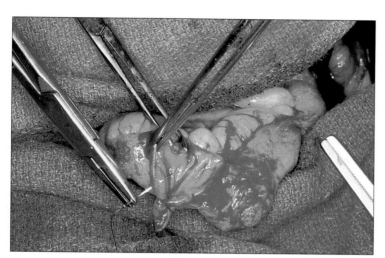

6.32 Placement of first suture layer.

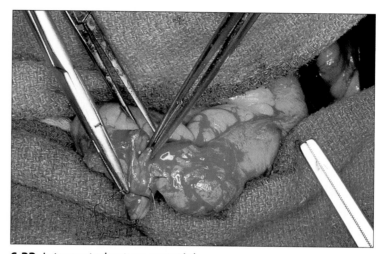

6.33 Interrupted suture material.

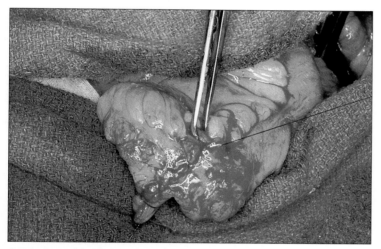

6.34 Completed suture line.

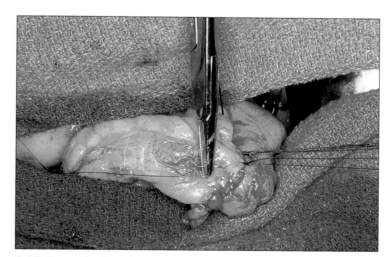

6.35 Second suture layer.

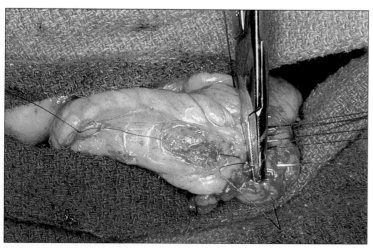

6.36 Completion of second suture line.

absorbable suture is placed in interrupted Lembert stitches (*Figs 6.37, 6.38*). It is important to remember that these sutures must approximate the serosal layer, not strangulate it (*Fig. 6.39*). This layer buries the absorbable suture layer. The last non-absorbable suture goes beyond the tagged absorbable suture at the end of the laceration (*Fig. 6.40*). All of the non-absorbable sutures are cut at this time. They are not cut earlier because they are used as traction sutures (*Fig. 6.41*).

Step 4

The patency of the small bowel lumen is tested at this time. This is accomplished by pressing together the thumb and forefinger on each side of the closure. The surgeon should be able to palpate a definite lumen in the middle of the suture layers (*Fig. 6.42*).

ALTERNATIVE PROCEDURES

The continuity of the gastrointestinal tract must be maintained. If circumstances and /or the condition of the gastrointestinal tract do not permit a simple repair, diversion of the fecal stream can be performed. This diversion may be by either various small-to-small or small-to-large bowel ananstomoses or by exteriorizing the faecal stream by a jejunostomy, ileostomy, or colostomy.

COMPLICATIONS

Complications can be divided into two broad categories: those that result from the soilage of the peritoneal cavity and those that are related to the surgical repair.

When a tear in the intestinal tract has occurred it is safe to assume that peritoneal contamination will follow. Consequently,

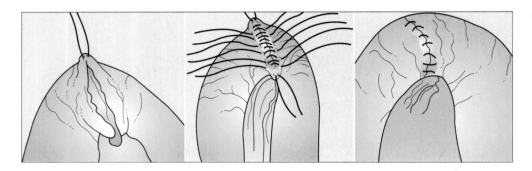

6.37 Illustration of bowel laceration repair.

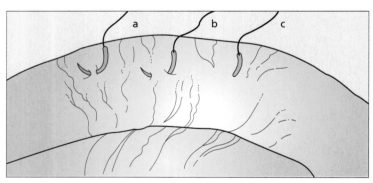

6.38 Needle **a** is through the serosa; **b** enters the muscularis; while **c** enters the submucosa.

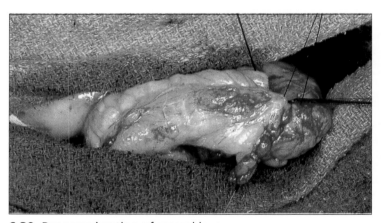

6.39 Reapproximation of serosal layer.

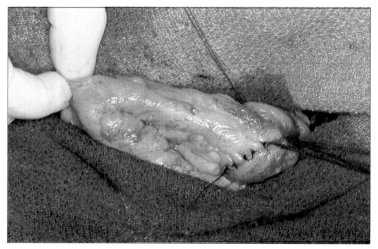

6.40 Non-absorbable layer goes beyond the absorbable layer.

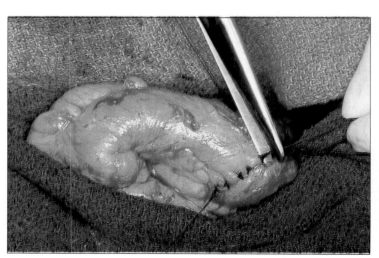

6.41 Cutting of suture.

the abdominal cavity must be irrigated with copious amounts of saline after repair. Treatment with antibiotics is usually begun at this time. If for some reason these measures are unsuccessful, the patient may develop an intra-abdominal abscess and/or peritonitis. If the repair leaks but is confined to the layers of the intestinal tract, an abscess may form that is confined to the wall of the intestine. These conditions should be suspected if symptoms so indicate, and appropriate measures should be taken to correct them.

Of course, complications can occur because of the operative procedure no matter how skilled the surgeon. If the patient has received intra-abdominal radiation, has Crohn's disease, or has an intra-abdominal malignancy, or should the laceration-repair and the abdominal incision end up in apposition to each other, an enterocutaneous fistula may develop. Caring for this complication requires considerable expertise on the part of the surgeon. As with all intra-abdominal surgery, an intestinal obstruction is always a possibility and should be dealt with by the usual means.

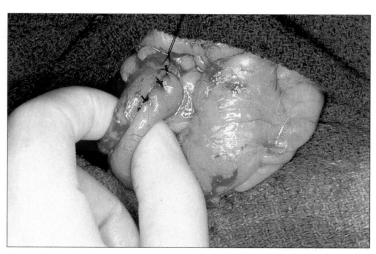

6.42 Completion of the procedure.

PRESACRAL NEURECTOMY

The first report of a presacral neurectomy appeared in the literature of 1899. Both Jaboulay and Ruggi independently reported using this procedure to relieve pelvic pain. The procedure gained prominence in 1924, when Cotte reported his extensive experience. Today, presacral neurectomy should be reserved for a limited number of carefully selected patients for whom all other methods of therapy have failed[16–20].

SURGICAL INDICATIONS

The most common indication has been secondary dysmenorrhea, usually associated with endometriosis or pelvic adhesions. Since the introduction of antiprostaglandins, this surgical procedure has had fewer indications. A literature review reveals that about 70–80% of the patients experience significant relief of midline pelvic pain and dysmenorrhea as a result of presacral neurectomy. *Fig. 6.43* outlines the indications for presacral neurectomy in the patient with central pelvic pain.

Indications for Presacral Neurectomy
Central pelvic pain due to:
Dysmenorrhea
Primary
Secondary
Endometriosis
Other
Sacral backache
Pelvic adhesions
Unknown etiology
Dyspareunia

6.43 Indications for presacral neurectomy.

SURGICAL PROCEDURE
Step 1
The type of abdominal incision used in this operation is chosen to allow easy access to the sacral promontory and aortic bifurcation region (*Fig. 6.44*). Either a Pfannenstiel or a midline incision can be used. The para-aortic area is best located by palpating the aorta. The patient should be placed in a steep Trendelenberg position to allow the bowel to be packed away from the operative site. The small intestine is then packed into the upper abdomen. This will be primarily the upper right quadrant, because the mesentery of the small intestine originates from the right of the aorta. The colon can usually be allowed to fall into the pelvis, where it will be out of the operative field (*Fig. 6.45*).

Step 2
The posterior peritoneum overlying the bifurcation is identified (*Fig. 6.46*). To understand why a presacral neurectomy is effective and how to minimize complications, the surgeon must be knowledgeable about the anatomy in this area. In 1899, Elaut described the anatomy of the presacral nerve in *Surgery Obstetrics and Gynecology*.

"The presacral nerve has its origin at the level of the superior mesenteric artery where it consists of two or three intermesenteric nerves which may cross over and communicate. They join at the bifurcation of the aorta to form the superior hypogastric plexus i.e. the presacral nerve."

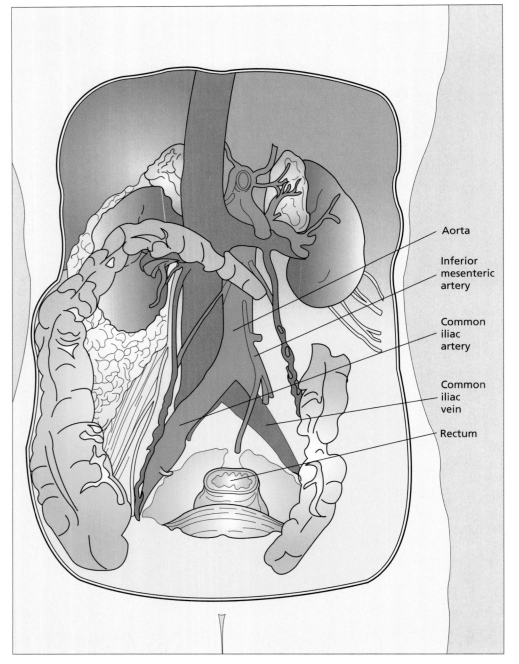

6.44 Illustration of the aortic bifurcation and sacral promontory.

Aorta

Inferior mesenteric artery

Common iliac artery

Common iliac vein

Rectum

Only about 24% of patients have a well-defined nerve. This is usually located in the triangular space formed by the common iliac arteries. Here it is situated above the promontory of the fourth and fifth lumbar vertebrae. The nerve is better described as a "plexus" (*Figs 6.47, 6.48*). Perhaps Elaut described this best

when he wrote, "the majority [of patients] had a definite intricate network of nerve fibres in the loose areolar subperitoneal tissue [which] becomes denser in the neighborhood of the plexus so as to form a rather compact covering membrane around the different nerve fibrils holding them together in a fanshaped ensemble."

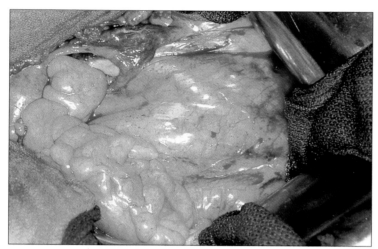

6.45 Operative field.

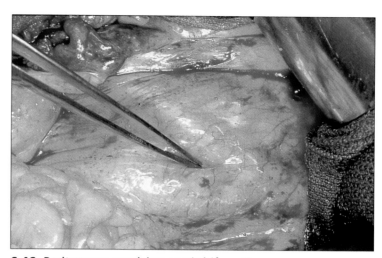

6.46 Peritoneum overlying aortic bifurcation.

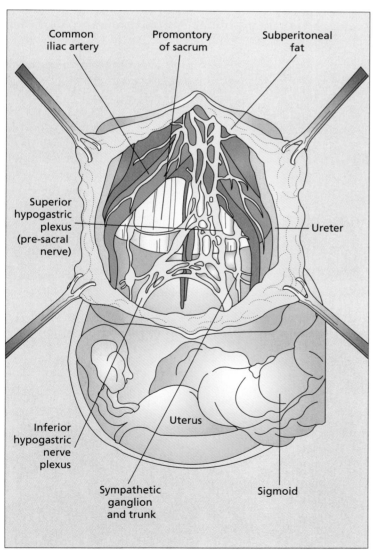

6.47 Illustration of anatomy in operative field.

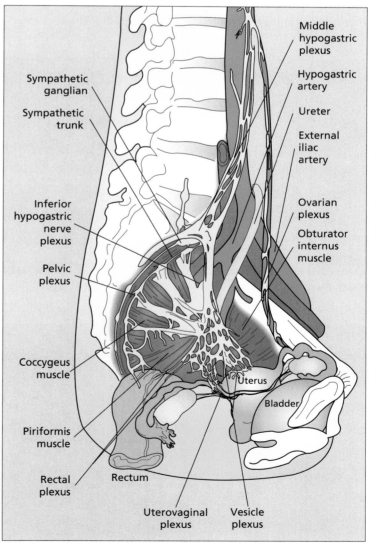

6.48 Illustration of pelvic nerve.

Step 3

The posterior peritoneum is elevated about 5 cm below and slightly to the right of the bifurcation (*Fig. 6.49*). The posterior peritoneum is incised (*Fig. 6.50*) about 10 cm from the previously described point to about 5 cm above and to the left of the aorta to the inferior mesenteric artery (*Fig. 6.51*).

Step 4

The borders of the dissection are left–the inferior mesenteric artery; right–the right ureter; cephalad–the aortic bifurcation; and caudal–the mid common iliac arteries (*Fig. 6.52*). The edges of the cut peritoneum are retracted. The dissection of the nerve plexus is begun on the side opposite the surgeon. On the right, all of the subperitoneal fibrofatty tissue is dissected free from the peritoneum down to the right ureter (*Figs 6.53, 6.54*). On the left, the procedure is repeated and the dissection is continued laterally to the inferior mesenteric artery. This should put the surgeon over the right and left common iliac arteries just beneath the bifurcation of the aorta.

Step 5

A right-angled clamp is passed beneath all of this fibrofatty tissue overlying the fourth and fifth lumbar vertebrae (*Fig. 6.55*). The clamp slides beneath this tissue over or just medial to one of the iliac arteries and exits over or medial to the opposite iliac artery.

The nerve fibrils lie in this fibrofatty tissue, and sometimes they can be easily identified, as seen in this patient; however, usually a definite nerve is not identifiable. The middle sacral artery is located between the nerve plexus and on the anterior surface of the vertebrae. It usually does not sustain injury because it is closely adherent to the vertebral bodies. This nerve plexus is cross-clamped and a 3- to 4-cm section is excised. This section of the fibrofatty tissue should be submitted to the pathologist for histologic identification of the nerve (*Fig. 6.56*). A hemaclip can be placed across both ends of the incised tissue (*Fig. 6.57*). The peritoneum can be closed with a running stitch of absorbable #3-0 suture.

ALTERNATIVE PROCEDURES

Several treatments exist for dysmenorrhea and/or dyspareunia, the main indications for a presacral neurectomy. Medical therapy consists of administering oral contraceptives and antiprostaglandins. If the patient has severe dysmenorrhea and/or dyspareunia, a hysterectomy may be acceptable if she has no further interest in bearing children.

COMPLICATIONS

To understand the potential complications, one must understand the nerve supply of the pelvis. The superior hypogastric plexus (i.e., the presacral nerve) divides into two branches, the right and

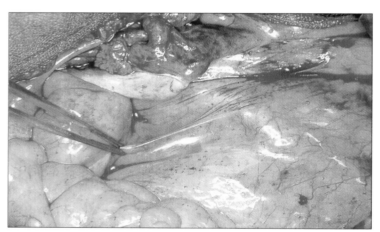

6.49 Elevation of posterior peritoneum.

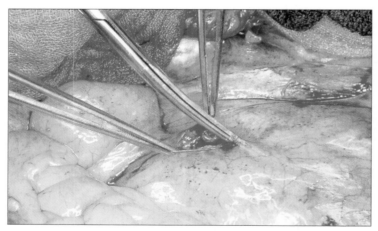

6.50 Incision of posterior peritoneum.

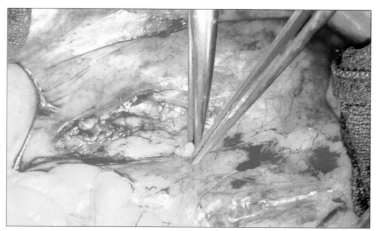

6.51 Completed incision of posterior peritoneum.

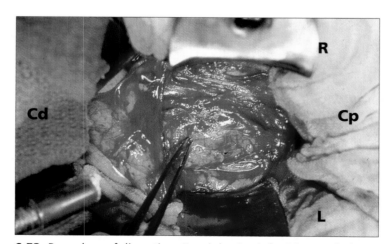

6.52 Boundary of dissection. R = right; L = left; Cd = caudad; Cp = cephalad.

left inferior hypogastric plexi, as it descends into the pelvis. These inferior hypogastric nerves descend laterally and downward into the sacral end of each uterosacral ligament. They then spread out into the pelvic plexi. The pelvic plexi pass forward over the lateral portion of the rectum and upper vagina. Pelvic plexi are sub-divided into secondary plexi. These include the rectal plexus to the rectum, the uterovaginal plexus to the uterus and vagina, and the vesical plexus to the bladder.

Although a number of surgeons have reported an absence of complications, some may arise due to this operative technique. The most common problem is injury to the middle sacral artery and/or vein. If this occurs, the bleeding should be stopped by whatever manner is appropriate. This could include cautery, ligation, and/or sterile thumbtacks.

The remaining reported complications relate to the relevant anatomy and occur during the postoperative period. Bowel complications such as constipation are believed to be due to interference of the pelvic plexus, specifically the rectal plexus. Constipation usually improves over time, and until it does the patient will need to take mild laxatives. A small bowel obstruc-tion may occur after this surgery as a result of adhesions, as it may after any surgery, and should be treated by standard methods.

Both urine retention and incontinence may result from this procedure. Both of these conditions are believed to be due to interruption of the pelvic nerve supply. They should be treated symptomatically until the organs have a chance to recover. Other complications thought to be due to the interrupted nerve supply include vaginal dryness and painless labor. Vaginal dryness should be treated with vaginal moisturizing agents as long as is necessary. Patients who might experience painless labor must be aware of this condition and monitor their pregnancy closely.

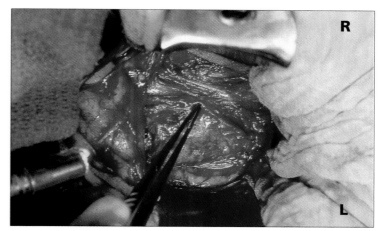

6.53 Removal of fibroadipose tissue.

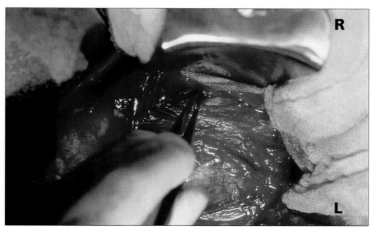

6.54 Completion of dissection.

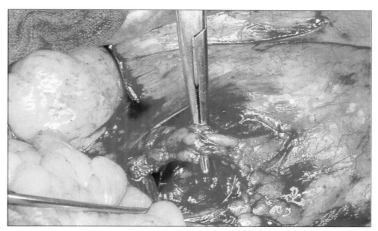

6.55 Removal of neural tissue.

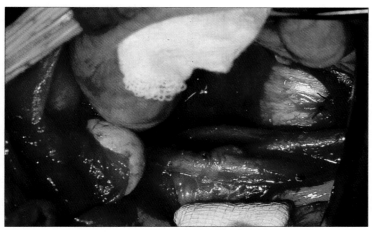

6.56 Completion of neural tissue removal.

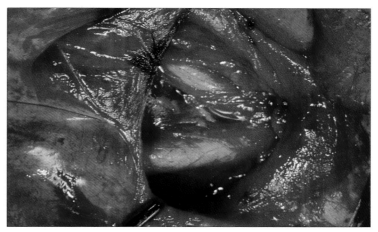

6.57 Placement of hemaclip.

REPAIR OF URETERAL INJURY

Injury to the ureter occurs in about 0.5–2.5% of gynecologic surgical procedures[21, 22]. The most effective way to avoid ureteral injury is to identify and expose the ureters at the time of surgery. Even when this is done consistently for all pelvic procedures, it is still possible to injure the ureter. This usually occurs when attempts are made to control hemorrhage, or when extensive endometriosis is encountered or the anatomy is altered by another pathologic process, such as remnant ovarian syndrome.

The most common sites of ureteral injury are: near the pelvic brim where the infundibulopelvic ligament is clamped; at the level of the uterine artery; and at the cervicovaginal junction. Of these, injury at the level of the uterine artery is most commonly seen.

INDICATIONS

If recognized, all urethral injuries should be repaired at the time of the surgical procedure. In general, most gynecologic surgery-related injuries involve only 1–2 cm of ureteral length, as they are secondary to suture ligation or a crush injury from clamp placement.

The type of procedure used to repair an injured ureter depends on the site and length of the injured segment. This section illustrates the two most common methods of ureteral repair, ureteroureterostomy and ureteroneocystostomy. If the gynecologic surgeon were familiar with these two techniques, almost all ureteral injuries that would be encountered could be successfully repaired.

Ureteroureterostomy is the procedure of choice when the injury occurs above the midplane of the pelvis (at the infundibulopelvic ligament or uterine artery), whereas ureteroneocystostomy is used for injuries that occur below the midplane of the pelvis (cardinal ligament or at the level of the cervix).

SURGICAL PROCEDURE: URETEROURETEROSTOMY
Step 1
The site of ureteral injury is identified and the damaged segment is mobilized so that an approximately 2 cm segment of ureter is cleared from its surrounding connective tissue sheath. This step is necessary so that minimal tension is placed on the anastomosis (*Fig. 6.58*).

Step 2
Both the cephalad and caudad damaged ends of the ureter are excised, so that the "freshened" ends can be reapproximated. The ends are then spatulated, which increases the circumference of the ureteral orifice (*Fig. 6.59*).

Step 3
A Silastic "double J" ureteral stent (*Fig. 6.60*) is inserted so that one end is placed in the renal pelvis and the other in the bladder (*Fig. 6.61*).

Step 4
Four interrupted #4-0 or #5-0 absorbable sutures are placed to reapproximate the cut ends of the ureter. These sutures are placed full-thickness through the serosa and mucosa. Thus, the reanastomosis is done over the ureteral catheter and should be free of tension (*Figs 6.62, 6.63*).

Step 5
A Silastic closed suction drain is placed through the lower quadrant of the abdomen on the side of the repair. The drain is placed in the retroperitoneal space adjacent to the anastomosis (*Fig. 6.64*) and is left in place until no urine is collected from it (usually 2 to 3 days).

Step 6
The Silastic ureteral catheter is left in place for about 2 weeks, and can be removed cystoscopically. An intravenous pyelogram is performed at 4–6 postoperative weeks to ensure that the ureter is patent and is not stenotic.

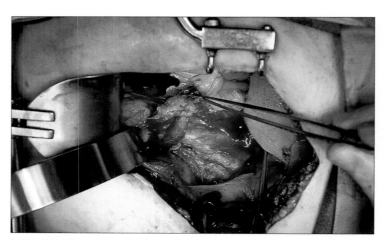

6.58 Mobilization of injury site.

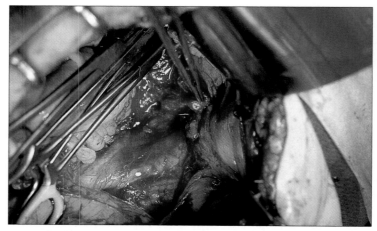

6.59 The injured site is "freshened".

SURGICAL PROCEDURE: URETERONEOCYSTOSTOMY
Step 1
The site of ureteral injury is identified and the damaged segment is mobilized so that a 2 cm segment is cleared from its surrounding connective tissue sheath. The distal ureteral segment is ligated with a permanent suture material so that there is no retrograde leakage of urine from the original insertion into the bladder (*Fig. 6.65*).

Step 2
The space of Retzius (retropubic space) is entered and the bladder mobilized. The posterior bladder wall must meet the proximal portion of the ureter that is to be implanted. Enough of the bladder is mobilized to ensure minimal tension at the site of repair.

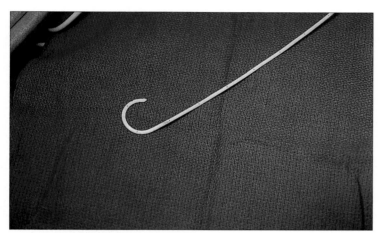

6.60 Silastic "double J" stent.

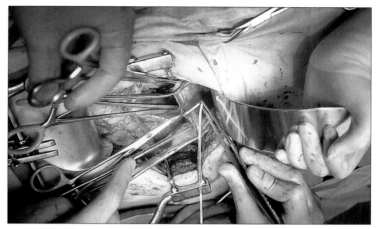

6.61 Placement of stent in ureter.

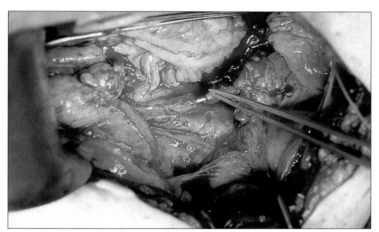

6.62 Stent placed in both proximal and distal segment.

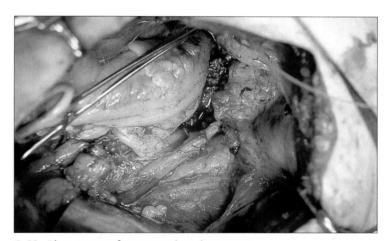

6.63 Placement of reapproximation suture.

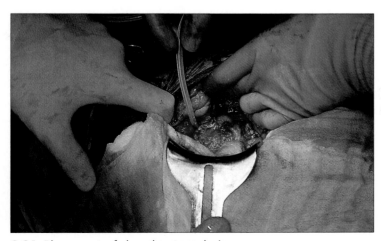

6.64 Placement of closed system drain.

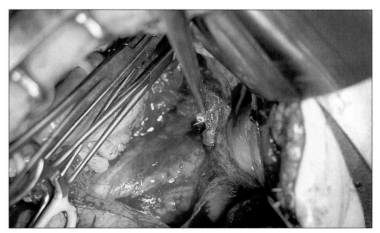

6.65 Identification of site of ureteral injury.

Step 3

A 3–4 cm cystotomy is performed in the dome of the bladder and the bladder trigone is identified. To facilitate the cystotomy, the bladder can be filled with 200–300 ml of sterile saline. The site at which the ureter will be reimplanted is chosen in the posterior bladder wall, and a Kelly clamp is used to tent the posterior wall of the bladder. A knife is used to incise the bladder wall at this point (*Fig. 6.66*).

Step 4

A #2-0 traction suture is placed in the distalmost end of the ureter so that it can be used to pull the ureter through the bladder wall. The cut portion of the ureter is then grasped and brought through the bladder wall. Lee and Symmonds[23] have shown that it is not necessary to tunnel the ureter through the submucosal layer of the bladder (*Figs 6.67, 6.68*).

Step 5

Once the ureter is brought through the bladder wall, the end is spatulated so that the ureteral orifice is enlarged. Four interrupted #4-0 or #5-0 absorbable sutures are placed through the entire thickness of the ureteral wall and the mucosal and muscularis layers of the bladder and superficially in the serosal layer of the ureter if any tension is encountered at the ureter (*Fig. 6.69*).

Step 6

A 6F or 8F "double J" Silastic ureteral catheter is inserted from the bladder into the newly created ureteral orifice so that one end of the stent rests in the renal pelvis with the opposite end in the bladder. The stent can be secured to the ureteral catheter. Therefore, when the ureteral catheter is removed, the ureteral stent is removed with it. Alternatively, the stent can be removed cystoscopically (*Fig. 6.70*).

Step 7

The cystotomy is repaired with either a continuous running suture or interrupted sutures of an absorbable suture material. Either a single-layer or a two-layer closure can be used (*Figs 6.70, 6.71*).

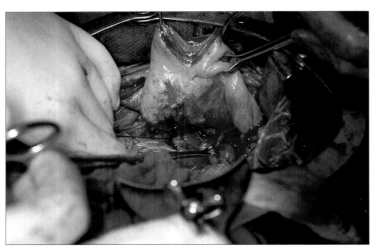

6.66 Cystotomy.

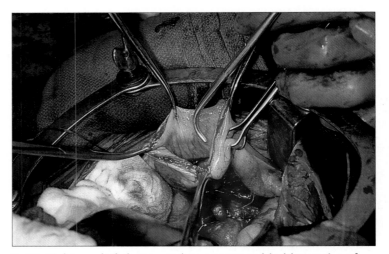

6.67 Right-angled clamp used to penetrate bladder at site of reimplantation.

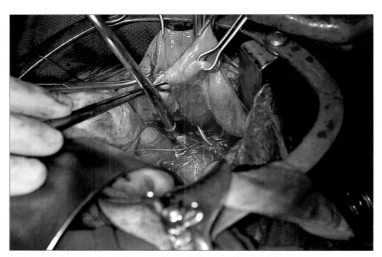

6.68 Right-angled clamp placed through bladder.

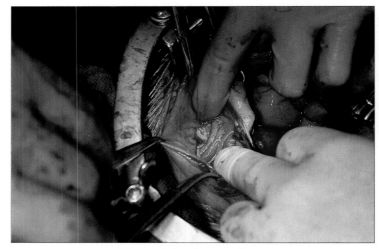

6.69 Ureter passed through bladder wall.

Step 8

To ensure that there is no tension on the repair, two or three synthetic absorbable sutures are placed in the dome of the bladder to incorporate the serosa and muscularis. These sutures are then attached to the fascia of the iliopsoas muscle. It is necessary to be certain that the genitofemoral nerve is not entrapped by these sutures.

Step 9

A Silastic closed suction drain is placed through the lower abdominal quadrant on the side of the repair and placed adjacent to the insertion point. The drain is left in place until no urine is collected from it (*Fig. 6.72*).

ALTERNATIVE PROCEDURES

Other types of ureteral repairs include transureteroureterostomy, cutaneous ureterostomy, and interposition of a bowel segment between two cut ureteral segments.

A bladder flap (Boari or Demel) can be created if the excised or damaged portion of the ureter is so extensive that end-to-end

anastomosis or neocystotomy is not possible. In these procedures, a portion of the bladder wall is formed into a tube, which allows creation of a conduit between the ureter and bladder.

If the ureteral injury is not recognized at the time of surgery, some controversy exists over the most prudent management plan. If the ureter is not completely occluded or transected, retrograde placement of ureteral stents may obviate the need for surgical repair. If this is not the case, percutaneous nephrostomy tubes can be inserted and left in place until the inflammation associated with the initial surgical procedure has subsided. The ureter can then be repaired using the techniques described above.

COMPLICATIONS

The most efficient way to prevent complications of ureteral repair is to prevent ureteral injury. This can be done in most instances by identifying the course of the ureter throughout the surgical procedure. However, despite these precautions, ureteral injury can and will sometimes occur.

Once repaired, complications specific to ureteral repair include lumen stenosis, urinoma formation, and devascularization. These potential complications can be prevented with the use of Silastic ureteral stents, operative site drainage, and careful attention to preserving the blood supply to the ureter. Although less common, additional complications that may be encountered include ureterovaginal[23] or vesicovaginal fistula formation.

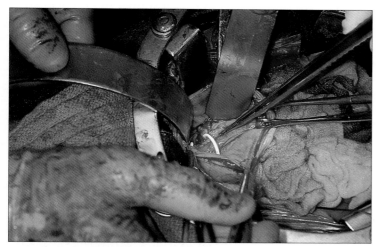

6.70 Ureteral stent in place in the newly created ureteral orifice.

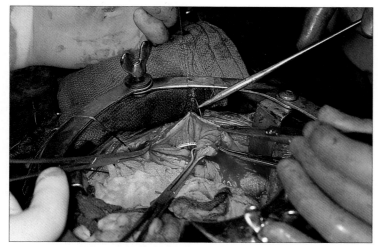

6.71 Suture closure of cystotomy.

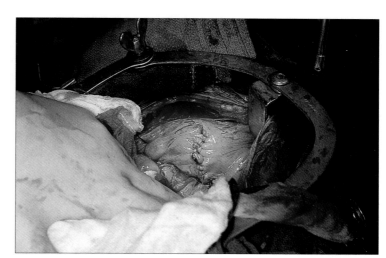

6.72 Bladder closure completed.

REPAIR OF CYSTOTOMY

Most surgical injuries to the bladder are supratrigonal and occur when an abdominal incision is made. Consequently, the gynecologic surgeon should be readily able to recognize the indications of surgical injury to the bladder and be very comfortable with the procedures necessary to repair a bladder laceration[24, 25].

SURGICAL INDICATIONS

The location of the laceration is important in determining the method of surgical repair. All bladder injuries should be repaired immediately by surgical reapproximation.

Reported situations that should alert the surgeon to the possibility of a bladder laceration include: any disease that will distort the bladder anatomy; any condition that makes a bladder incision necessary to complete the dissection; any operation that utilizes the bladder peritoneum; and previous pelvic surgery that affects the bladder anatomically.

SURGICAL PROCEDURE

The surgical procedure detailed below emphasizes important considerations in the repair of bladder laceration – knowledge of existing conditions that may increase the possibility of a bladder laceration, diagnosis, and repair of the laceration.

Step 1

During an abdominal hysterectomy, the dissection of the bladder off the vesicovaginal fascia proved to be very difficult because of extensive adhesions resulting from previous cesarean sections. A bladder laceration occurred. *Fig. 6.73* shows a clearly visible intravesical Foley balloon indicating bladder laceration.

Step 2

The surgeon must be certain of the extent of the laceration. This is more difficult if there are extensive adhesions that may require additional dissection to clearly determine the full extent of the tear. In this instance, an Allis clamp is placed at each end of the tear. This serves to identify not only the extent of the tear but also the full thickness of the bladder wall (*Fig. 6.74*).

Step 3

The laceration can be closed in two or three layers. The technique of closure is more important than the number of layers. The first-layer closure is accomplished by using a #3-0 delayed absorbable suture. Beginning at one end of the laceration, a running stitch penetrates all layers of the bladder wall (*Fig. 6.75*). To be certain all layers are penetrated, the mucosa can be rolled out for good visualization. This layer should invert the mucosa of the bladder (*Fig. 6.76*). The suture should be left long at each end of the incision to aid in identifying the laceration for the next-layer closure.

Step 4

Tension should be placed on the sutures located at each end of the laceration. When extensive adhesions are present, dissection may be necessary to adequately identify the layers of the bladder for second-layer closure (*Fig. 6.77*).

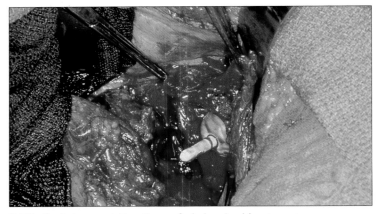

6.73 Cystotomy at the time of abdominal hysterectomy.

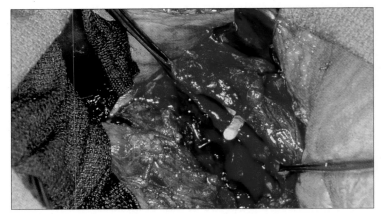

6.74 Identification of extent of laceration.

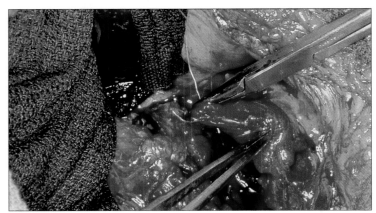

6.75 First layer of bladder closure.

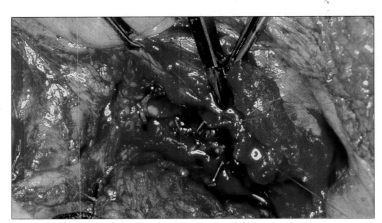

6.76 Closure of bladder with tension.

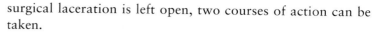

Step 5

A second layer of #3-0 delayed absorbable suture in either running or interrupted stitches should be placed in the bladder serosa and muscularis (*Fig. 6.78*). This should invert the first layer (*Fig. 6.79*) and produce a water-tight closure of the bladder laceration (*Fig. 6.80*).

ALTERNATIVE PROCEDURES

The majority of bladder lacerations are recognized and closed at the time of surgery. Occasionally one may escape detection. If a surgical laceration is left open, two courses of action can be taken.

When the laceration is minor and small, successful treatment can be expected. The majority of these minor injuries will heal if continuous bladder drainage is maintained. For a major bladder laceration, there is no acceptable alternative other than bladder drainage and immediate repair.

COMPLICATIONS

Complications can be divided into two major categories: those that are not recognized intraoperatively; and those that result from a failed closure attempt. In either case, re-exploration and repair are mandatory.

Complications from an untreated extraperitoneal laceration result in urine extravasation forming a urinoma, which may become infected. Operative drainage of the infected urinoma and closure of the laceration are necessary. Appropriate antibiotic coverage is also mandatory.

The urinoma may drain extra-abdominally and result in the formation of a vesicocutaneous fistula. When the bladder is repaired, the fistula tract must be identified and removed. Complications of a laceration that drains intraperitoneally also result from urine extravasation. A generalized chemical and/or infectious peritonitis can result. The laceration must be repaired immediately and the peritonitis treated.

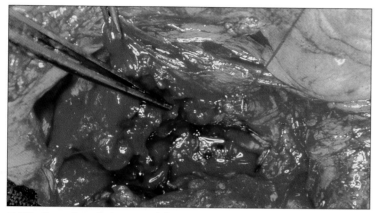

6.77 Completed closure of first suture layer.

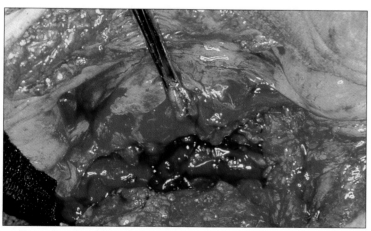

6.78 Second layer of suture closure.

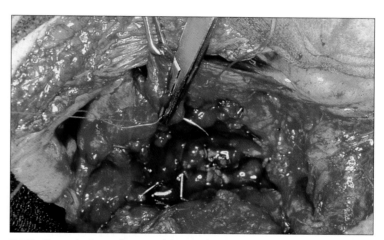

6.79 Completion of second-layer closure.

6.80 Illustration of bladder closure.

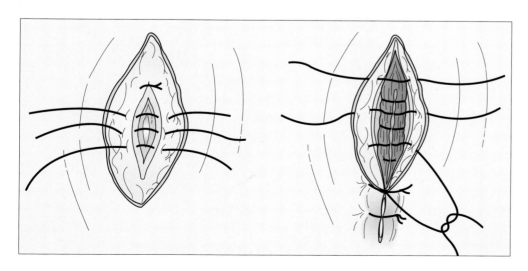

FULL-THICKNESS SKIN GRAFT

In 1989, Nichols and Randall[26] described the use of a full-thickness skin graft in gynecology. Many authors have described the use of this procedure to repair various types of vaginal stenosis[27]. The stated advantages of the procedure include the elimination of contraction, which may occur with split-thickness grafts, and the simplicity of the procedure.

SURGICAL INDICATIONS

The indications for the use of a full-thickness skin graft are outlined in *Fig. 6.81*.

The patient illustrates the typical indications for this procedure. She is a 28-year-old who developed two areas of vaginal stenosis secondary to childbirth, which resulted in apareunia. It was decided to use this procedure for the reasons previously listed.

SURGICAL PROCEDURE

Step 1

Physical examination revealed an external genitalia of normal appearance. The introitus could barely admit one finger.

Speculum examination revealed a midvaginal stenosis (*Figs 6.82–6.84*).

Step 2

A relaxing vaginal incision is made at the 3 or 9 o'clock position. This incision should be enlarged so that an area of full-thickness vaginal epithelium down to the subcutaneous tissue is removed (*Fig. 6.85*). All bleeding in these sites must be meticulously controlled. The margins of the incision should be undermined enough to have a vaginal lip to which the graft can be sewn. Enough of the vaginal tissue should be removed to enlarge the vaginal introitus sufficiently to accept two or three fingers (*Fig. 6.86*).

Step 3

The midvaginal stenosis is identified. A similar elliptical incision(s) is made at this level, sufficient to allow entry of two or three fingers. The surgeon must be certain the incision is long enough to extend front to back of the stenotic ring. Again, hemostasis must be ensured (*Fig. 6.87*).

Indications for Full-Thickness Skin Graft
Congenital anomalies
Menopausal atrophy
Stricture secondary to a surgical procedure

6.81 Indications for a full-thickness skin graft to correct a small or stenotic vagina.

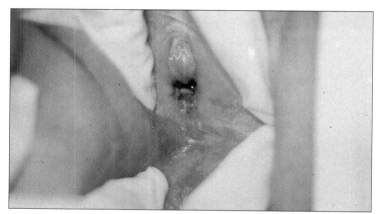

6.82 External genitalia.

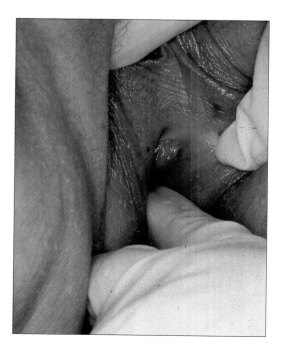

6.83 Introitus barely admits one finger.

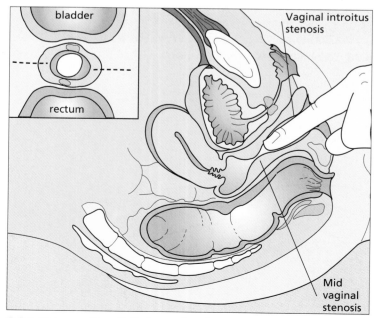

6.84 Preoperative digital examination.

Step 4

Next, the graft is harvested. The authors prefer to remove the skin from an area near the iliac crest. By flexing the patient's knees, a skin fold between the thigh and anterior abdominal wall can be identified. We prefer an incision beginning at the superior iliac crest and posteriorly following the skin fold for the required distance. This will hide the incision under most swimwear, and it will appear similar to the skin fold, thus being cosmetically acceptable. An elliptical piece of full-thickness skin, large enough to cover the defects created by the vaginal elliptical incisions, is removed (*Figs 6.88, 6.89*).

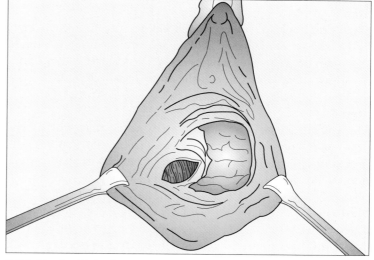

6.85 Vaginal Introitus.

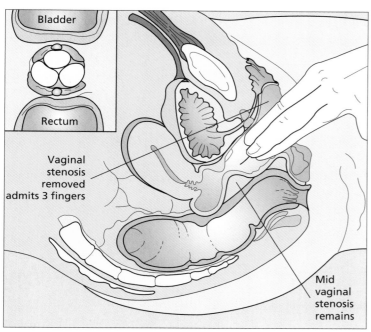

6.86 Illustration of midvaginal stenosis.

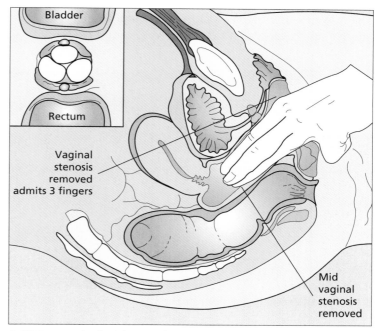

6.87 Removal of midvaginal stenosis.

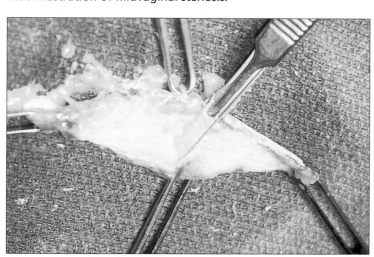

6.88 Preparation of donor skin graft.

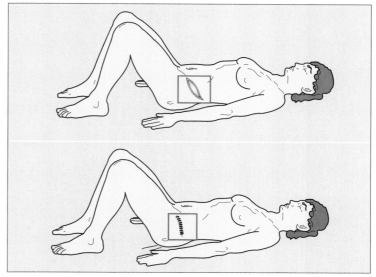

6.89 Donor site incision (top) and the closed donor site (bottom).

Step 5
Small skin hooks or towel clips should be placed on each angle of the excised skin and the skin is then stretched tight. A small, sharp curette, scalpel, or scissors is used to remove all of the fatty tissue from the dermal side of the graft (*Figs 6.90, 6.91*).

Step 6
The full-thickness graft is cut into pieces that will fit the previously made elliptical vaginal incisions (*Figs 6.92, 6.93*). The first graft is sutured, with #3-0 interrupted absorbable sutures, into the previously prepared midvaginal area.

Step 7
The remainder of the full-thickness graft is cut to fit the elliptical areas previously prepared at the vaginal introitus (see *Fig. 6.92*). This graft is positioned with #3-0 interrupted absorbable sutures.

Step 8
The site of the full-thickness graft is closed in a single layer with interrupted stitches of #3-0 absorbable suture (*Fig. 6.94*). A previously fashioned sponge-rubber mold covered with two condoms is inserted into the vagina. The surgeon must be certain that the mold can be inserted without disturbing the grafts; it is secured by sewing it to the lips of the labia. This mold is left in place for 7 days, during which time the patient is confined to bed. On the seventh day the mold is removed and the vagina inspected. The patient may be discharged, but she should use a soft plastic sponge-rubber mold intravaginally until postoperative examination at 4 to 6 weeks.

COMPLICATIONS
There are three categories of possible complications: infections, graft failure, and restenosis.

Infection may occur in the graft donor or recipient site. The donor site will demonstrate the characteristic signs of infection: redness, swelling, and tenderness. Treatment should consist of antibiotics, incision, and drainage. Since the recipient site is not obvious, diagnosis may not be as readily made as for the donor site. The patient may have a fever, a malodorous vaginal discharge, and/or sloughing of the graft. She should receive anti-

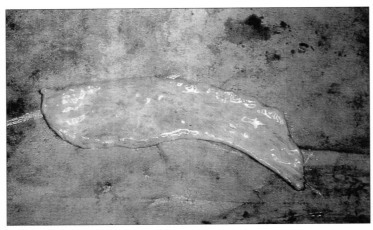

6.90 Full-thickness skin graft removed.

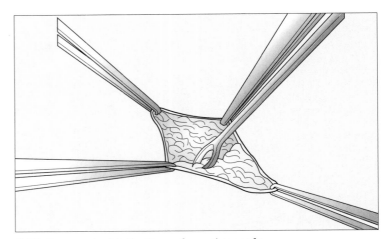

6.91 Removal of fatty tissue from the graft.

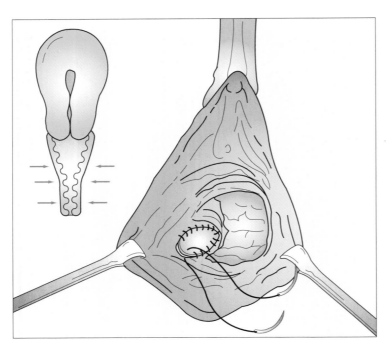

6.92 Illustration of graft placement.

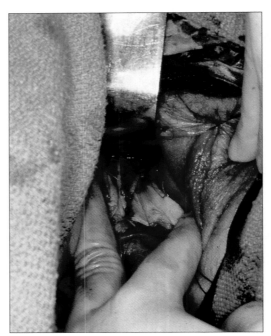

6.93 Graft placement in the vagina.

biotics, if appropriate. Vaginal douching will remove the infected graft and help to clean the vagina for a future graft when and if appropriate.

The graft may slough for several reasons. It may be positioned with the epidermis next to the vaginal stroma instead of the dermis. The recipient site may not be completely hemostatic, resulting in the collection of a hematoma beneath the graft. This prevents contact between the graft and the vaginal stroma, and an adequate graft blood supply will not form. If the graft site becomes infected, the graft will almost certainly be rejected.

Restenosis is perhaps the most unfortunate complication. The patient has recovered without incident, yet at least part of the original problems and symptoms still exist. The surgeon and patient must decide if an additional attempt is worth while.

ALTERNATIVE PROCEDURES

Alternative procedures which can be used as surgical adjunct or replacement procedures are outlined in *Fig. 6.95*.

NEOVAGINA: USE OF AN OMENTAL GRAFT

The omentum has been used for a variety of reasons (*Fig. 6.96*)[28–32]. The rich vascular supply is one reason for its versatility, as is its potential to be expanded to cover large areas. Additional advantages include its ready availability and the fact that its use does not interfere with any other known function. The gynecologic surgeon would be well advised to become familiar with this structure and its many uses, because the body offers few structures with such versatility associated with so few potential complications.

SURGICAL INDICATIONS

This procedure can be used for patients with either vaginal atresia or vaginal agenesis. The patient should be positioned in the dorsal lithotomy position and should be draped to allow access to both the abdomen and the vagina. The incision must allow access to both the upper abdomen and pelvis. A midline incision is preferable.

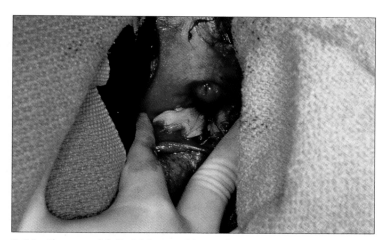

6.94 Closure of full-thickness skin graft.

Alternative Procedures
Split-thickness skin graft
Tissue flaps
Vaginal dilators
Lateral relaxing incisions
Sliding skin graft with a vertical incision
Estrogen cream
Reverse perineorrhaphy
Z-plasty

6.95 Alternative procedures to full-thickness skin graft.

Omental Uses
1. Intestinal sling or pelvic hammock
2. Bed for split-thickness skin graft
3. Protects intestinal anastomosis
4. Fills abdominal wall defects
5. Reconstruction in irradiated areas
6. Absorption of extracellular body fluids
7. Helps develop normal body contours
8. Helps repair R-V and V-V fistulae
9. Covers peritoneal defects
10. Covers inert material in wounds
11. Vaginal construction or lengthening

6.96 Uses of the omental graft.

SURGICAL PROCEDURE

Step 1

The omentum is identified and any adhesions are removed. The omentum is brought out onto the abdomen (*Fig. 6.97*). The blood supply is evaluated and the size and mobility of the omentum are determined. The blood supply arises from the gastroepiploic arcade, and is composed of the right and left gastroepiploic arteries. The middle omental artery, arising from the gastro-epiploic arcade, extends the length of the omentum and divides it in half. This artery helps to form a rich vascular arch in the distal portion of the omentum, known as Haller's arch. This arch is formed by an anastomosis between the middle, right and left omentum, and accessory omental arteries. This arch allows lengthening of the omentum as necessary (*Figs 6.98, 6.99*).

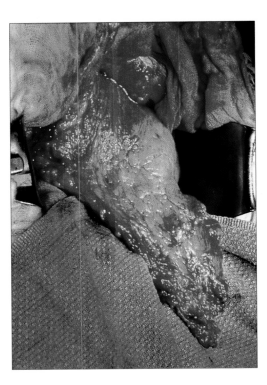

6.97 Identification of Omentum.

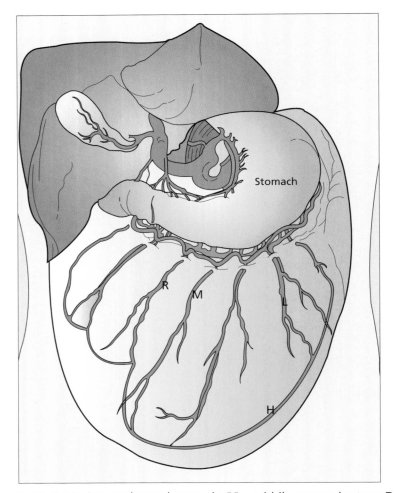

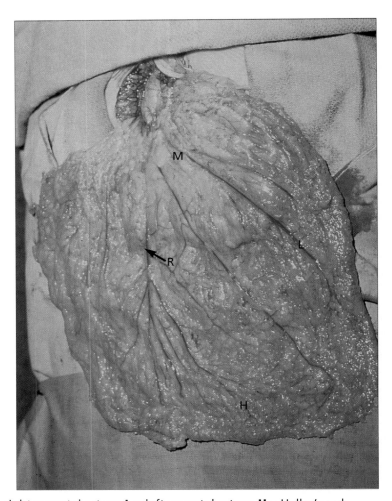

6.98, 6.99 Omental vascular supply. **M** = middle omental artery; **R** = right omental artery; **L** = left omental artery; **H** = Haller's arch.

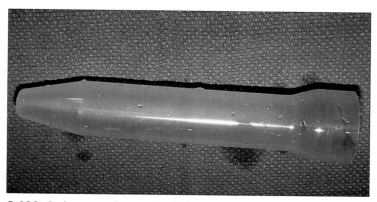

6.100 Syringe used as vaginal obturator.

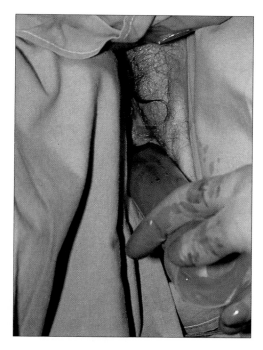

6.101 Placement of vaginal obturator in vagina.

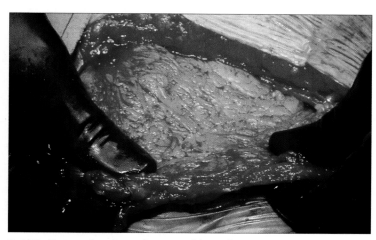

6.102 Determination of omental length.

Step 2

In a patient with vaginal shortening and dyspareunia after a hysterectomy, a vaginal obturator will be useful in surgery to help identify the vaginal apex. The authors prefer to use a 50 ml syringe casing as a vaginal obturator (*Fig. 6.100*). It should be inserted into the vagina (*Fig. 6.101*). At this stage the vagina is very short and will allow the obturator to be inserted only a few centimeters.

Step 3

The length of the omentum is determined by the surgeon, who must decide if it must be lengthened or if it is long enough naturally to reach into the pelvis (*Fig. 6.102*).

Step 4

If the omentum is too short, its blood supply must be determined so that an appropriate lengthening procedure can be performed. The gastroepiploic arch must be identified and divided. The various vascular arches are investigated to determine which is of sufficient length to be used (*Fig. 6.103*).

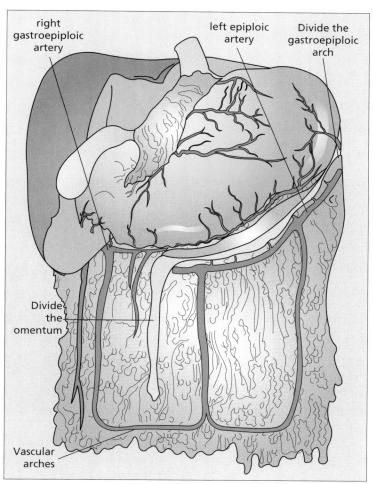

6.103 The omental anatomy.

Step 5

The omentum is rolled into a cylinder. With a #2-0 delayed absorbable suture, the outside edges are sutured together, thus forming the cylinder. The surgeon must be certain not to include either of the accessory omental arteries. Occlusion of these arteries might result in an inadequate blood supply to the distal portion of the omentum, causing necrosis of this important area. The cylinder should have a diameter of at least 6–10 cm (*Fig. 6.104*). The depth of the cylinder is determined by suturing with the #2-0 delayed absorbable suture perpendicular to the long axis of the omental cylinder at the desired depth (*Fig. 6.105*).

Step 6

The omental cylinder is brought into the pelvis. This is usually done via the left paracolic gutter (*Figs 6.106, 6.107*).

Step 7

The previously placed vaginal obturator is advanced, thus identifying and expanding the vaginal apex (*Figs 6.108, 6.109*). The angles of the vaginal apex are grasped with Allis clamps (*Fig. 6.110*).

Step 8

With both sharp and blunt dissection, the vaginal cavity is entered. Hemostasis of the vaginal cuff is secured (*Figs 6.111, 6.112*).

Step 9

Delayed absorbable #2-0 sutures are placed at 1 cm intervals around the circumference of the vaginal apex. The sutures with the needles still attached are tagged and placed in an orderly fashion around the pelvic brim (*Fig. 6.113*).

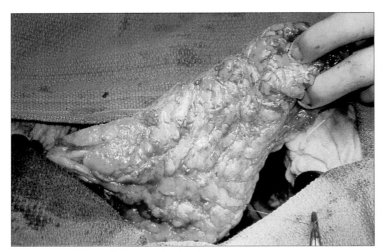

6.104 Creation of omental cylinder.

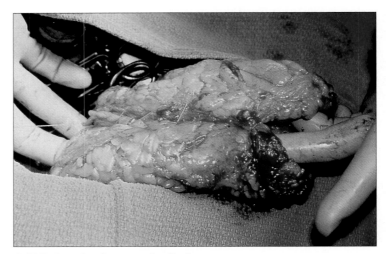

6.105 Depth of omental cylinder.

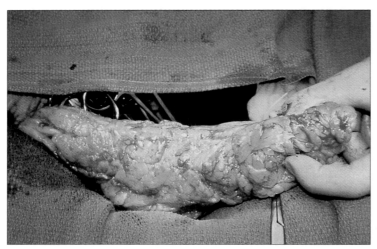

6.106 Completion of omental cylinder.

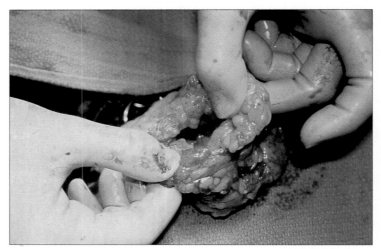

6.107 Opening of omental cylinder.

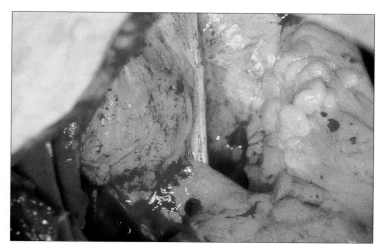

6.108 Identification of vaginal apex.

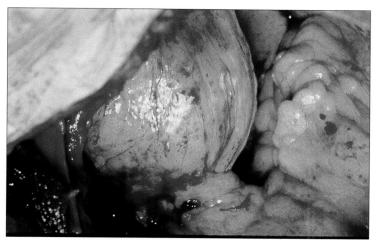

6.109 Vagina extended by obturator.

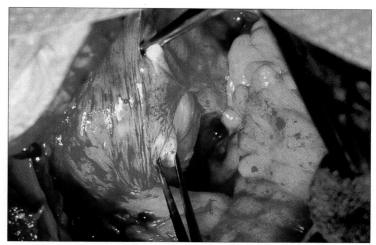

6.110 Opening of vaginal cavity.

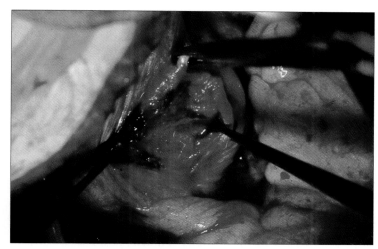

6.111 Hemostasis of vaginal opening.

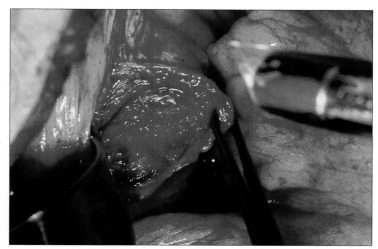

6.112 Completion of vaginal opening.

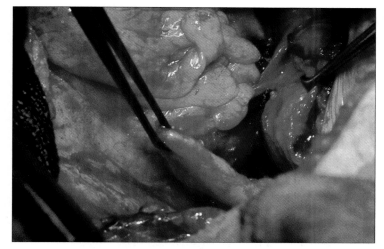

6.113 Suture placement for securing graft.

Step 10

The omental cylinder is placed in the pelvis with the open end of the cylinder in contact with the apex. The omental cylinder is sutured to the vaginal apex. This will create a vagina or lengthen the shortened vagina (*Figs 6.114, 6.115*).

Step 11

While the abdomen is still open and under direct vision, a foam-rubber mold is placed in the vagina. The surgeon should be certain the mold extends beyond the omental vaginal anastomosis and into the omental cylinder (*Figs 6.116, 6.117*).

Step 12

Our experience with the omentum leads us to consider it unnecessary to use a skin graft. The omentum will epithelize without the potential complication of a split-thickness skin graft. This potential complication consists primarily of constriction, thus decreasing the size of the neovagina. The vaginal speculum is inserted to the maximal depth at the 2-week postoperative visit. The sutures at the omental vaginal anastomosis are still visible. Epithelization of the omentum has begun. This can be appreciated by the smoothness of the omental surface in contrast to the usual irregular appearance (*Fig. 6.118*).

ALTERNATIVE PROCEDURES

Vaginal atresia or agenesis may be corrected by either surgical or non-surgical techniques (*Fig. 6.119*).

COMPLICATIONS

These can be divided into complications specific to the omentum and those that are common to any abdominal surgery. Those that may be directly related to the omentum include constriction

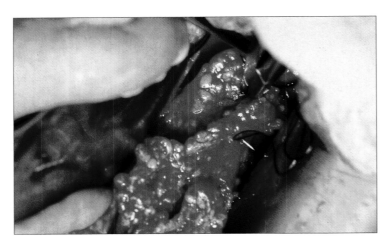

6.114 Omental cylinder placed in pelvis.

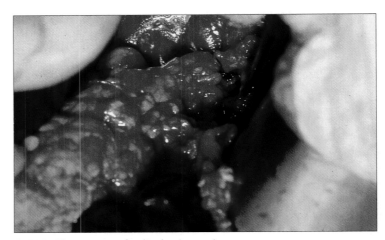

6.115 Placement of cylinder in vagina.

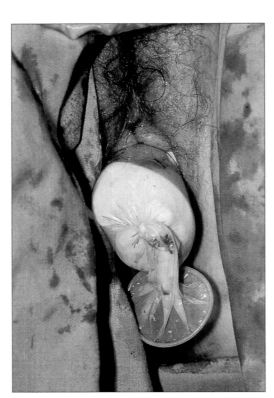

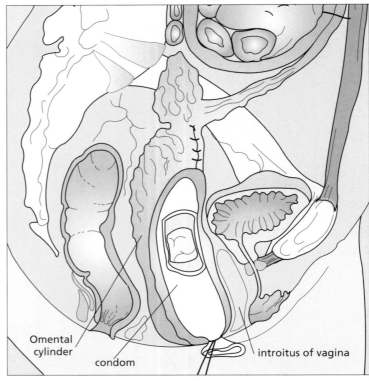

6.116 Placement of faom-rubber mold.

Omental cylinder
condom
introitus of vagina

6.117 The completed procedure.

ring formation at the anastomosis site, omental necrosis, and omental constriction.

A constriction ring at the anastomosis site is probably the most common potential complication. The best method of treating this is prevention. This can be best accomplished by inserting the vaginal mold while the healing process is occurring. A mold should continue to be worn until the patient resumes sexual intercourse as construction can reoccur even if the healing process is complete.

Should necrosis of the omentum occur, the vaginal apex should be allowed to seal itself. It is unlikely that this will become obvious until the time of the first examination, when no omentum will be visible. The patient and her physician will have to decide if further surgery is desired.

Omental constriction is best prevented by the continuous use of the vaginal mold until sexual activity resumes. Should constriction occur, the vagina can be lengthened by the pressure of frequent intercourse.

MARTIUS PROCEDURE

In 1942, Martius[33] first described using the bulbocavernosus muscle and fat pads as a transposition graft. Since that time, the Martius procedure has been closely associated with the closure of rectovaginal and vesicovaginal fistulae.

The procedure provides tissue in which sutures can be secured, tissues that can fill in dead space, and an excellent blood supply. The fact that this operation does not alter the anatomy of the vulva and is cosmetically pleasing is also important.

SURGICAL INDICATIONS

Fig. 6.120 summarizes the indications for use of the Martius procedure for repair and/or reconstruction of the vagina.

SURGICAL PROCEDURE

This operation demonstrates the use of the bulbocavernosus muscle and fat pad to replace the missing tissue[34]. The procedure can be divided into three main stages: identifying and obtaining the muscle; identifying the anal sphincter and preparing the vestibule to receive the muscle and its fat pad; and positioning the muscle and fat pad and closing the wound.

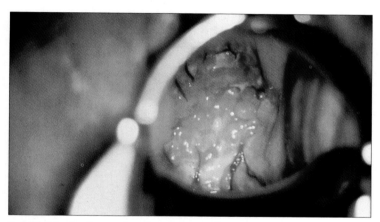

6.118 Vaginal examination two weeks post-op.

Alternative Procedures	
I. Non-surgical	II. Surgical
A. Intermittent pressure	Intestine
a. Ingram	A. Small
b. Frank	a. Baldwin
	B. Large
	a. Turner–Warwick
	b. Pratt
	c. Wagner–Baldwin

6.119 Alternative procedures to correct vaginal atresia or agenesis.

Surgical Indications	
Repair	**Construction**
Rectovaginal fistula	Vagina
Vesicovaginal fistula	Perineal body
Perineal laceration	
Postradiation necrosis	

6.120 Surgical indications for Martius procedure.

IDENTIFYING AND OBTAINING THE MUSCLE
Step 1
Examination of the patient depicted in *Figs 6.121, 6.122* reveals three distinct problems that must be corrected by this procedure. First, this patient has no perineal body. Second, there is a U-shaped defect in the rectovaginal tissue at the perineal body. Third, the anal sphincter is separated superiorly.

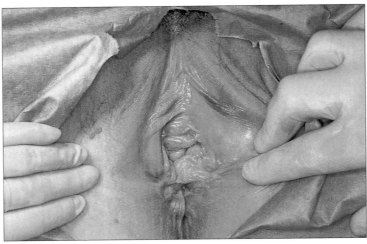

6.121 Examination of external genitalia.

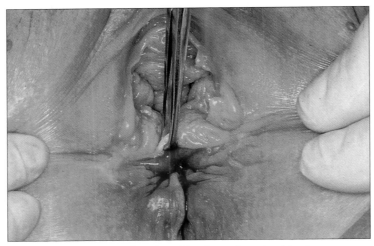

6.122 Examination of perineal body and anal sphincter.

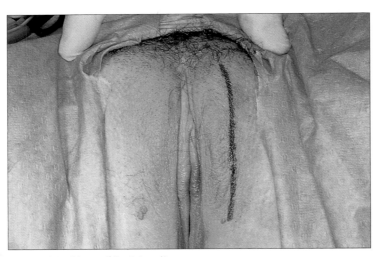

6.124 Marking of incision line.

Step 2
The bulbocavernosus muscle and fat pad, which are responsible for the greater part of the labia majora, are identified (*Fig. 6.123*). A 10 cm incision is made parallel to the long axis of this muscle in the center of the labia majora (*Fig. 6.124*). The surgeon must always be aware of the location of the blood supply to the muscle, which arises from the internal pudendal artery and enters the muscle and fat pad inferolaterally (*Figs 6.125, 6.126*).

Step 3
The incision is made through the skin just as far as the underlying tissue (*Fig. 6.127*). The bulbocavernosus muscle and fat pad are sharply dissected from the medial and lateral sides of the labia majora (*Fig. 6.128*). Care should be taken not to buttonhole the skin and to leave some fat on the skin to ensure its survival (*Fig. 6.129*). The tissue fuses caudal with the transverse perineal muscle and the anal sphincter. The cranial end terminates in the midline beneath the symphysis pubis (*Fig. 6.130*). Since the blood supply enters inferolaterally, the cranial end of the muscle and fat pad can be incised, thus freeing the muscle so it can be rotated to the desired location. In this patient, that location is the perineal body (*Fig. 6.131*).

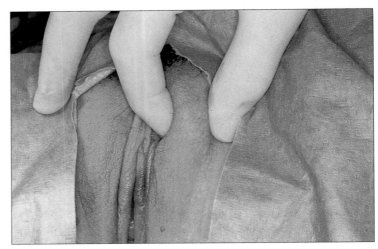

6.123 Demonstration of bulbocavernosus muscle.

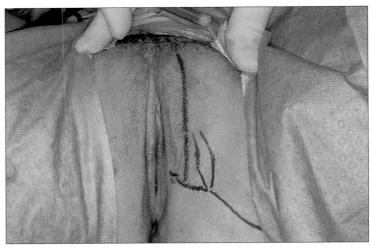

6.125 Illustration of vascular supply.

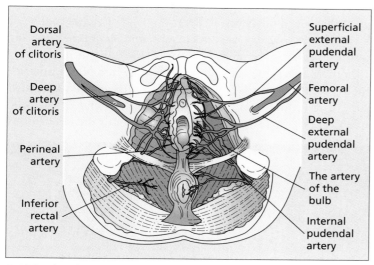

6.126 Blood supply to the muscle.

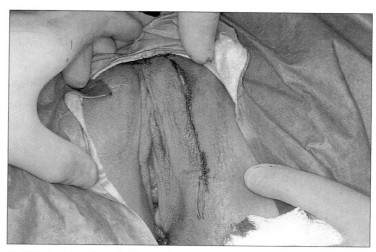

6.127 Incision into labia majora.

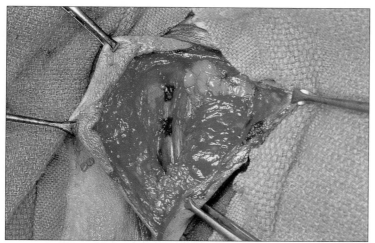

6.128 Dissection of bulbocavernous muscle.

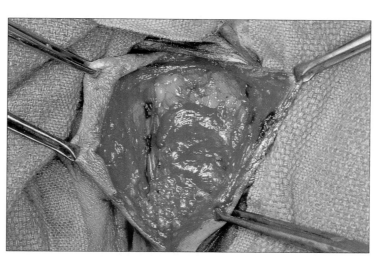

6.129 Completion of dissection.

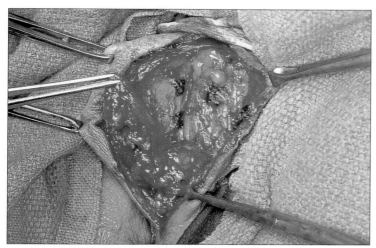

6.130 Hemostasis secured.

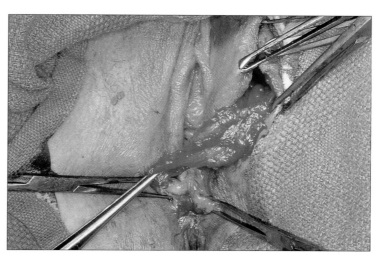

6.131 Bulbocavernosus fat pad graft.

IDENTIFYING THE ANAL SPHINCTER AND PREPARING THE VESTIBULE TO RECEIVE THE MUSCLE AND ITS FAT PAD

Step 4

A moist pad is placed over the bulbocavernosus muscle, and the edges of the labia majora are approximated and held in place by Allis clamps (*Fig. 6.132*). Additional Allis clamps are then placed on both sides of the perineal defect (*Fig. 6.133*). Either saline or a hemostatic solution, such as vasopressin, is injected into the rectovaginal space to identify it (*Fig. 6.134*).

In this patient, the vagina is sharply dissected off the anterior surface of the rectum (*Fig. 6.135*). This dissection is extended laterally to allow identification of the right end of the anal sphincter (*Figs 6.136, 6.137*). This dissection is then performed

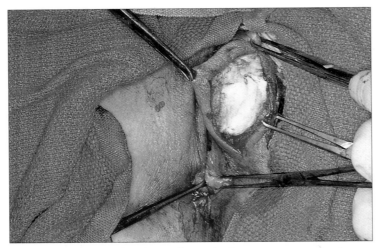

6.132 Placement of moist pad over bulbocavernosus muscle.

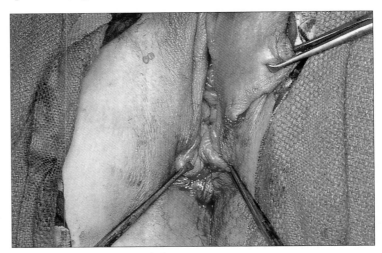

6.133 Clamping of the defect.

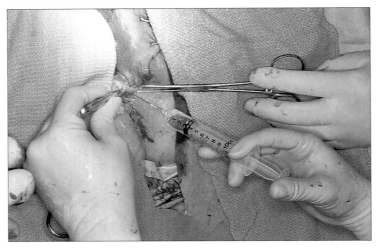

6.134 Identification of rectovaginal space.

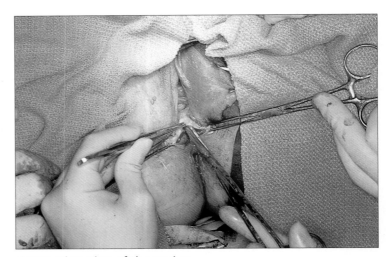

6.135 Dissection of the vagina.

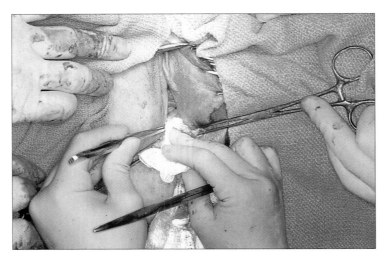

6.136 Extending the dissection laterally.

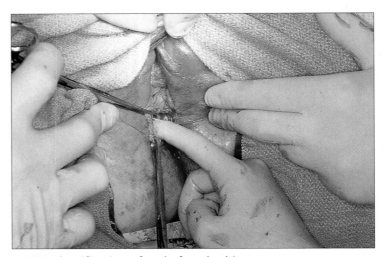

6.137 Identification of end of anal sphincter.

on the left side to identify the other end of the anal sphincter (*Fig. 6.138*). The ends of the anal sphincter are dissected free (*Fig. 6.139*) sufficiently to allow them to meet in the midline with minimal tension (*Fig. 6.140*).

A 2.5 cm incision is made in the medial side of the labia majora (*Fig. 6.141*) at the base of the bulbocavernosus muscle. An Allis clamp is passed medially through this incision, and the cranial end of the muscle is grasped and gently pulled through this incision (*Fig. 6.142*). The muscle is positioned to be certain it will fill the space for which it is intended (*Fig. 6.143*). Once this has been determined, the muscle is returned to its original location.

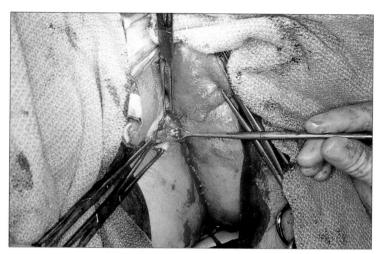

6.138 Identification of other end of anal sphincter.

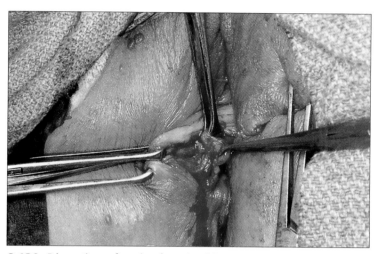

6.139 Dissection of ends of anal sphincter.

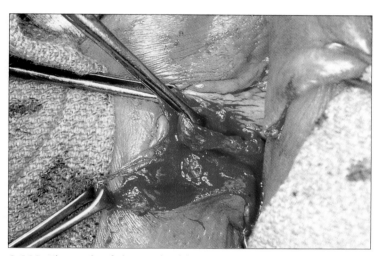

6.140 The ends of the anal sphincter are allowed to meet in the middle.

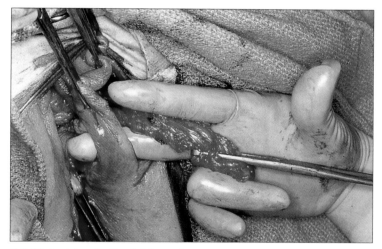

6.141 Incision in the labia majora.

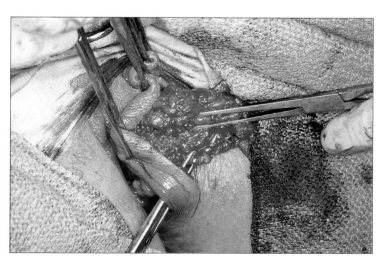

6.142 Pulling the muscle through the incision.

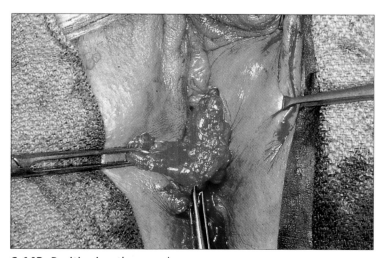

6.143 Positioning the muscle.

POSITIONING THE MUSCLE AND FAT PAD AND CLOSING THE WOUND

Step 5

The apex of the rectal mucosa is identified, and a #3-0 absorbable suture is placed at the apex (*Fig. 6.144*). The rectal mucosa is then closed with this suture in a running stitch (*Fig. 6.145*). The previously identified ends of the anal sphincter are approximated in the midline, using Allis clamps (*Fig. 6.146*). These muscles are sutured together (*Fig. 6.147*) with #3-0 absorbable suture, thus re-establishing the anal sphincter's integrity (*Fig. 148*).

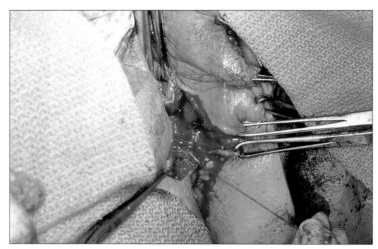

6.144 Placement of suture at apex of the rectal mucosa.

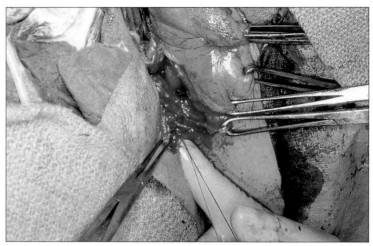

6.145 Closure of rectal mucosa.

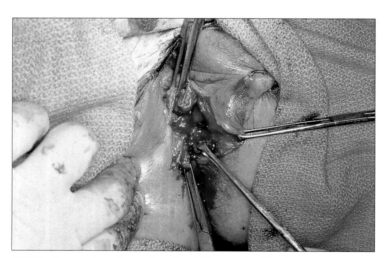

6.146 Approximation of ends of the anal sphincter.

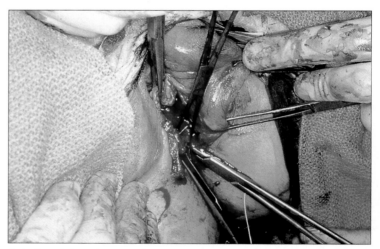

6.147 Joining the muscles together.

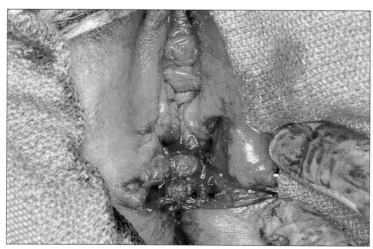

6.148 Anal sphincter re-established.

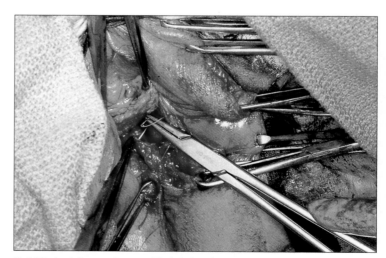

6.149 Incision at base of left labia major.

Step 6

The bulbocavernosus muscle and fat pad are pulled through the incision at the base of the left labia majora (*Figs 6.149–6.151*), and are sutured over the approximated anal sphincter (*Fig. 6.152*). The muscle adds bulk to the perineal body, and the neovascularization helps the sphincter to heal (*Fig. 6.153*).

Step 7

The incision in the left labia is closed with interrupted stitches, using a #3-0 absorbable suture (*Figs 6.154–6.156*). Some physicians prefer to place a drain in the site from which the bulbocavernosus muscle was removed.

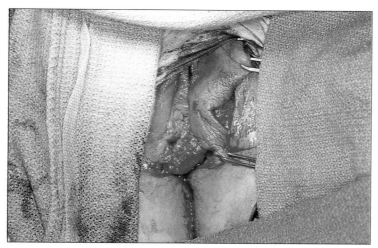

6.150 Muscle and fat pad pulled through the incision.

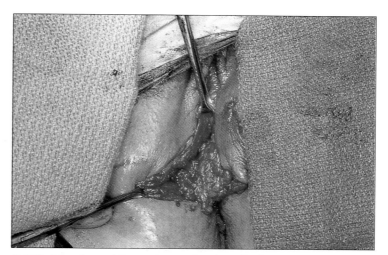

6.151 Muscle and fat pad completely pulled through the incision.

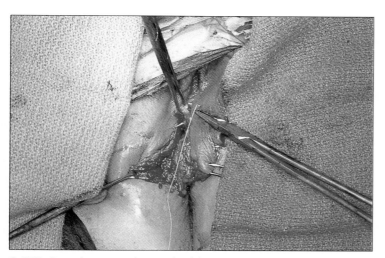

6.152 Suturing over the anal sphincter.

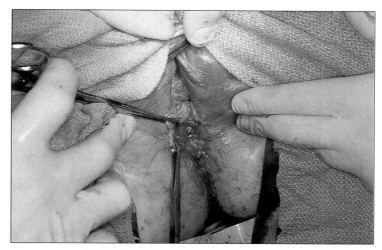

6.153 Completed vaginal reconstruction.

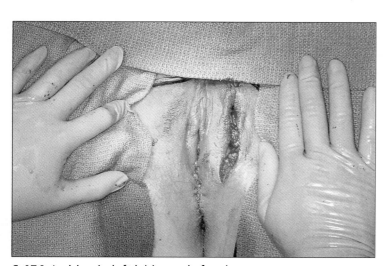

6.154 Incision in left labia ready for closure.

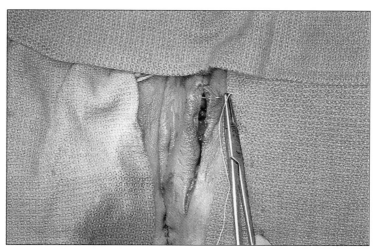

6.155 Suture of incision.

ALTERNATIVE PROCEDURES

Fig. 6.157 lists several alternative procedures and grafts that can be used for vaginal reconstruction.

COMPLICATIONS

The potential complications after this surgical procedure are primarily those that may occur after any flap rotation. The nonflap complication is primarily infection. In this example, infection is a real consideration because of the rectal involvement.

If infection should occur, the triad of redness, swelling, and tenderness will be present. This does not necessarily mean that all is lost. The surgeon must decide if this triad represents cellulitis or if pus has formed. In the first situation antibiotics may be the only treatment required. If pus is present, as with any infection, incision and drainage should be performed in addition to administration of antibiotics. It should be remembered that the neovascularization is provided by the muscle, and with any luck,

the muscle will survive. Should the muscle be completely lost, the opposite bulbocavernosus muscle can be used at a later date to complete the repair.

The flap complications are mainly a compromise of the blood supply. This may occur because the flap is too long for the amount of blood reaching the muscle. In this instance, only that portion of the muscle with an inadequate blood supply will be lost. The surgeon will have to debride the necrotic muscle until an adequate blood supply is established. At this point, healing will begin and the patient should be observed to evaluate the healing process. If healing is adequate, then nothing else needs to be done. If healing is inadequate and the flap fails to achieve the desired effect, the opposite bulbocavernosus muscle can be used. Should the muscle become twisted during the rotation, the entire blood supply is compromised. In this event, the entire muscle may be lost. The, healing must be allowed to occur and another approach used.

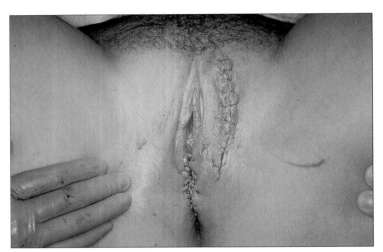

6.156 Completion of closure of left labia.

Alternative Procedures
Ingelman–Sundberg repair
Graham procedure
Simple layered repair
Franz procedure
Myocutaneous–Gracilius flap
Rectus abdominus flap
Tensor fascia lata flap

6.157 Alternative procedures for vaginal reconstruction.

REFERENCES

1. Kelly HA. Ligation of both internal iliac arteries for hemorrhage in hysterectomy for carcinoma uteri. *Bull Johns Hopkins Hosp* April 1894;5:53–4.

2. Burchell RC. Internal iliac artery ligation: hemodynamics. *Obstet Gynecol* 1964;737–9.

3. Mattingly RF, Thompson JD. *Telinde's Operative Gynecology*. 6th ed. St. Louis, MO: JB Lippincott & Co. 1985:95–7.

4. Reich WJ, Nechtow MJ. Ligation of the internal iliac (hypogastric) arteries: a life-saving procedure for uncontrollable gynecologic and obstetric hemorrhage. *J Int Coll Surg* 1961;36:157–68.

5. Sciarra JJ, Droegemueller W. *Obstetrics and Gynecology*. Vol 1. St. Louis, MO: JB Lippincott & Co. 1988;73:1–21.

6. Siegel P, Mengert WF. Internal iliac artery ligation in obstetrics and gynecology. *JAMA* 1961:178:1059–62.

7. Voitk AJ, Lowry JB. Is identical appendectomy a safe practice. *Can J Surg* 1988;31:448–51.

8. Waters EG. Elective appendectomy with abdominal and pelvic surgery. *Obstet Gynecol* 1977;50:511.

9. Westerman C, Mann WJ, Chumas J, Rochelson B, Stone ML. Routine appendectomy in extensive gynecologic operations. *Surg Gynecol Obstet* 1986;162:307–12.

10. Rose PG, Reale FR, Fisher A, Hunter RE. Appendectomy in primary and secondary staging operations for ovarian malignancy. *Obstet Gynecol* 1991;77:116–18.

11. Krebs HB. Intestinal injury in gynecologic surgery: a ten-year experience. *Am J Obstet Gynecol* 1986;155:509–13.

12. Hunt WG, Dunn LJ. Complications of gynecological surgery. In: Greenfield W, ed. *Complications in Surgery and Trauma*. 2nd ed. Philadelphia, PA: JB Lippincott & Co. 1984:790–9.

13. Kaser O, Ikle FA, Hirsch HA. *Atlas of Gynecological Surgery*. New York, NY: Thieme–Stratton, Inc. 1985:11–15.

14. Masterson BJ. *Manual of Gynecologic Surgery*. New York, NY: Springer-Verlag. 1979:215.

15. Ridley JH. *Gynecologic Surgery Errors, Safeguards, Salvage*. Baltimore: Williams & Wilkins. 1974:108–13.

16. Elaut L. The surgical anatomy of the so called presacral nerve. *Surg Gynecol Obstet* 1932;55:581–9.

17. Flienger JRH, Umstad MP. Presacral neurectomy – a reappraisal. *Aust NZ J Obstet Gynaecol* 1991;31:76–9.

18. Lee RB, Stone K, Magelsse D, Belts RP, Benson WL. Presacral neurectomy for chronic pelvic pain. *Obstet Gynecol* 1986;68:517–21.

19. Malinak LR. Operative management of pelvic pain. *Clin Obstet Gynecol* 1980;32:191–200.

20. Polan ML, DeCherney A. Presacral neurectomy for pelvic pain in infertility. *Fertil Steril* 1980;34:557–60.

21. Mann WJ, Arato M, Pastner B, Stone M. Ureteral injuries in an obstetrics and gynecology training program: etiology and management. *Obstet Gynecol* 1988;72:82.

22. Carlton CE Jr, Scott R Jr, Guthrie AG. The initial management of ureteral injuries: a report of 78 cases. *J Urol* 1971;105:335.

23. Lee RA, Symmonds RE. Ureterovaginal fistula. *Am J Obstet Gynecol* 1971;109:1032.

24. Nichols DH. *Clinical Problems, Injuries and Complications of Gynecologic Surgery*. 2nd ed. Baltimore, MD: Williams & Wilkins Co. 1988;54:161–4, 188–9.

25. Knapstein PG, Friedberg V, Sevin BU. *Reconstructive Surgery in Gynecology*. New York, NY: Thieme–Stratton Inc. 1990:28–9, 206–8.

26. Nichols DH, Randall CL. *Vaginal Surgery*. 3rd ed. Baltimore, MD: Williams & Wilkins. 1989:403–12.

27. Morley GW, DeLaney JOL. Full-thickness skin graft vaginoplasty for treatment of the stenotic foreshortened vagina. *Obstet Gynecol* 1991;77:485–9.

28. Alday ES, Goldsmith HS. Surgical technique for omental lengthening based on arterial anatomy. *Surg Gynecol Obstet* 1972;13:103–7.

29. Burger RA, Riedmiller H, Knapstein PG, Friedberg V, Hohenfellner R. Ileocecal vaginal construction. *Am J Obstet Gynecol* 1989;161:162–7.

30. Petie JY, Lacour J, Margulis A, Reed WP. Indications and results of omental pedicle grafts in oncology. *Cancer* 1979;44:2343–8.

31. Turner-Warwick R, Kirby RS. The construction and reconstruction of the vagina with the colocecum. *Surg Gynecol Obstet* 1990;170:132–6.

32. Wheeless CR. Neovagina constructed from an omental J flap and a split thickness skin graft. *Gynecol Oncol* 1989;35:224–6.

33. Martius H. Zur Auswahl der Harnfestelund Inkontinenz-Operationaen. *Zentralbl Gynaekol* 1942;66:1250–2.

34. Betson JR. Bulbocavernous fat-pad transplant. *Obstet Gynecol* 1965;26:135–41.

7

Hysterectomy and Related Procedures

Thomas G. Stovall

Robert L. Summitt, Jr.

Peter R. Casson

VAGINAL HYSTERECTOMY

Vaginal hysterectomy offers significant advantages over other approaches to hysterectomy in the patient who can successfully undergo vaginal surgery. Among the advantages are decreased intraoperative and postoperative morbidity, decreased cost, decreased recovery time, and the ability to perform the procedure on an outpatient basis.

SURGICAL INDICATIONS

The majority of vaginal hysterectomies are performed for what should be considered elective indications. Rarely is a vaginal hysterectomy performed for life-saving purposes. Therefore, the indications for vaginal hysterectomy are typically those operations that cannot be or have not been managed successfully with more conservative medical or surgical therapy. Common indications for vaginal hysterectomy are listed in *Fig. 7.1*.

Indications for Vaginal Hysterectomy
Abnormal or dysfunctional uterine bleeding
Symptomatic leiomyomata
Symptomatic pelvic organ prolapse
Dysmenorrhea and/or dyspareunia
Cervical intraepithelial neoplasia or microinvasive carcinoma of the cervix
Complex endometrial hyperplasia

7.1 Indications for vaginal hysterectomy.

SURGICAL PROCEDURE
Step 1

The most important observation in determining the feasibility of a vaginal hysterectomy is the demonstration of uterine mobility. In patients with no apparent prolapse, poor pelvic support can often be demonstrated by observing descent of the uterus with a series of Valsalva maneuvers. Some gynecologists advocate the application of a tenaculum to the anterior cervical lip with subsequent traction as the patient bears down. However, this technique is uncomfortable and it is not necessarily predictive of successful vaginal hysterectomy.

Ideally, the angle of the pubic arch should be 90° or greater (*Fig. 7.2*), the vaginal canal ample, and the posterior vaginal fornix wide and deep. The surgeon can use a closed fist to measure the bituberous diameter, which should exceed 10 cm (*Fig. 7.3*). The size and shape of the gynecoid pelvis contribute to easier accessibility to the operative site and increased exposure.

Step 2

Once the patient has been given appropriate regional or general anesthesia, she is placed in the dorsal lithotomy position, with the buttocks positioned just over the table edge (*Fig. 7.4*). Several stirrup types are available, although we prefer the "candy-cane" type. Adequate padding should be used, and marked flexion of the thigh and pressure points should be avoided. The Trendelenburg position (10–15°) aids in intravaginal visualization. Variable-intensity lamps are positioned to direct light over the operator's shoulder. Although not routinely used, a headlight can be worn to provide direct horizontal lighting.

Step 3

The vagina is prepped with a povidone–iodine solution and the bladder drained. The catheter is removed rather than being left in place during the procedure. Several methods for draping are available, including use of individual or single-piece drapes; the method chosen is at the surgeon's discretion. There is no need to shave or clip the pubic hair.

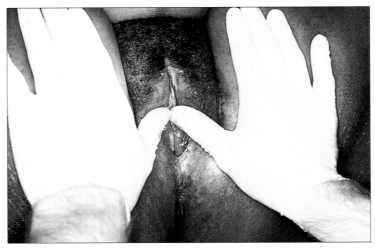

7.2 Estimation of pubic arch angle.

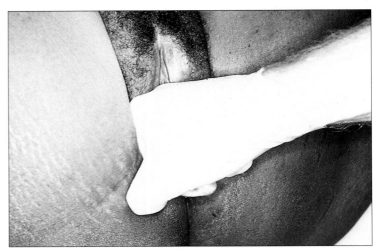

7.3 Estimation of bituberous diameter.

Step 4

The examination under anesthesia is performed to confirm prior findings of the office examination and to assess uterine mobility and descent. The anterior and posterior lips of the cervix are grasped with a single- or double-toothed tenaculum (*Fig. 7.5*).

Step 5

The peritoneal reflection of the posterior cul-de-sac can be identified by putting the vaginal mucosa and underlying connective tissue on stretch with forceps (*Fig. 7.6*). The vaginal mucosa and the peritoneum are opened with Mayo scissors, and an interrupted suture is placed to approximate the peritoneum and vaginal cuff. A weighted speculum is then placed into the posterior cul-de-sac. The posterior pelvic cavity is examined for pathologic alterations of the uterus or adhesive disease.

Step 6

With retraction of the lateral vaginal wall and countertraction on the cervix, the uterosacral ligaments are clamped, with the tip of the clamp incorporating the lower portion of the cardinal ligaments. The clamp is placed perpendicular to the uterine axis (*Fig. 7.7*). The pedicle is cut close to the clamp but should not be cut past the tip of the clamp. The pedicle is sutured with a synthetic absorbable suture material. Once ligated, the uterosacral ligaments can be transfixed to the posterolateral vaginal mucosa.

The suture is held with a hemostat to facilitate location of any bleeding at the completion of the procedure and to aid in closure of the vaginal mucosa.

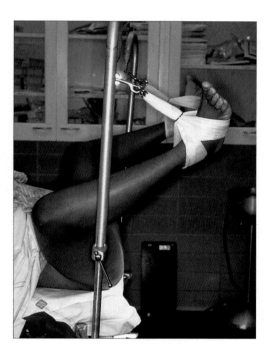

7.4 Positioning for vaginal surgery.

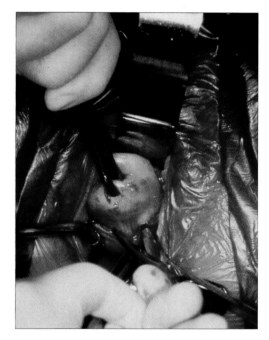

7.5 Cervix grasped with tenaculum.

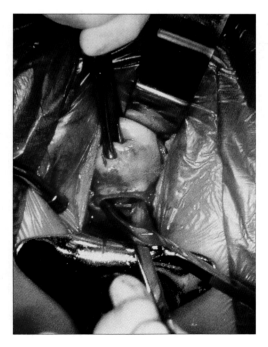

7.6 Posterior cul-de-sac entry.

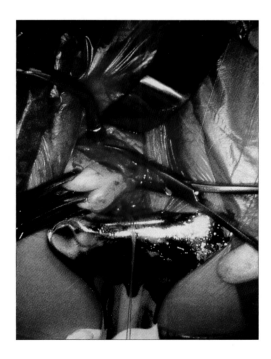

7.7 Clamping of uterosacral ligaments.

Step 7

The anterior vaginal mucosa is incised at the junction of the cervix, and the epithelium is dissected sharply from the underlying tissue or can be pushed back bluntly with an open sponge (*Fig. 7.8*).

The use of paracervical and submucosal epinephrine prior to incision of the vaginal mucosa is not indicated as it has been shown to increase the postoperative infection rate.

Step 8

With continued traction on the cervix, the cardinal ligaments are identified, clamped, cut, and ligated with sutures (*Fig. 7.9*).

Step 9

Downward traction is applied to the cervix. The bladder is advanced sharply or bluntly with an open moistened 4 × 8 gauze sponge. Unless the vesicovaginal peritoneal reflection is easily

identifed at this point, entry can be delayed. There is no danger in doing so as long as the operator has ascertained that the bladder has been advanced.

Opening of the anterior peritoneal cavity should not be done blindly, as this increases the risk of bladder injury. The peritoneum is grasped with the forceps, tented, and opened with scissors, with the tips pointed towards the uterus (*Fig. 7.10*). A Deaver retractor is then placed and the peritoneal contents are identified. The retractor also serves to keep the bladder out of the operative field.

Step 10

Contralateral and downward traction is applied to the cervix. The anterior and posterior leaves of the visceral peritoneum and the uterine vessels are incorporated into the clamp (*Fig. 7.11*). The pedicle is cut and suture-ligated. A single-suture and single-

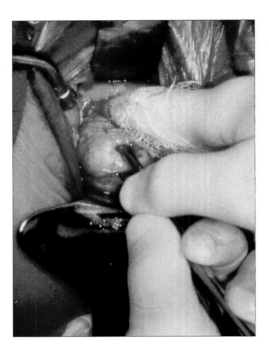

7.8 Mobilization of anterior vaginal mucosa.

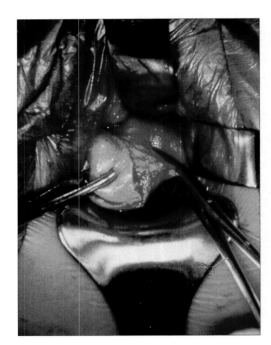

7.9 Clamping of cardinal ligament.

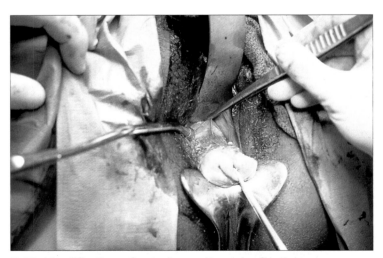

7.10 Identification of anterior peritoneal reflection.

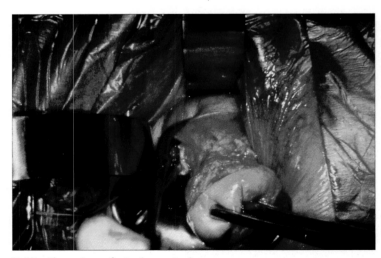

7.11 Clamping of uterine arteries.

clamp technique is adequate and decreases the potential risk of injury to the ureter.

If not previously entered, the peritoneal fold is usually readily identified before or just after clamping and suture ligation of the uterine arteries.

Step 11

A tenaculum is placed onto the uterine fundus in a successive fashion to deliver the fundus posteriorly (*Fig. 7.12*). The operator's index finger is used to identify the utero-ovarian ligament and aid in clamp placement. The remainder of the broad ligament and utero-ovarian ligaments are clamped, cut, and ligated. A single clamp is used, but the pedicle is double-ligated with a suture tie, followed by suture ligature distal to the first (*Fig. 7.13*). A hemostat is placed on the second suture to aid in identification of any bleeding.

Step 12

Traction is applied to the utero-ovarian pedicle. The ovary is drawn into the operative field by grasping it with a Babcock clamp. A Heaney clamp is placed across the infundibulopelvic ligament and the ovary and tube are excised (*Fig. 7.14*). A transfixion tie and suture ligature are placed on the infundibulopelvic ligament. If this is not practicable, a pre-tied surgical loop suture can be used to ligate the vascular pedicle.

Step 13

A lap-strip is placed into the peritoneal cavity, and each pedicle is visualized and inspected for hemostasis (*Fig. 7.15*). If additional sutures are required, they should be placed precisely to avoid damage to the ureter or bladder.

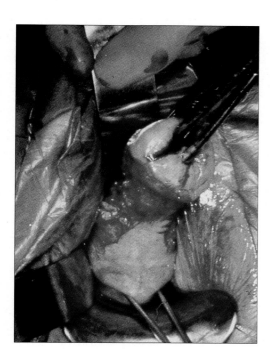

7.12 Delivery of uterine fundus.

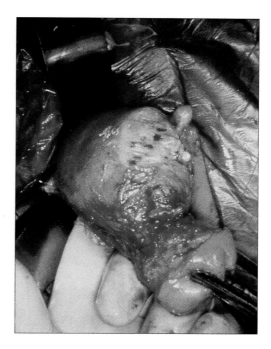

7.13 Clamping of utero-ovarian ligament.

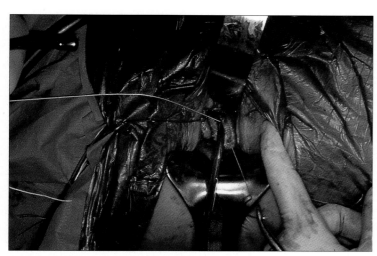

7.14 Clamping of infundibulopelvic ligament.

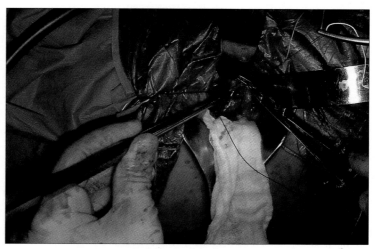

7.15 Inspection for hemostasis.

Step 14
Although it is commonly done, we do not routinely reapproximate the hemoperitoneum. If this is to be carried out, a continuous absorbable purse-string suture is inserted to incorporate the distal portion of the upper pedicle and the uterosacral ligaments. It also incorporates the posterior peritoneum and vaginal mucosa (*Fig. 7.16*).

If a McCall-type culdoplasty is performed, an absorbable suture is placed through the full thickness of the posterior vaginal wall at a point where the highest portion of the vaginal vault will be. The patient's left uterosacral ligament pedicle is grasped and the suture passed through. The suture incorporates the posterior peritoneum between the uterosacral ligaments, then the right uterosacral ligament. The suture is completed by passing the needle from the inside to the outside at the same point that it was begun. The suture is tied, thereby approximating the uterosacral ligaments and posterior peritoneum (*Fig. 7.17*).

The vaginal mucosa can be reapproximated in a vertical or horizontal manner, using either interrupted or continuous sutures. In this case, the vaginal mucosa is reapproximated horizontally with interrupted absorbable sutures (*Fig. 7.18*).

ALTERNATIVE PROCEDURES
Since most of the conditions for which vaginal hysterectomy is used are not life-threatening, medical and less invasive surgical alternatives should be recommended. Examples of this include hormonal manipulation, endometrial curettage, pessary use, endometrial ablation, and conservative treatment options for cervical intraepithelial neoplasia.

SURGICAL COMPLICATIONS
Complications of vaginal hysterectomy can be divided into intraoperative and postoperative and are similar to those complications that can occur with abdominal hysterectomy. *Fig. 7.19* lists the more commonly encountered complications.

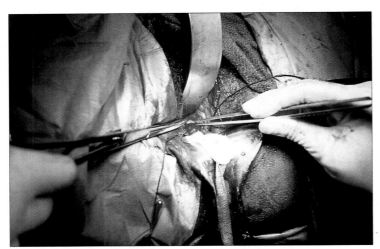

7.16 Peritoneal closure.

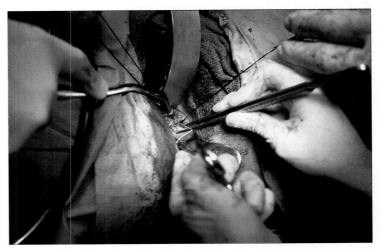

7.17 McCall-type culdoplasty.

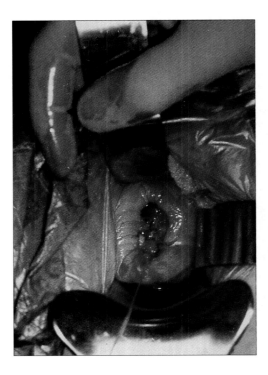

7.18 Closure of vaginal mucosa.

Complications of Vaginal Hysterectomy	
Intraoperative Complications	**Postoperative Complications**
Bladder injury	Hemorrhage
Bowel injury	Infection
Hemorrhage	Adnexal abscess
Inability to complete the surgical procedure	Urinary retention
	Vesicovaginal fistula
	Bowel fistula
	Fallopian tube prolapse
	Evisceration
	Vaginal cuff granulation tissue

7.19 Complications encountered at the time of vaginal hysterectomy and in the subsequent postoperative period.

ABDOMINAL HYSTERECTOMY

Hysterectomy is one of the most common surgical procedures performed by the gynecologic surgeon. Much has been written about this surgical procedure, its indications, and its results. We will not attempt to review these data, but instead will concentrate on the surgical technique.

SURGICAL INDICATIONS

Except in the case of some types of genital cancer, a less invasive form of therapy can be employed for most conditions in which hysterectomy might be used as therapy. More so than with other major operations, quality of life is an important consideration when hysterectomy is contemplated. The gynecologist and the patient should not elect hysterectomy without due consideration of alternative medical therapies and/or less invasive surgical procedures. *Fig. 7.20* lists the commonly cited indications for

---

Indications for Abdominal Hysterectomy

Leiomyomata uteri greater than 14–16 weeks' gestational size

Endometriosis

Adnexal pathology

Pelvic pain unresponsive to conservative therapy

Pelvic inflammatory disease/tubo-ovarian abscess not responsive to medical therapy

Hysterectomy indicated in the presence of pelvic adhesive disease

Obstetric hemorrhage

Endometrial carcinoma

Ovarian carcinoma

Fallopian tube carcinoma

7.20 Commonly cited indications for abdominal hysterectomy.

---

hysterectomy. An abdominal approach is usually indicated when a vaginal approach is contraindicated. In general, this occurs when adnexal or other forms of pelvic pathology are suspected, or when the uterus is greater than 14–16 weeks', gestational size. If the hysterectomy is being performed for genital prolapse, conversely, the vaginal approach is usually preferable.

SURGICAL PROCEDURE
Step 1

The patient is placed in the dorsal supine position. After receiving adequate anesthesia, the patient's legs are placed in a frog-leg position and a pelvic examination is performed to validate the pelvic findings. The vagina is cleansed with a solution of betadine and a Foley catheter is placed in the bladder. The legs are then extended and the patient reassumes the dorsal supine position.

Step 2

A variety of methods are available for skin cleaning. The most common of these methods is a 5-min betadine scrub, followed by application of betadine solution. Other commonly used methods include betadine scrub followed by alcohol, with application of an iodine-impregnated occlusive drape (*Fig. 7.21*), or the use of an iodine/alcohol combination (Dura-Prep) with or without application of an iodine-impregnated occlusive drape (*Fig. 7.22*).

Step 3

The type of incision is determined by several factors including: simplicity of the incision; the need for exposure; the potential need for enlarging the incision; the strength of the healed wound; cosmesis of the healed incision; and the location of previous surgical scars.

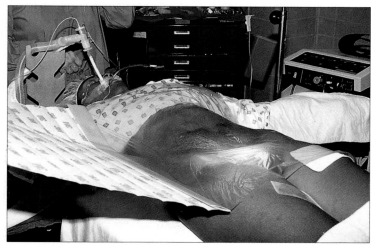

7.21 Occlusive drape.

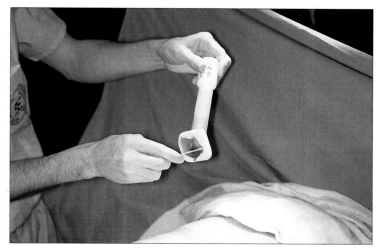

7.22 Optional type prep solution.

The skin is opened with the scalpel and the incision extended through the subcutaneous tissue and fascia (*Fig. 7.23*). With traction applied to the lateral edges of the incision, the knife's belly is used to divide the fascia and the peritoneum is opened. These steps can also be completed with electrocautery.

The upper abdomen and then the pelvis are systematically explored. If cytologic sampling of the peritoneal cavity is required, the sample should be obtained before abdominal exploration.

Step 4

A variety of retractors have been designed for pelvic surgery. The Balfour retractor, the O'Connor–O'Sullivan, or the Bookwalter retractor are the most commonly used. The Bookwalter retractor has a variety of adjustable blades which can be helpful, particularly in the obese patient. It is advisable to protect the wound edges with moist laps before placing the retractor blades.

Step 5

The uterus is elevated by placing broad ligament clamps at each cornua, such that the tips enclose the round ligament (*Fig. 7.24*). This placement allows uterine traction and prevents back-bleed-ing when the round ligament is cut.

Before proceeding with the bulk of the surgical procedure, any anatomic obscurations should be corrected so that the normal pelvic anatomy is restored.

Step 6

The uterus is deviated to the patient's left, placing the right round ligament on traction. With the proximal portion held by the broad ligament clamp, the distal portion of the round ligament is ligated with a suture ligature (*Fig. 7.25*). The round ligament is then cut, separating the anterior and posterior leaves of the broad ligament. The anterior leaf of the broad ligament is incised with Metzenbaum scissors along the vesico-uterine fold separating the peritoneal reflection of the bladder from the lower uterine segment (*Fig. 7.26*).

Step 7

The retroperitoneum is entered by extending the incision cephalad on the posterior leaf of the broad ligament. Care must be taken to remain lateral to both the infundibulopelvic ligament and iliac vessels. The ureter should remain attached to the medial leaf of the broad ligament to protect its blood supply (*Fig. 7.27*).

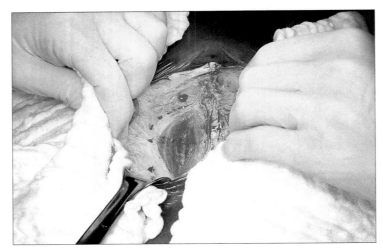

7.23 Abdominal incision.

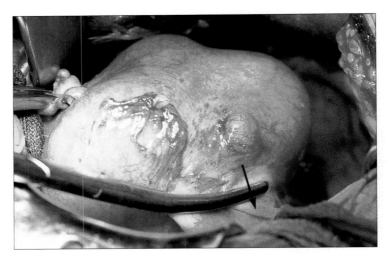

7.24 Method of uterine elevation. Right round ligament is arrowed.

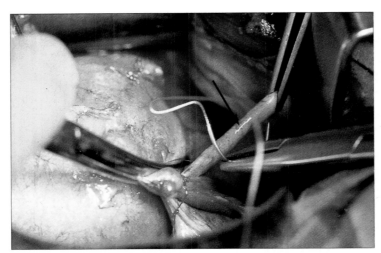

7.25 Suture ligation of round ligament. Right round ligament is arrowed.

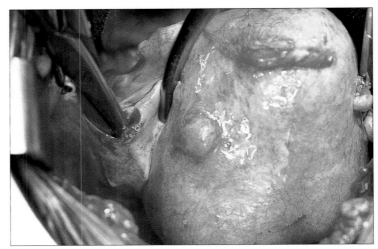

7.26 Opening of vesico-uterine fold.

If the ureter cannot be identified in this manner, the external iliac artery can be followed cephalad to the bifurcation of the common iliac artery. At this point, the ureter can be identified crossing the common iliac artery.

Step 8

If the ovaries are to be preserved, the uterus is retracted towards the pubic symphysis and deviated to one side, subjecting the contralateral infundibulopelvic ligament, tube, and ovary to tension. With the ureter under direct visualization, an opening is created in the peritoneum of the posterior leaf of the broad ligament under the utero-ovarian ligament and Fallopian tube. The tube and the utero-ovarian ligament on each side are clamped with a curved Heaney or Ballentine clamp and ligated with both a free tie and suture ligature (*Fig. 7.28*). The medial clamp at the uterine cornu should control back-bleeding.

If the ovaries are to be removed, the peritoneal opening is enlarged and extended cephalad to the infundibulopelvic ligament and caudad to the uterine artery. This allows proper exposure of both the uterine artery and the infundibulopelvic ligament. In addition, the ureter is released from its close proximity to the uterine vessels and the infundibulopelvic ligament.

A curved Heaney or Ballentine clamp is placed lateral to the ovary, making certain that the entire ovary is included in the surgical specimen. The infundibulopelvic ligament on each side is cut and doubly ligated (*Fig. 7.29*).

Step 9

Using Metzenbaum scissors with the tips pointed towards the uterus, the bladder is sharply dissected off the lower uterine segment and cervix. An avascular plane (the vesicocervical space) exists between the lower uterine segment and bladder. Tonsil forceps can be placed on the bladder edge to provide counter-traction and easier dissection.

Step 10

The uterus is then retracted cephalad and deviated to one side of the pelvis, subjecting the lower ligaments to stretch. The uterine vasculature is skeletonized, and any remaining areolar tissue is removed. A curved Heaney clamp is placed perpendicular to the uterine artery at the junction of the cervix and the body of the uterus. Its tip should be clamped adjacent to the uterus at the anatomic narrowing of the uterus (*Fig. 7.30*). The same procedure is repeated on the opposite side.

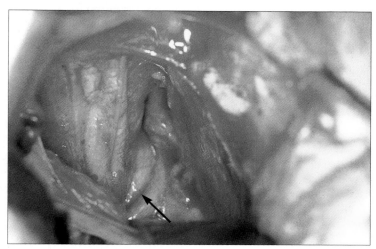

7.27 Utereral identification (arrowed).

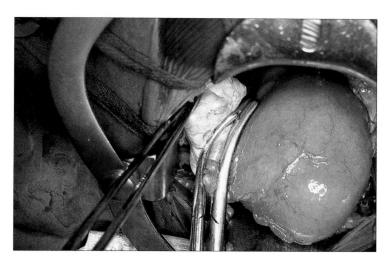

7.28 Clamping of utero-ovarian ligament.

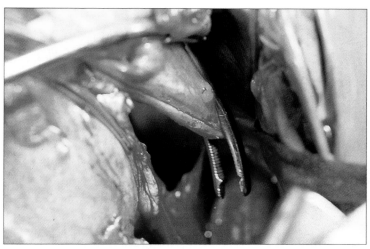

7.29 Clamping of infundibulopelvic ligament.

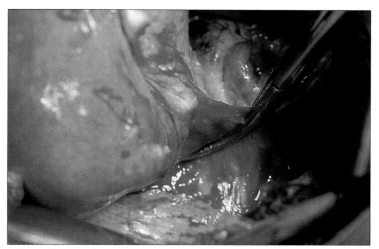

7.30 Ligation of the uterine artery pedicle.

Step 11

If the rectum requires mobilization from the posterior cervix, the posterior peritoneum between the uterosacral ligaments, just beneath the cervix, can be incised. A relatively avascular tissue plane exists in this area and allows mobilization of the rectum inferiorly (*Fig. 7.31*).

Step 12

The cardinal ligament is divided by placing a straight Heaney clamp medial to the uterine vessel pedicle for a distance of 2–3 cm parallel to the uterus. The ligament is then cut and the pedicle suture ligated. This step is repeated on each side until the junction of the cervix and vagina is reached (*Fig. 7.32*)

Step 13

The uterus is subjected to traction cephalad and the tip of the cervix is palpated. Curved Heaney clamps are placed bilaterally, incorporating the uterosacral ligament and the upper vagina just below the cervix. No excess vagina needs to be removed. The uterus is then removed with heavy curved scissors (*Fig. 7.33*).

Step 14

Several techniques have been described. A synthetic absorbable suture is placed between the tips of the two clamps. This suture is used for both traction and hemostasis. A separate suture is placed at the tip of each clamp and the pedicles are sutured in a Heaney manner, thereby incorporating the uterosacral and cardinal ligament at the angle of the vagina.

Another technique for cuff closure uses a running locking suture for hemostasis around the cuff edge. The vaginal cuff is then left open to heal secondarily.

Although not recommended by the authors, absorbable staples can be used for vaginal cuff closure (*Fig. 7.34*).

Step 15

The pelvis is thoroughly irrigated with saline or Ringer's lactate solution. Meticulous care is taken to ensure hemostasis throughout the pelvis, particularly of the vascular pedicles.

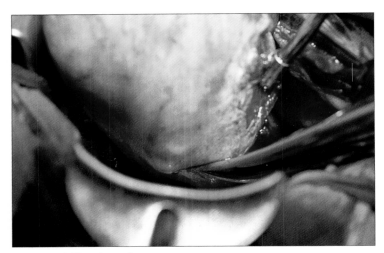

7.31 Mobilization of rectum.

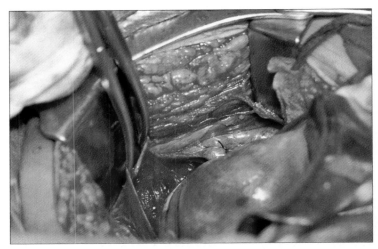

7.32 Clamping of cardinal ligament.

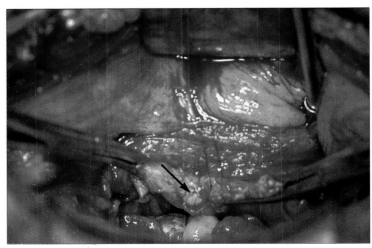

7.33 Closure of vaginal cuff (arrowed).

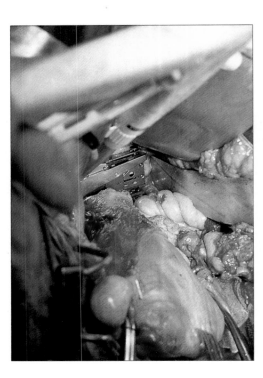

7.34 Staple closure of vaginal cuff.

Step 16

The pelvic peritoneum is not reapproximated. Research suggests that this may increase tissue trauma and promote adhesion formation. If the ovaries are not removed, some suggest ovarian suspension to the pelvic sidewall to minimize the risk that they will become retroperitoneal or adherent to the vaginal cuff.

Step 17

The parietal peritoneum is not reapproximated as a separate layer. Fascial closure can be accomplished with interrupted or continuous methods (see above). The subcutaneous tissue is irrigated and hemostasis is obtained. Staples, sutures, or skin tapes can be used to reapproximate the skin.

ALTERNATIVE PROCEDURES

The procedure as described should not be used to treat a condition that could otherwise be managed with medical therapy or more conservative surgical therapy. Medical management for many conditions for which medical therapy is considered an alternative treatment is often very successful.

COMPLICATIONS

The complications surrounding hysterectomy can be divided into intraoperative and postoperative ones (*Fig. 7.35*). Most intraoperative complications are preventable with appropriate surgical technique. However, there will be an irreducible number of operative injuries that cannot be avoided by even the most skilled surgeons.

LAPAROSCOPY-ASSISTED VAGINAL HYSTERECTOMY

Since its first description in 1989, laparoscopy-assisted vaginal hysterectomy (LAVH) has grown in popularity. Although it should not be used to replace traditional vaginal hysterectomy or even abdominal hysterectomy in all instances, there are potential advantages. A major potential advantage of this procedure is the possibility of conversion from an abdominal to a vaginal approach for hysterectomy in a patient who would otherwise require a laparotomy.

SURGICAL INDICATIONS

At present, consistent benefits of this surgical technique have not been shown for any single indication for hysterectomy. It is clear that if traditional vaginal hysterectomy can be accomplished, it should be the operative approach of choice. However, if the vaginal approach is not possible, operative laparoscopic assistance might offer an advantage. *Fig. 7.36* summarizes the potential indications for use of the laparoscopic approach for hysterectomy.

SURGICAL PROCEDURE

The procedure has been described using a variety of techniques, including electrocautery, endoscopic stapling, and suturing. Various methods have also been described that allow completion of specific parts of the procedure laparoscopically. It is, indeed, possible to perform the entire procedure laparoscopically,

Intraoperative and Postoperative Complications after Abdominal Hysterectomy
Intraoperative complications
Ureteral injury
Bladder injury
Bowel injury
Hemorrhage
Postoperative complications
Infection
Hemorrhage
Urinary tract infection
Vesicovaginal fistula
Bowel fistula formation
Pulmonary complications
Wound complications
Thrombophlebitis
Fascial dehiscence
Ileus and small bowel obstruction

7.35 Intraoperative and postoperative complications after abdominal hysterectomy.

Potential Indications
Patients with a contraindication to vaginal hysterectomy
Peritonitis
Ileus or bowel obstruction
Acute pelvic inflammatory disease
Ovarian carcinoma
Tubo-ovarian abscess
Patients with one or more relative contraindications to vaginal hysterectomy
Nulliparity
Chronic pelvic pain
Endometriosis
Severe pelvic adhesive disease
Uterine size greater than 14 weeks' gestational size
Adnexal pathology requiring hysterectomy
Uterine immobility

7.36 Potential indications for laparoscopy assisted vaginal hysterectomy.

including closure of the vaginal cuff. In the authors' experience, this requires prolonged operative time compared with completing the procedure via the vagina. The procedure depicted here describes a three-puncture technique that completes the majority of the procedure laparoscopically while the posterior colpotomy, ligation of the uterosacral ligaments, and vaginal cuff closure are performed vaginally.

ENDOSCOPIC PART
Step 1
After the induction of general anesthesia, the patient is placed in the dorsal lithotomy position. The "candy-cane" stirrups allow adequate exposure during the vaginal approach. Setting the stirrups at their lowest adjustment point keeps the thighs out of the operative field during the laparoscopic part of the operation (*Fig. 7.37*).

The perineum, vagina, and lower abdomen are draped with a combination of laparoscopy and vaginal drapes.

Step 2
A Hulka tenaculum is attached to the cervix through a side-open Graves' speculum, making certain to antevert the uterus. A Foley catheter is inserted into the bladder and remains in place throughout the surgical procedure (*Fig. 7.38*).

Step 3
Three 12 mm trocars are inserted into the abdomen by a direct insertion technique. Initially the umbilical trocar is placed, followed by gas insufflation of the abdomen. Two additional 12 mm trocars are placed in the right and left lower quadrants 6–8 cm above the pubic rami, taking care to avoid the inferior epigastric vessels (*Fig. 7.39*). If one elects to use sutures or cautery, the trocar sizes can be reduced to a 10 mm periumbilical trocar along with either two 5 mm or two 10 mm trocars in the lower quadrants.

Step 4
A full abdominal survey is performed, paying particular attention to the presence of adhesions or upper abdominal pathology.

Beginning at the left round ligament, the peritoneum is lifted at the level of the vesico-uterine fold and incised with scissors (*Fig. 7.40*). The incision is continued across the lower uterine segment to the opposite round ligament, using sharp dissection and electrocautery.

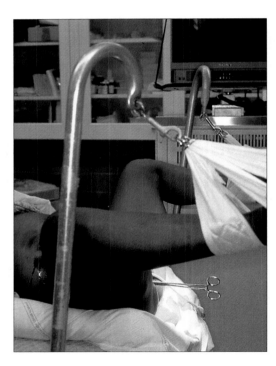

7.37 Patient positioning for LAVH.

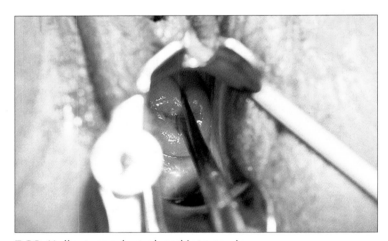

7.38 Hulka tenaculum placed into cervix.

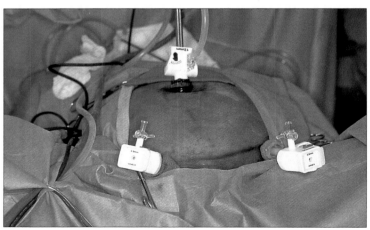

7.39 Trocar placement for LAVH.

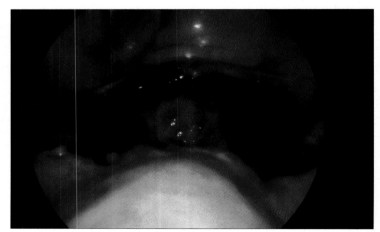

7.40 Incision of vesico-uterine fold.

The bladder flap is dissected from the lower uterine segment and cervix by both sharp and blunt dissection. To maintain hemostasis, the unipolar cautery attached to the scissors is activated before cutting.

Step 5

The uterus is anteverted and moved to the side opposite the ureter that is to be dissected. The peritoneum above the ureter is elevated with grasping forceps and then incised with scissors (*Fig. 7.41*). The ureter is visualized and dissected to a level inferior to the cardinal ligaments. The same procedure is repeated on the opposite side.

Step 6

If the ovaries are to be removed, a peritoneal window is made in the pelvic sidewall just superior to the ureter. This peritoneal edge is cut cephalad to the infundibulopelvic ligament and cauded to the uterine artery. This step allows the ureter to drop away from the uterine artery and functions to skeletonize the uterine and ovarian vessel complex. An endoscopic multifire stapler is then placed across the infundibulopelvic ligament distal to the ovary.

If the ovary is to be preserved, the stapler is placed across the utero-ovarian pedicle proximal to the ovary (*Fig. 7.42*). The size of the stapler to be used is determined by use of the Endo-Gauge. Once the stapling unit is properly positioned, it is closed and locked in place. The closed position is inspected, paying particular attention that no bowel is enclosed and that the ureter is free. Once cut, the cut and stapled edges are inspected for hemostasis. The same procedure is repeated on the opposite side.

Step 7

The uterus is pushed upward and to the opposite of the side to be ligated. This subjects the uterine artery pedicle to tension. The Endo-GIA is aligned vertically along the uterus, incorporating the uterine artery. A White 3.0 V stapling unit is typically used for this step. The endoscopic stapler is pushed down to the apex of the previously cut pedicle and the stapling unit is closed. The position of the ureter can be inspected to make certain that it is not within the stapling unit (*Fig. 7.43*).

Step 8

In most cases, the endoscopic portion of the surgery is completed after ligation and division of the uterine arteries. However, the surgeon can also apply an endoscopic stapler to the cardinal ligaments on both sides (*Fig. 7.44*). If one elects to stop at this point, the remainder of the surgical procedure is completed vaginally. A second alternative is to make an anterior colpotomy incision using the unipolar cautery and scissors. This can usually be readily accomplished.

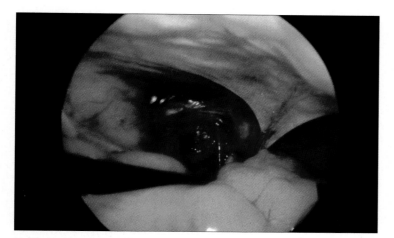

7.41 Ureteral exposure.

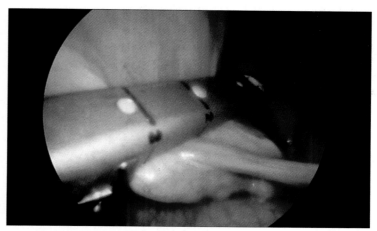

7.42 Ligation of utero-ovarian ligament.

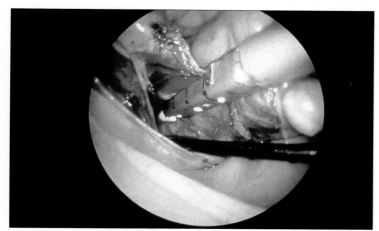

7.43 Ligation of uterine artery.

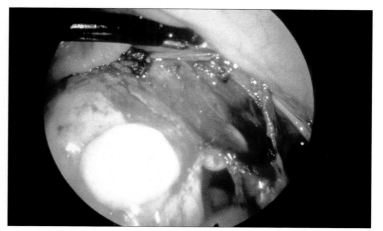

7.44 Ligation of cardinal ligament.

VAGINAL PART

Step 9

The vaginal portion of the procedure is begun by placing a weighted speculum into the vagina to obtain exposure. The Hulka tenaculum is removed and a suitable tenaculum is applied to the cervix.

The posterior cul-de-sac is entered with scissors and a suture is placed to attach the posterior cul-de-sac peritoneum to the vaginal mucosa (*Fig. 7.45*). A long-blade weighted speculum is then placed into the posterior cul-de-sac.

Step 10

If the anterior peritoneum had already been incised, a Dever retractor is placed into the anterior cul-de-sac. If not, the uterosacral ligaments are clamped directly.

Haney-type clamps are used to clamp the uterosacral ligament, which is then transected with scissors and sutured with a synthetic absorbable suture (*Fig. 7.46*). The same procedure is repeated on the opposite side.

If the anterior peritoneum has not been incised laparoscopically, the anterior vaginal mucosa is circumscribed and blunt and sharp dissection is used to separate the anterior peritoneum from the vaginal mucosa. The anterior cul-de-sac is then entered sharply.

Step 11

One additional pedicle is usually all that is required at this point. It is helpful to palpate the next pedicle, feeling the staple line from below, to direct clamp placement. Once divided, the uterus is removed and the pedicle is suture-ligated for hemostasis (*Fig. 7.47*).

Step 12

After ensuring hemostasis, the vaginal mucosa is closed with a series of interrupted sutures. The vaginal angles are reapproximated to the uterosacral–cardinal ligament complex, with the remainder of the vagina being closed with interrupted sutures (*Fig. 7.48*).

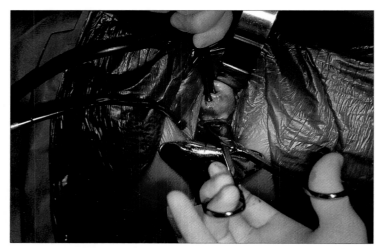

7.45 Posterior cul-de-sac entry.

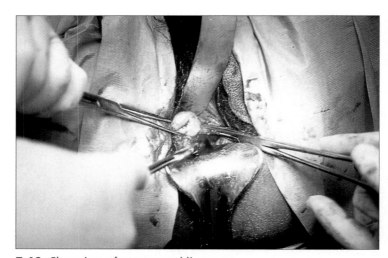

7.46 Clamping of uterosacral ligament.

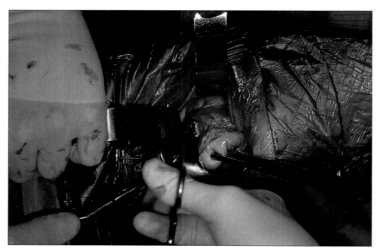

7.47 Ligation of uterine artery.

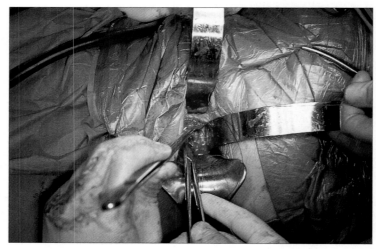

7.48 Vaginal cuff closure.

Step 13

The abdomen is insufflated with the laparoscope. The pelvis is irrigated with saline and hemostasis is ensured. The trocar incisions are closed with subcuticular stitches.

ALTERNATIVE PROCEDURES

The procedure as described should not be used to replace traditional vaginal hysterectomy, but should be used only in an effort to replace abdominal hysterectomy. One must always remember, when planning a hysterectomy, that medical management for many conditions is well tolerated and controls the patient's problems.

COMPLICATIONS

Complications reported with this surgical procedure can be classified into those that are related to the laparoscopy, those related to vaginal hysterectomy, and those related to stapling or electrosurgery (*Fig. 7.49*).

UTERINE MORCELLATION

Uterine morcellation is a well-known but often underutilized surgical procedure, whereby the uterus is removed piecemeal. This technique is used as an adjunct during vaginal hysterectomy. Several methods of uterine morcellation have been described, including hemisection or bivalving, wedge resection, or intramyometrial coring/Lash procedure. Uterine morcellation allows increased utilization of the vaginal approach in patients with leiomyomata uteri.

INDICATIONS

Uterine morcellation can be used in combination with vaginal hysterectomy in patients with enlarged uteri secondary to leiomyomata. It should not be used by the inexperienced gynecologic surgeon, but it is a technique that can be easily taught and learned.

SURGICAL PROCEDURE

No method of uterine morcellation is applicable to all surgical situations; therefore, one or more of the methods presented here can be used.

Step 1

Before beginning any morcellation procedure, the uterine vessels must be ligated and the peritoneal cavity entered (*Fig. 7.50*). Although it is helpful to have entered both the anterior and the posterior cul-de-sac, this is not mandatory.

Complications Reported	
Laparoscopy related	**Stapling device related**
Uterine perforation	Functional failure
Preperitoneal insufflation	Disassembly
Gas embolism	Hemorrhage
Inferior epigastric artery injury	Ureteral injury
Bladder injury	Bladder injury
Bowel injury	Bowel injury
Major vessel injury	**Electrosurgery related**
Vaginal hysterectomy related	Thermal injury
Cystotomy	Hemorrhage
Hemorrhage	
Rectal injury	
Ureteral injury	
Vesicovaginal fistula	

7.49 Complications reported with laparoscopy-assisted vaginal hysterectomy.

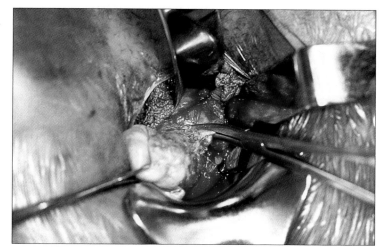

7.50 Clamping of uterine vessels.

UTERINE HEMISECTION

Bivalving the uterus is the least-used morcellation technique, but seems best-suited for the fundal, midline leiomyomata. The procedure is begun by incising the cervix in the middle (*Fig. 7.51*), with the incision extending in the midline to divide the uterine fundus. One side of the uterus and cervix is removed and then the other (*Fig. 7.52*).

WEDGE MORCELLATION

This technique of uterine morcellation is best suited for anterior or posterior fibroids or for fibroids in one or the other broad ligaments, i.e., when the fibroids are away from the midline. The cervix is amputated and the myometrium grasped with clamps. Wedge-shaped portions of myometrium are removed from the anterior and/or posterior uterine wall (*Fig. 7.53*). The apex of the wedge is kept in the midline, thereby reducing the bulk of the myometrium. This process is repeated until the uterus can be removed or until a pseudocapsule of a fibroid is reached. The fibroid can be grasped with a Leahy clamp or towel clip; traction is applied, and a "myomectomy" performed. The uterine volume is reduced enough to allow clamping and ligation of the utero-ovarian ligament, thereby allowing uterine removal. The final specimen is made up of morsels of uterine muscle, which are submitted for histologic analysis (*Fig. 7.54*).

INTRAMYOMETRIAL CORING

The coring or Lash technique is best utilized for the uterus composed predominantly of midline leiomyomata. The myometrium above the ligated uterine vessels is incised parallel to the axis of the uterine cavity and serosa (*Fig. 7.55*). The incision is continued around the full circumference of the myometrium in a symmetrical fashion beneath the uterine serosa. Traction is maintained on the cervix and the avascular myometrium is cut

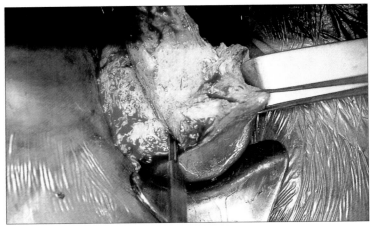

7.51 Uterine hemisection.

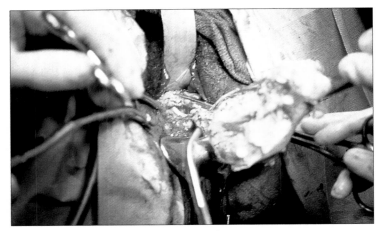

7.52 Uterine hemisection completed.

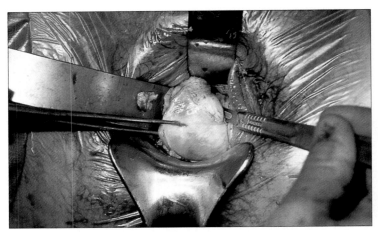

7.53 Wedge morcellation of uterus.

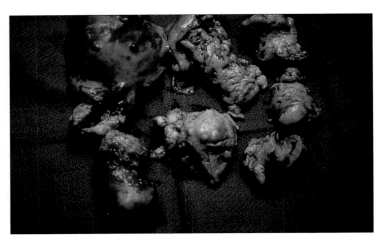

7.54 Surgical specimen after morcellation.

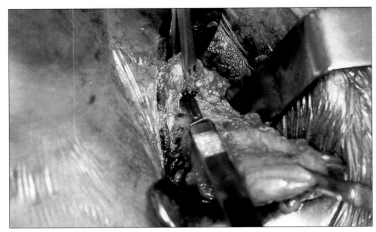

7.55 Intramyometrial coring.

so that the endometrial cavity is not entered. The knife should not be held perpendicular to the uterine serosa, as this will lead to amputation of the cervix (*Fig. 7.56*). When done correctly, the coring technique converts the uterus from a globular to an elongated tissue mass (*Figs 7.57, 7.58*). The uterus and cervix are delivered as a single specimen. Incision of the lateral portions of the myometrium medial to the remaining attachment of the broad ligament results in considerable additional descent of the uterus and greatly increases the mobility of the uterine fundus. The cored uterus is removed by clamping the utero-ovarian pedicle and Fallopian tubes.

ALTERNATIVE PROCEDURES

When the uterus is large, a decision must be made by the gynecologic surgeon to proceed with an abdominal or a vaginal approach to hysterectomy. Uterine morcellation allows the vaginal removal of larger uteri than would otherwise be possible. A gonadotrophin-releasing hormone agonist can also be used before hysterectomy to reduce the overall uterine volume. However, even with this approach, uterine morcellation may be necessary.

COMPLICATIONS

There are no complications that apply to uterine morcellation that are not also complications seen with hysterectomy.

ABDOMINAL MYOMECTOMY

Myomectomy, defined as the surgical removal of uterine leiomyomata with conservation of the uterus, is a procedure more prone to hemorrhage and other operative complications than hysterectomy. When carefully done, myomectomy provides a valuable alternative for treatment of symptomatic leiomyomata in women who wish to retain their fertility. When the presence of leiomyomata may be contributing to fetal wastage (or, rarely, infertility), myomectomy may significantly enhance the outcome of pregnancy. Meticulous surgical technique is necessary to avoid intraoperative hemorrhage that might require hysterectomy and to maintain the functional integrity of the uterus and the adnexa.

Adequate preoperative preparation is important in optimizing the outcome. A hysterosalpingogram (with oblique views) delineates the position of the tumor(s) and the degree to which the endometrial cavity is distorted. Ultrasound (both vaginal and abdominal) defines the location, number, and surgical accessibility of the leiomyomata. A significant reduction in tumor size can be achieved by treatment with GnRH analogues, progestins, or Danazol. The latter also has an additional androgenic stimulatory effect on hematopoiesis. In addition to preoperative iron therapy, the most prudent part of the preoperative preparation in these patients is storage of two units of autologous blood in all but the simplest cases.

Opinions vary regarding the necessity for elective cesarean section in pregnancies conceived after myomectomy. Some authorities advocate cesarean section only if the uterine cavity has been transected, whereas others suggest a more conservative approach.

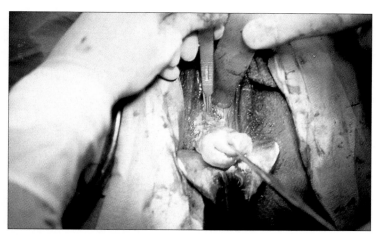

7.56 Demonstration of inappropriate angle for coring technique.

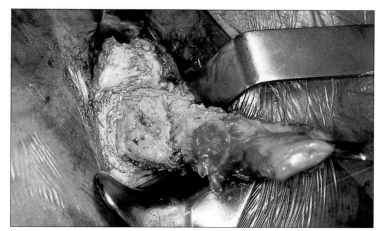

7.57 Elongation of uterine fibroid.

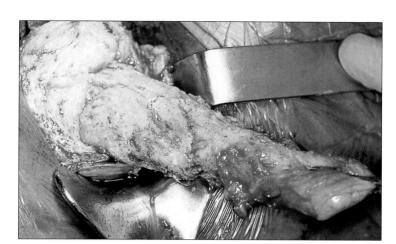

7.58 Conversion of globular uterine size to elongated size.

SURGICAL INDICATIONS

The surgical indications for myomectomy are given in *Fig. 7.59*.

SURGICAL PROCEDURE

Step 1

In this case, a 39-year-old woman with primary infertility, endometriosis, and a previous right salpingo-oophorectomy presented for *in vitro* fertilization. Gross distortion of the uterine cavity was evident on the hysterosalpingogram. Diagnostic hysteroscopy or even laparoscopy is often performed to delineate the location of leiomyoma (*Fig. 7.60*). Hysteroscopy is especially useful for

determining whether the myoma arises posterior or anterior to the uterine cavity; judicious use of this technique can avoid inadvertent transection of the cavity.

Step 2

After hysteroscopy, a No.10 or No.12 pediatric Foley catheter is placed in the uterine cavity. It is attached to a 50 ml catheter-tip syringe filled with dilute indigo carmine dye. The catheter balloon is first tested (*Fig. 7.61*) and, after insertion, traction is placed on the catheter to ensure good intrauterine placement (*Fig. 7.62*).

Step 3

The abdomen is then opened in the usual fashion. For all but the smallest myoma, a midline vertical or Malyard incision is preferable. Retraction is obtained with a Kirschner retractor (*Fig. 7.63*), and a wound protector used, minimizing blood leakage into the pelvic cavity. The bowel is carefully packed away and the myoma is exposed (*Fig. 7.64*).

Myomectomy	
Indications	**Alternative procedures**
Symptomatic leiomyomata	*Medical management*
Menorrhagia, metamenorrhagia	Progestins
Pelvic pressure/pain	GnRH analogues
Size or enlargement	Danazol
(>12–14 week size)	*Hysteroscopic removal* (submucous leiomyomata)
Fetal wastage	
Recurrent miscarriage	Hysterectomy
Second trimester loss	Myoma coagulation
Infertility	
To normalize uterine cavity before IVF	
To resolve cornual fallopian tube block	
In absence of other causes*	
*Controversial	

7.59 Surgical indications and alternatives for myomectomy.

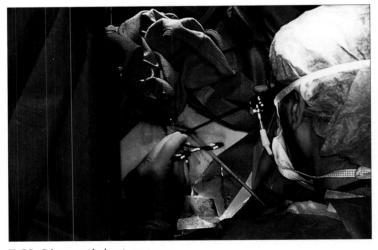

7.60 Diagnostic hysteroscopy.

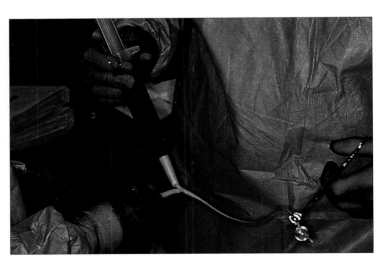

7.61 Testing of uterine balloon.

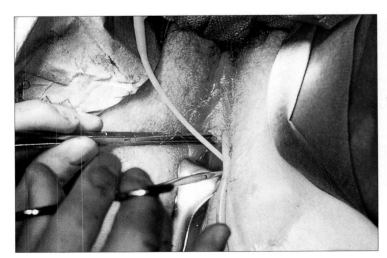

7.62 Placement of intrauterine catheter.

Step 4

With unipolar electrocautery, a midline incision is made in the thinnest area of myometrium overlying the myoma (*Fig. 7.65*) or, alternatively, in the optimal location in the midline to remove more than one myoma. The incision is extended through the myometrium using the coagulation and cutting currents until the pseudocapsule of the leiomyoma is identified and incised (*Fig. 7.66*). Meticulous hemostasis is essential, and copious irrigation

is performed throughout the procedure (*Fig. 7.67*) using 50 ml syringes with 20-gauge intravenous catheters and heparinized lactated Ringer's solution (5000 units/l).

Step 5

The myometrium overlying the myoma is then grasped with Allis forceps (*Fig. 7.68*) and the myoma is further exposed by careful

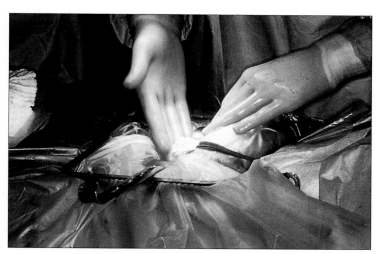

7.63 Placement of self-retaining retractor.

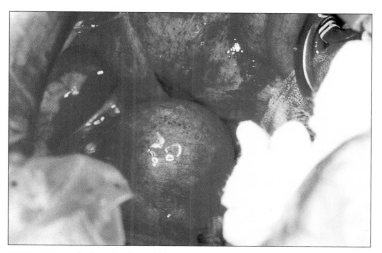

7.64 Intra-abdominal packing.

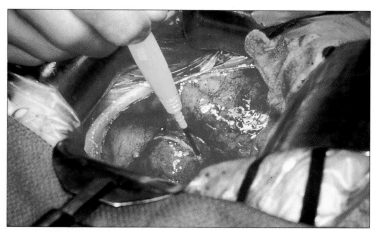

7.65 Myometrial incision.

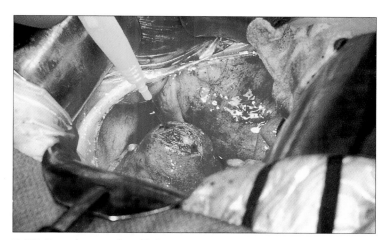

7.66 Pseudocapsule of leiomyomata.

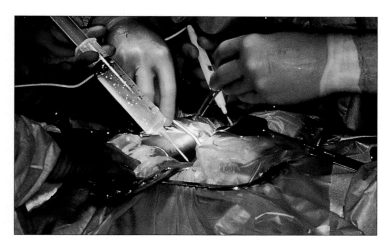

7.67 Irrigation of operative site.

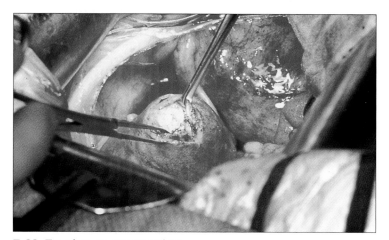

7.68 Traction on myometrium.

electrosurgical dissection and retraction (*Fig. 7.69*). Vessels in the pseudocapsule overlying the myoma should be identified and hemostasis obtained while the leiomyoma is *in situ*. Bleeding is far more troublesome to deal with in the enucleated tumor bed. Another common mistake is to stray from the surface of the myoma into the more vascular myometrium. To prevent this problem, a #2-0 or #3-0 polyglycolic acid stay suture is placed through the core of the myoma and gentle traction applied during dissection (*Fig. 7.70*). The myoma is then gradually enucleated (*Fig. 7.71*).

Step 6

It is imperative to stay on the tumour surface (*Fig. 7.72*) to avoid transecting the uterine cavity and the adjacent vessels. Any filament of adherent myometrium that appears to have a vascular supply to the myoma should be carefully clamped and suture ligated. Particular attention must be paid to this principle as the myoma becomes more mobile. Placing a clamp across the broad base of the myoma to hasten its removal is not recommended. As the endometrial cavity is often very close, premature clamping of the pedunculated base may result in endometrial compromise.

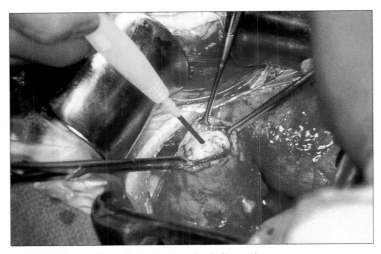

7.69 Continuation of electrosurgical dissection.

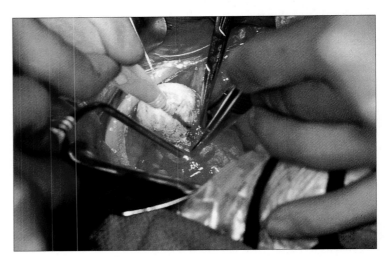

7.70 Dissection of myoma.

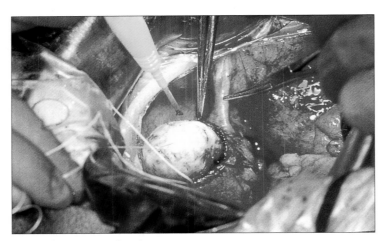

7.71 Myoma enucleation.

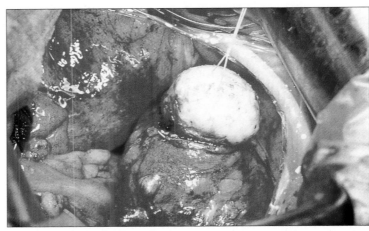

7.72 Myoma removal.

Step 7

After the myoma has been removed (*Fig. 7.73*), any remaining hemostats in the bed of the tumor are ligated (*Fig. 7.74*) and hemostasis ensured (*Fig. 7.75*). Sutures of #3-0 delayed absorbable material are then placed deeply across the myoma bed in either simple interrupted or figure-of-eight fashion, to obliterate any dead space (*Fig. 7.76*); care must be taken to avoid the uterine cavity. A second layer of sutures may be required to approximate the edges of the defect. Delayed #4-0 absorbable subcuticular suture is then placed along the length of the incision, resulting in effective closure with a minimum of surface suture material exposed (*Fig. 7.77*).

Step 8

The abdomen is copiously irrigated and hemostasis once again ensured. Antiadhesion prophylaxis using barrier adjuvants can be considered if hemostasis is complete (*Fig. 7.78*). The abdomen is then closed in the usual fashion.

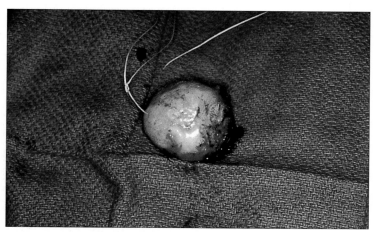

7.73 Specimen for hystologic analysis.

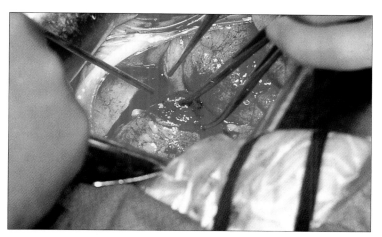

7.74 Hemostasis in fibroid bed.

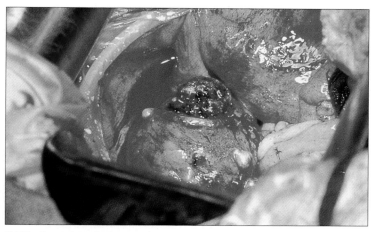

7.75 Complete hemostasis.

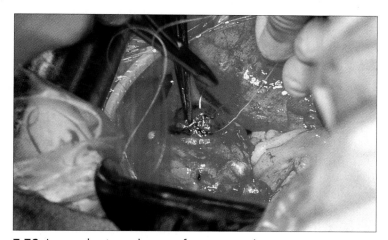

7.76 Layered suture closure of myoma cavity.

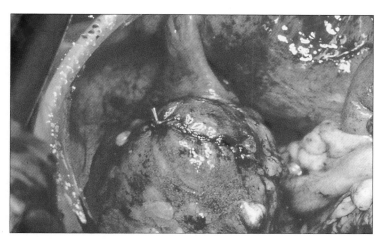

7.77 Closure of myoma cavity.

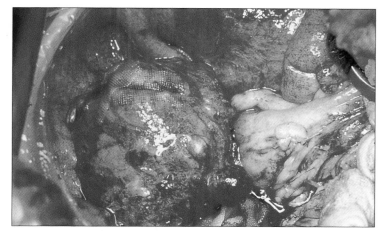

7.78 Placement of adhesive barrier.

COMPLICATIONS

Bleeding

Extensive myomectomy can result in significant blood loss. Techniques to reduce intraoperative hemorrhage include intra-myometrial injection of a dilute solution of Pitressin (a synthetic derivative of antidiuretic hormone). Ten units are diluted to 100 ml with physiologic saline and injected diffusely around the myoma before incision. The risk of delayed postoperative hemorrhage and the rare but spectacular cardiac side effects of this drug have dissuaded us from its use; we prefer to rely solely on meticulous hemostasis. Others advocate the use of lower uterine segment and infundibulopelvic ligament tourniquets to maintain hemostasis.

Postoperatively, intra-abdominal hemorrhage is characterized by falling serial hematocrits and by signs and symptoms of a persistent acute abdomen. With evidence of continuing hemorrhage, repeat operation should not be delayed. Although attempts of conservative management at reoperation to save the uterus may be entertained, in life-threatening cases hysterectomy should be performed. It is therefore wise to obtain consent for hysterectomy before every significant abdominal myomectomy. This will codify the discussion of this eventuality in the process of informed consent.

Pelvic adhesions

Adhesions are a common complication of myomectomy. To minimize the incidence of adhesions, intraoperative hemostasis and irrigation are important, as is leaving a minimum of exposed reactive suture material on the serosal surface of the uterus. Finally, the use of intraoperative antiadhesion prophylaxis, barrier or otherwise, although somewhat controversial, may be appropriate. The presence of infertility in a postmyomectomy patient should raise the suspicion of iatrogenic pelvic adhesions.

Intrauterine adhesions

In any myomectomy in which the uterine cavity is transected, there exists the possibility of intrauterine adhesion formation. An interval postoperative hysterosalpingogram is appropriate to rule out this event. This complication highlights the need for operative recognition of uterine cavity transection, a somewhat subtle finding due to distortion of the uterus. It is therefore important to have the ability to inject dye into the uterine cavity. Management of such intrauterine adhesions requires a subsequent hysteroscopic lysis under laparoscopic guidance.

Endometritis and myometritis

Although the chances of the development of postoperative endometrial or myometrial infection are small, the possibility does exist. Persistent postoperative fever necessitates aggressive intravenous antibiotic therapy after a work-up for other causes of infection. This situation, again, mandates interval postoperative hysterosalpingography to rule out intra- or extrauterine adhesions.

RETROPERITONEAL DISSECTION

Familiarity with the retroperitoneal anatomy is a must for any gynecologic surgeon. Entry into this space is necessary for almost all intra-abdominal gynecologic procedures and for prevention and management of many complications that can arise during gynecologic surgery.

SURGICAL INDICATIONS

Retroperitoneal dissection as a "stand-alone" procedure is rarely performed as part of a benign gynecologic procedure, but rather is done in conjunction with other procedures such as hysterectomy, oophorectomy, or management of hemorrhage or ureteral dissection.

SURGICAL PROCEDURE

The procedure depicted here demonstrates retroperitoneal dissection during hysterectomy and salpingo-oophorectomy. The procedure can be divided into two steps: entry into the retroperitoneal space and identification of anatomic landmarks.

Step 1

Entry into the retroperitoneal space is accomplished by suture ligation of the round ligament (*Fig. 7.79*), and then cutting the round ligament with scissors (*Fig. 7.80*).

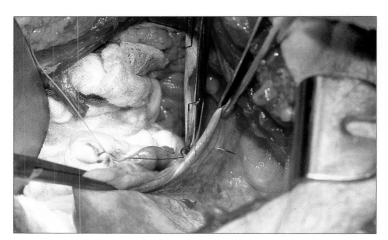

7.79 Suture ligation of round ligament.

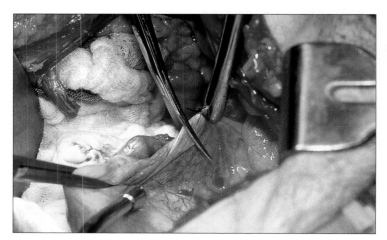

7.80 Cutting of round ligament.

Step 2

Both blunt and sharp dissection can be used to facilitate separation of the anterior and posterior leaves of the broad ligament. Once separated, blunt dissection can be used to facilitate mobilization of the loose areolar tissue in the retroperitoneal space (*Fig. 7.81*). This can also be accomplished after a hysterectomy by proceeding similarly with the stump of the round ligament.

Step 3

The ureter is identified on the medial leaf of the broad ligament. It initially passes over the bifurcation of the internal and external iliac arteries, where it generally first becomes important in gynecologic surgery. The ureter remains attached to the medial leaf of the broad ligament (*Fig. 7.82*) after the retroperitoneal space is opened and then crosses under the uterine artery and pierces the cardinal ligament. It then lies adjacent to the anterolateral surface of the cervix, and lies on the anterior vaginal wall before entering the bladder.

Step 3

The common iliac arteries are direct branches from the aorta. Division of the internal and external iliac vessels occurs in the area of the sacroiliac joint (*Fig. 7.83*). It is at this level that the ureter crosses the common iliac artery (*Fig. 7.84*).

The external iliac artery becomes the femoral artery with its accompanying vein, and near the inguinal ligament it gives off the deep inferior epigastric and deep circumflex iliac vessels.

The internal iliac artery and vein supply the pelvic viscera and muscles of the pelvic wall and gluteal area. The internal artery usually divides into an anterior and posterior division about 3–4 cm from the bifurcation of the common iliac artery. Ligation of the internal iliac artery (hypogastric artery) can be helpful in the management of pelvic hemorrhage and should be performed distal to the anterior division bifurcation. The internal iliac veins are lateral and posterior to the artery and have a complex and variable branching pattern.

ALTERNATIVE PROCEDURES

There are no surgical procedures that can replace retroperitoneal dissection and identification of the major anatomic landmarks that have been described. This type of dissection is always necessary when extensive adhesive disease, endometriosis, or another disease process is encountered that alters the normal pelvic anatomy.

COMPLICATIONS

The potential complications arising during retroperitoneal dissection include damage to the ureter or to major vessels of the pelvis. However, it is likely that these structures will remain undamaged if properly identified and mobilized out of the surgical field.

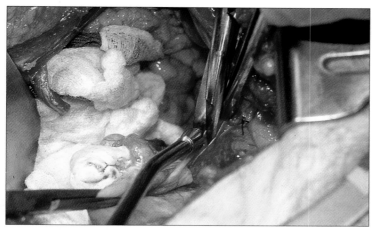

7.81 Sharp dissection into retroperitoneal space.

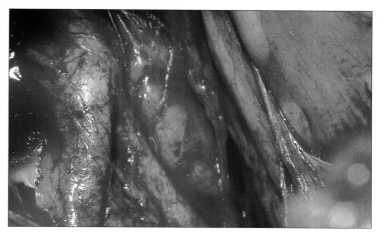

7.82 Identification of ureter.

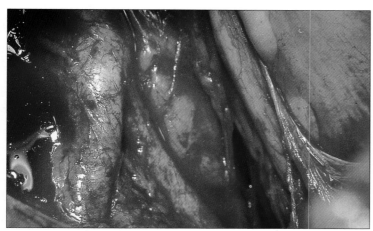

7.83 Common iliac artery bifurcation.

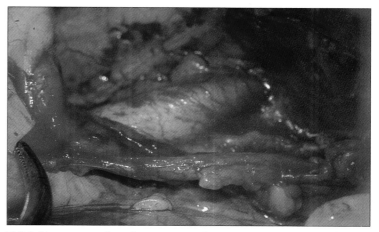

7.84 Ureter crossing the common iliac artery.

FURTHER READING

Copeland LJ, ed. *Textbook of Gynecology*. Philadelphia: WB Saunders, 1993.

Cruikshank SH. Methods of vaginal cuff closure during vaginal hysterectomy. *South Med J* 1988; 81:1375–8.

Dicker RC, Greenspan JR, Strauss LT, *et al*. Complications of abdominal and vaginal hysterectomy among women of reproductive age in the United States: the collaborative review of sterilization. *Am J Obstet Gynecol* 1982; 144:841–8.

Dillon TF. Control of blood loss during gynecologic surgery. *Obstet Gynecol* 1962; 19:428–35.

Esterday CL, Grimes DA, Riggs JA. Hysterectomy in the United States. *Obstet Gynecol* 1983; 62:203–12.

Grody MHT. Vaginal hysterectomy: the large uterus. *J Gynecol Surg* 1989; 5:301–12.

Herbst AL, Mishell DR, Stenchever MA, Droegemueller W, eds. *Comprehensive Gynecology*, 2nd ed. St Louis: Mosby Year Book, 1992.

Hurst BS. Uterine leiomyomas. Schlaff WP, Rock JA, eds. In: *Decision making in reproductive endocrinology*, Boston: Blackwell Scientific Publications, 1993: 129–34.

Kistner RW, Patton GW. *Atlas of infertility surgery*. Boston: Little Brown, 1975.

Kovac SR. Intramyometrial coring as an adjunct to the vaginal hysterectomy. *Obstet Gynecol* 1986; 67:131–6.

Lash AF. A method for reducing the size of the uterus in vaginal hysterectomy. *Am J Obstet Gynecol* 1941; 42: 452–9.

Masterson BJ. Total abdominal hysterectomy. In: *Manual of gynecologic surgery*, 2nd ed. New York: Springer–Verlag, 1986: 53–76.

McCall ML. Posterior culdoplasty. *Obstet Gynecol* 1957; 10:595–602.

Nezhat F, Nezhat C, Gordon S, Wilkins E. Laparoscopic versus abdominal hysterectomy. *J Reprod Med* 1992; 37: 247–50.

Nezhat C, Nezhat F, Silfen SL. Laparoscopic hysterectomy and bilateral salpingo-oophorectomy using multifire GIA surgical stapler. *J Gynecol Surg* 1990; 6:287–8.

Nichols DH, Randall CL, eds. *Vaginal Surgery*, 3rd ed. Baltimore: Williams & Wilkins, 1989.

Reich H, DeCaprio J, McGlynn F. Laparoscopic-hysterectomy. *J Gynecol Surg* 1989; 5: 213–16.

Stovall TG. Abdominal and vaginal hysterectomy for uterine myomas: surgery combined with medical therapy. *Sem in Reprod Endocrinol* 1992; 10: 385–9.

Stovall TG, Ling FW, Henry LC. A randomized trial evaluating leuprolide acetate prior to hysterectomy for leiomyomata. *Am J Obstet Gynecol* 1991; 164: 1420–5.

Stovall TG, Ling FW, Henry LC, Woodruff MR. A randomized trial evaluating leuprolide acetate prior to hysterectomy for leiomyomata. *Am J Obstet Gynecol* 154: 1991; 1420–5.

Stovall TG, Summitt RL, Bran DF, Ling FW. Outpatient vaginal hysterectomy: a pilot study. *Obstet Gynecol* 1992; 80:145–9.

Summitt RL, Stovall TG, Lipscomb GH, Ling FW. Randomized comparison of laparoscopic-assisted vaginal hysterectomy versus standard vaginal hysterectomy in an outpatient setting. *Obstet Gynecol* 1992; 80:895–901.

Thompson JD, Rock J, eds. *TeLinde's Operative Gynecology*, 7th ed. Philadelphia: JB Lippincott, 1992.

Tulandi T, Murray C, Guralnick M, *et al*. Adhesion formation and reproductive outcome after myomectomy and second look laparoscopy. *Obstet Gynecol* 1993; 82:213–15.

Wiskind AK, Thompson JD. Abdominal myomectomy: reducing the risk of hemorrhage. *Semin Reprod Endocrinol* 1992; 10:358–86.

Woodland MB. Ureter injury during laparoscopy-assisted vaginal hysterectomy with the endoscopic linear stapler. *Am J Obstet Gynecol* 1992; 167: 756–7.

8

Surgical Incision

Javier F. Magrina

This chapter includes the basic knowledge needed for performing incisions in the anterior abdominal wall, as well as management of incisional complications.

ANATOMY OF THE ANTERIOR ABDOMINAL WALL

MUSCLES

There are four major muscles, with their corresponding fascial layers: rectus, external oblique, internal oblique, and transverse. Their overall function is flexion and torsion of the abdomen, abdominal respiration, and protection of the abdominal viscera. A fifth accessory muscle is the pyramidalis.

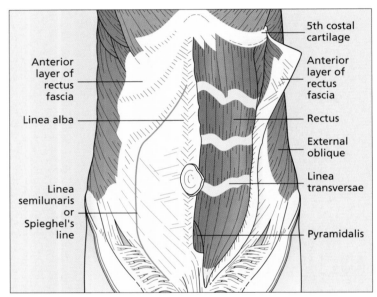

8.1 Rectus and pyramidalis muscles, and fascial lines of the anterior abdominal wall.

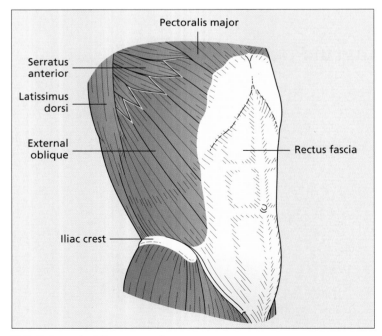

8.2 External oblique muscle.

Rectus

The rectus muscles (*Fig. 8.1*) are located in the midline of the anterior abdominal wall and extend from the pubic symphisis to the fifth through seventh ribs and xyphoid process. They are divided into four sections by the linea transversae that consist of three transverse tendinous attachments to the anterior rectus fascia. They are separated in the midline by the linea alba (see below).

External oblique

The fibers of the external oblique muscles (*Fig. 8.2*) run at a 45° angle to the midline, extending from the lower eight ribs to the iliac crests (alternating with digitations of the serratus anterior and latissimus dorsi), and lateral edges of the rectus muscles. They cover the anterolateral aspects of the anterior abdominal wall.

Internal oblique

The fibers of the internal oblique muscle (*Fig. 8.3*) lie immediately beneath and at a perpendicular angle to the fibers of the external oblique muscle. They extend from the iliac crest and thoracolumbar fascia (*Figs 8.4, 8.5*) to the lower three ribs and lateral edges of the rectus muscles.

Transverse

The fibers of the transverse abdominal muscles (*Fig. 8.5*) run immediately beneath the internal oblique muscle and extend from the internal aspect of the lower six ribs, cartilage, thoracolumbar fascia (*Fig. 8.4*) and iliac crest to the lateral edge of the rectus muscle in a perpendicular fashion.

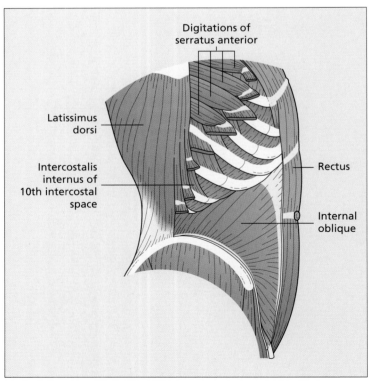

8.3 Internal oblique muscle. The external oblique has been removed to show the internal oblique, but its digitations from the ribs have been preserved. The anterior layer of the rectus fascia has been removed.

Pyramidalis

The pyramidalis muscles are two small muscles extending in a triangular fashion from the symphisis pubis to the lower few centimeters of the linea alba. They are absent in a small percentage of individuals. They are useful to the gynecologic surgeon as an aid in identification of the midline.

Fascia

Each of the four major muscles of the anterior abdominal wall lies within an anterior and a posterior fascial layer (*Fig. 8.6*).

External oblique

Both fascial layers pass anteriorly to the rectus muscle and insert in the linea alba.

Internal oblique

The fascial layers fuse at the medial edge of this muscle. There, it divides and extends anteriorly and posteriorly to the rectus muscle to insert in the linea alba, with the exception of the lower portion of the rectus muscle at which it extends only anteriorly to the muscle. This lower edge of the internal oblique fascia

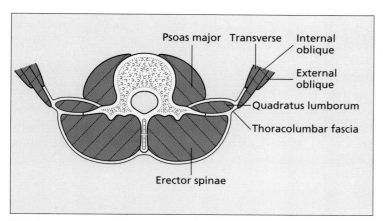

8.4 Transverse section through the posterior abdominal wall, showing disposition of the thoracolumbar fascia. Note that all other connective tissue layers have been omitted.

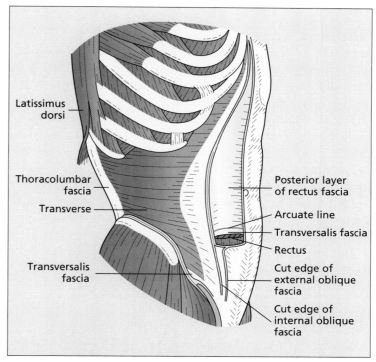

8.5 Transverse muscle. The external and internal oblique muscles have been removed.

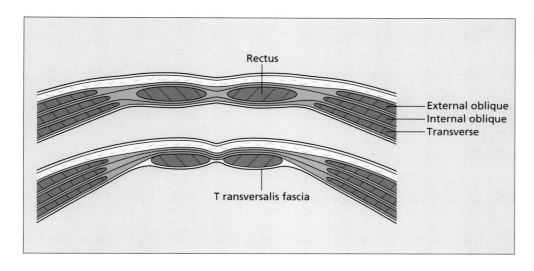

8.6 Fascial layers of anterior abdominal wall muscles. Superior, above arcuate line; inferior, below arcuate line.

constitutes, together with the transverse muscle fascia, the arcuate or semicircularis line (see below) (*Fig. 8.7*).

Rectus

The rectus fascia (*Fig. 8.6*) is different above and below the arcuate line. Above the arcuate line anteriorly, it is constituted by the fascia of the external oblique and the anterior layer of the internal oblique. Posteriorly, it is formed by the posterior fascia of the internal oblique and the transverse fascia. Below the arcuate line anteriorly, it includes the fascia of the external oblique, both layers of the internal oblique, and the transverse fascia. Posteriorly, there is no rectus fascia, constituting the weakest area in the anterior abdominal wall. This accounts for the higher incidence of ventral hernias noted in lower midline as compared with transverse incisions.

Fascial lines

Arcuate or semicircularis line (see *Fig. 8.7*) is formed by the lower edge of the posterior fascial layer of the internal oblique and the transverse fascia. It is usually found midway between the umbilicus and the pubic symphisis.

The linea alba (see *Fig. 8.1*) is located in the midline and is formed by the internal and external oblique and transverse fasciae.

The semilunaris or Spieghel's line (see *Figs 8.1, 8.7*) is a slightly curved line located near the lateral border of each rectus muscle. It is constituted by the fusion of the internal and external oblique fasciae. It represents an area of the anterior abdominal wall at which there is no muscle.

The linea transversae (see *Fig. 8.1*) is composed of three transverse tendinous attachments of each rectus muscle to the anterior rectus fascia.

BLOOD SUPPLY

The blood supply of the anterior abdominal wall (*Figs 8.8, 8.9*) is derived from the circumflex, epigastric, intercostal, subcostal, and superficial external pudendal vessels. The circumflex arteries include the superficial and deep vessels; the epigastrics include the superior, inferior, and superficial arteries. An extensive collateral system provides an excellent blood supply to all the layers of the anterior abdominal wall. The poorest blood supply is found at the linea alba.

Superficial circumflex

The superficial circumflex is derived from the femoral artery at the fossa ovalis in the femoral triangle. It is distributed in the subcutaneous tissue of the lower and lateral anterior abdominal wall, supplying blood to the fascia and skin. It is sectioned during groin node dissections, gridiron incisions, and long transverse incisions.

Deep circumflex

The deep circumflex originates from the external iliac just before the inguinal ligament. It ascends, first, below the transverse muscle and then between the transverse and internal oblique muscles, to which it supplies blood. It may be sectioned during pelvic node dissections and lateral abdominal incisions.

Superior epigastric

The superior epigastric is the terminal branch of the internal thoracic mammary artery (which is a branch of the subclavian artery). It is distributed throughout each of the upper rectus muscles and anastomoses freely with the inferior epigastric. It is divided during fashioning of a rectus muscle flap for vaginal reconstruction.

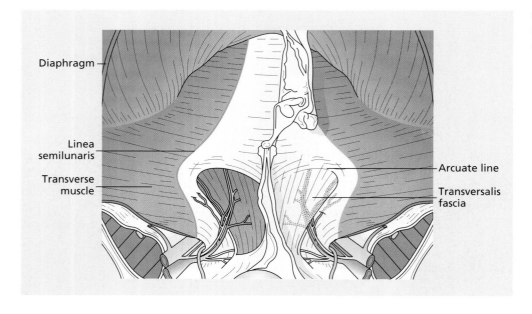

8.7 The arcuate or semicircularis line, as seen in the posterior aspect of the anterior abdominal wall.

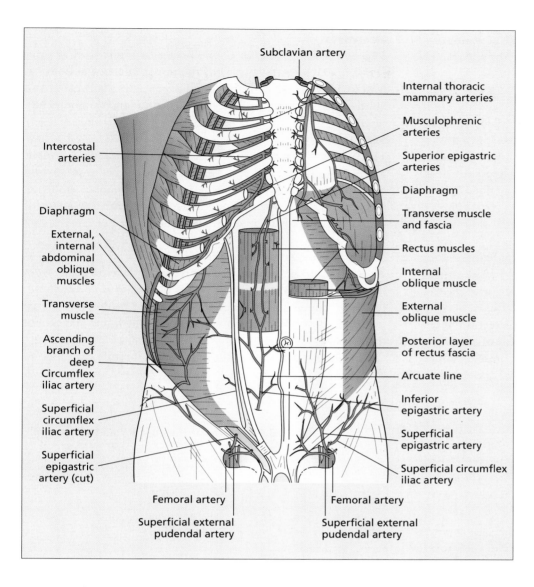

8.8 Arteries of the anterior abdominal wall.

Subclavian artery

Internal thoracic
mammary arteries

Musculophrenic
arteries

Superior epigastric
arteries

Diaphragm

Transverse muscle
and fascia

Rectus muscles

Internal
oblique muscle

External
oblique muscle

Posterior layer
of rectus fascia

Arcuate line

Inferior
epigastric artery

Superficial
epigastric artery

Superficial circumflex
iliac artery

Intercostal
arteries

Diaphragm

External,
internal
abdominal
oblique
muscles

Transverse
muscle

Ascending
branch of
deep
Circumflex
iliac artery

Superficial
circumflex
iliac artery

Superficial
epigastric
artery (cut)

Femoral artery

Superficial external
pudendal artery

Femoral artery

Superficial external
pudendal artery

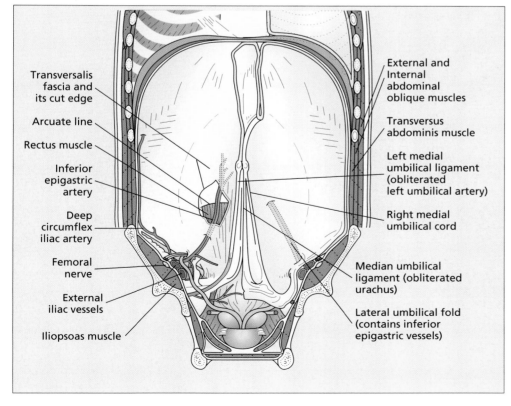

8.9 Arteries of the anterior abdominal wall located on its posterior aspect (internal view).

Transversalis
fascia and
its cut edge

Arcuate line

Rectus muscle

Inferior
epigastric
artery

Deep
circumflex
iliac artery

Femoral
nerve

External
iliac vessels

Iliopsoas muscle

External and
Internal
abdominal
oblique muscles

Transversus
abdominis muscle

Left medial
umbilical ligament
(obliterated
left umbilical artery)

Right medial
umbilical cord

Median umbilical
ligament (obliterated
urachus)

Lateral umbilical fold
(contains inferior
epigastric vessels)

The musculophrenic branch of the internal thoracic mammary artery also supplies blood to the upper portion of the abdominal muscles.

Superficial epigastric

The superficial epigastric originates from the femoral artery, close to the upper border of the fossa ovalis of the groin. It ascends in the subcutaneous tissue of the medial and lower anterior abdominal wall, supplying blood to the fascia and skin. It is sectioned during low transverse incisions and groin node dissections.

Inferior epigastric

The inferior epigastric branches from the external iliac just before the inguinal ligament and ascends towards the posterior aspect of the rectus muscle, anastomosing with the superior epigastric and lower posterior intercostal arteries. These arteries may be injured during the placement of drains through the rectus muscle with an abdominal wall retractor or by placement of accessory laparoscopic trocars. They are divided by rectus muscle-cutting incision (Maylard incision). They may be sectioned during pelvic node dissection.

Intercostal

The two lower branches of the posterior intercostal arteries (T8–L1) extend anteriorly into the upper anterior abdominal wall to anastomose with the superior epigastric, subcostal, and lumbar arteries. They provide muscle, fascia, and skin branches.

Subcostal

The subcostal arteries are in series with the intercostal arteries and below the twelfth rib. They pass through the transverse muscle and run between this and the internal oblique, supplying blood to both of them. They anastomose with the superior epigastric, intercostal, and lumbar arteries.

Superficial external pudendal artery

The superficial external pudendal artery originates medially from the femoral artery at the fossa ovalis of the groin. It distributes in the subcutaneous tissue of the lower and medial abdominal wall and labia majora, supplying blood to the fascia and skin of these areas.

The venous drainage of the anterior abdominal wall follows the pathway of the arteries.

8.10 Nerves of the anterior abdominal wall.

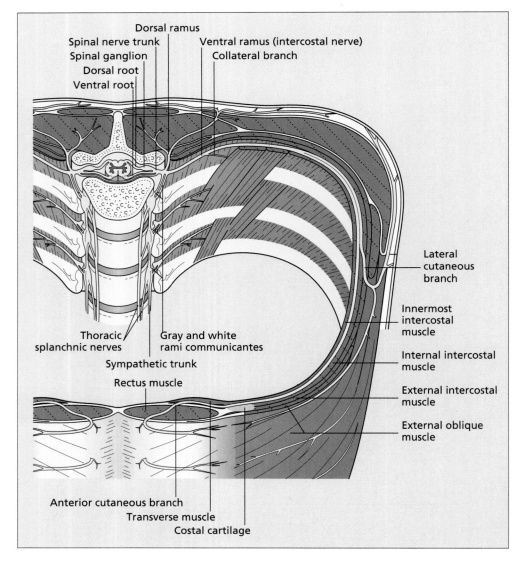

Dorsal ramus
Spinal nerve trunk
Spinal ganglion
Dorsal root
Ventral root
Ventral ramus (intercostal nerve)
Collateral branch

Lateral cutaneous branch
Innermost intercostal muscle
Internal intercostal muscle
External intercostal muscle
External oblique muscle

Thoracic splanchnic nerves
Gray and white rami communicantes
Sympathetic trunk
Rectus muscle
Anterior cutaneous branch
Transverse muscle
Costal cartilage

NERVES

The nerve supply of the anterior abdominal wall is provided by the seventh to twelfth thoracic ventral rami of the spinal nerves and the first lumbar ventral ramus (T7–L1).

There are twelve pairs of thoracic ventral rami of the spinal nerves (T1–T12). They are all intercostal and are known as intercostal nerves (T1–T11), except for the twelfth (T12) which lies subcostally and is known as a subcostal nerve. Each ramus is connected with the adjacent sympathetic ganglion by gray and white rami communicantes.

The lower six rami (T7–T12) extend to the anterior abdominal wall, providing innervation to muscles and skin (*Fig. 8.10*). Each ramus gives off a lateral and an anterior cutaneous branch. These branches pierce the adjacent muscles and provide segmental innervation to the skin of the anterior and posterior abdominal walls (*Fig. 8.11*). Because of the existence of collateral branches, significant overlap occurs between cutaneous adjacent segments.

The external and internal oblique, transverse, and rectus muscles are all innervated by the lower six ventral rami of the spinal nerves. In addition, the internal oblique and transverse muscles also receive innervation from the first lumbar ventral ramus (L1). The pyramidalis is supplied by the ventral rami of the twelfth spinal nerve (subcostal nerve).

The innervation of the muscles of the anterior abdominal wall follows that of the skin, an important consideration in protection of the abdominal viscera. Immediate reflex contraction of the muscles provides protection against a forceful blow.

The lower intercostal nerves are connected with the sympathetic thoracic ganglia by white and grey rami communicantes. The sympathetic ganglia provide the splanchnic nerves, which innervate the abdominal viscera, thus forming a communication between the abdominal viscera and the abdominal wall muscles. For example, in the presence of acute infection of the abdominal viscera, such as peritonitis, a persistent contraction of the muscles of the abdominal wall (guarding) develops. This serves to protect the affected part of the body.

The first lumbar ventral rami (L1) usually receive a branch from the twelfth thoracic (subcostal nerve). It bifurcates into iliohypogastric and ilioinguinal nerves (*Fig. 8.12*), which provide innervation to the skin of the lower abdominal wall (*Fig. 8.13; see also Fig. 8.10*).

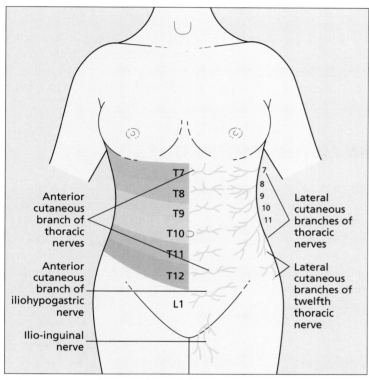

8.11 Cutaneous innervation of the anterior abdominal wall.

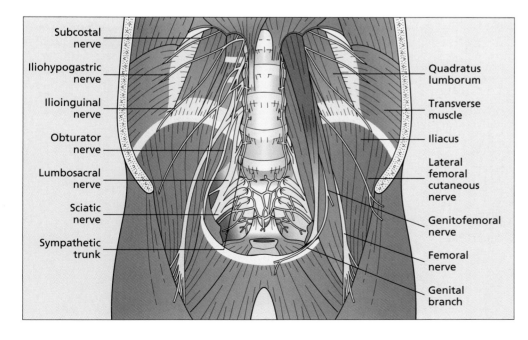

8.12 Origination of iliohypogastric nerve and ilioinguinal nerve (L1).

The iliohypogastric nerve (L1) gives off an anterior cutaneous branch which provides innervation to the skin of the suprapubic area. The lateral cutaneous branch innervates the skin of the posterolateral gluteal area. The ilioinguinal nerve (L1) supplies the skin of the mons pubis and labia majora.

Because of the transverse course of these nerves in the lower part of the abdominal wall, they may be sectioned during low transverse incisions (resulting in sensory deficits of the tributary areas) or they may be incorporated into the sutures during closure of a transverse incision (resulting in the nerve entrapment syndrome; see below).

LYMPHATICS

The lymphatics of the anterior abdominal wall are located above (superficial to) and below (deep to) the deepest fascial layer of the anterior abdominal wall.

The superficial lymphatic channels follow the subcutaneous blood vessels. Those located inferiorly to the umbilicus follow the superficial circumflex iliac and the epigastric vessels (see *Fig. 8.8*) and drain in the superficial inguinal nodes. The lymphatics superior to the umbilicus run in an oblique course to the pectoral and subscapular axillary lymph nodes. A few drain to the parasternal nodes.

The deep lymphatics follow the deep blood vessels. Those inferior to the umbilicus follow the deep circumflex iliac and inferior epigastric vessels (see *Fig. 8.8*) to the external iliac nodes. Those superior to the umbilicus follow the superior epigastric vessels and drain in the parasternal nodes.

TENSION LINES OF THE SKIN

The elastic fibers of the skin provide a state of "elasticity" or constant tension of the skin. They are found in bundles in the dermis and adjacent to the collagen fibers and connective tissue. Their course is perpendicular to the underlying muscles[1]. Because the skin is constantly pulled and stretched by the movement of the underlying muscles and joints, lines of minimal tension develop, such as skin folds and creases. An incision parallel to these lines is subjected to minimal tension during healing and will result in a fine, narrow, slightly visible scar. An incision perpendicular to the lines of minimal tension will be under constant tension and will result in a hypertrophic, noticeable scar.

In the anterior abdominal wall, because of the flexion movement of the abdominal muscles, the lines of minimal tension develop in a transverse fashion. Therefore, transverse incisions are less noticeable and more cosmetic than vertical incisions.

This concept has replaced the original "Langer lines," which have been discovered to have little practical application since they do not take into consideration the effect of dynamic skin tension, due to movement, on a healing wound[1]. If a cosmetic result is desired, incisions should follow the normal creases, folds, and skin flexion lines.

INCISION TECHNIQUES

SKIN

Traction–countertraction is necessary to perform an even, straight (epidermis and dermis) skin incision with a single pass of the scalpel (*Fig. 8.14*). If additional passes are needed, it is important to follow the previous one to avoid jagged edges, which result in inadequate apposition for skin closure (*Fig. 8.15*). When passing the scalpel, the knife should be put down to prevent injury and possible disease transmission. Electrocautery (cut setting, blend 1) can replace the scalpel for performance of the incision from

8.13 Iliohypogastric and ilioinguinal nerves (L1) – superficial innervation of the skin.

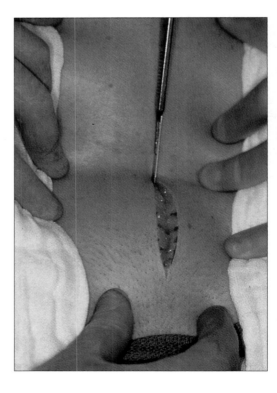

8.14 Vertical lower midline incision. Traction–countertraction are necessary to perform an even straight cut of the skin until the subcutaneous tissue can be seen.

the skin to the peritoneum. This may also be a helpful technique in the patient with AIDS, as it reduces the potential for injury to the surgeon or assistants.

A No. 10 blade is adequate for most gynecological incisions. Mini-incisions, such as for minilaparotomy tubal ligation, are best performed with a No. 15 blade. Puncture incisions, such as for placement of drains or laparoscopy, are best accomplished with a No. 11 blade (*Fig. 8.16*).

SUBCUTANEOUS TISSUE

Traction and countertraction are again necessary. The scalpel used for the skin is used to perform as few passes as possible to divide the subcutaneous tissue. Each pass of the scalpel should follow the same vertical plane to avoid creating jagged edges and devitalized areas of fatty tissue, which may predispose to delayed

healing, seroma formation, and infection (*Fig. 8.17*; see also *Fig. 8.15*).

The skin scalpel may be used for the subcutaneous tissue. Changing scalpels has not been shown to decrease wound infection in prognostic studies[2].

The electrocautery (cut setting, blend 1) is preferred by some surgeons for the subcutaneous tissue to save time and reduce blood loss. However, animal studies have demonstrated delayed healing and decreased tensile strength at 2 to 4 weeks in wounds produced by electrosurgery or laser compared with scalpel wounds[3,4].

It is preferable to delay coagulation of the small bleeding points until the incision has been completed through all layers of the abdominal wall. Most of the bleeders will have stopped by then and only the significant ones will require coagulation.

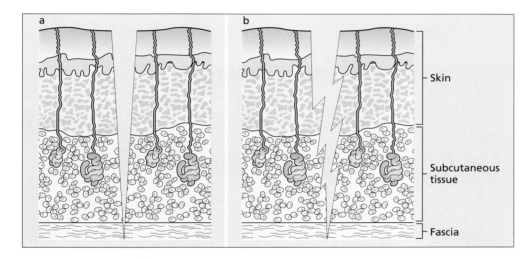

8.15 Technique of incision. A: Desired perpendicular cut allows adequate wound approximation. B: Jagged edges result from repeat passes of the knife blade through different planes.

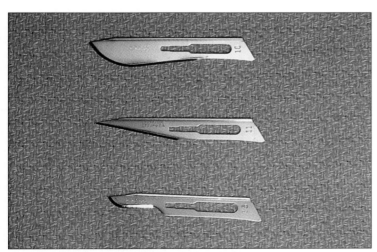

8.16 Types of scalpel blades commonly used for gynecologic operations. Upper, No. 10; middle, No. 11; lower, No. 15.

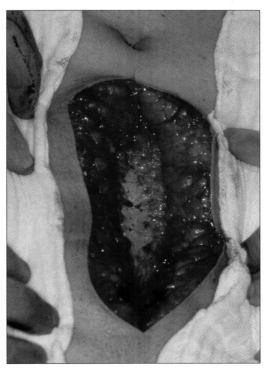

8.17 Vertical lower midline incision. Each pass of the scalpel through the subcutaneous tissue should follow the same vertical plane to avoid creating jagged edges. The superficial external pudendal vessels have been coagulated in the lowermost part of the incision.

FASCIA

The same skin scalpel is ideal to provide a straight, clean-cut fascial incision. Traction–countertraction and simultaneous elevation of the skin and subcutaneous tissue facilitate exposure of the fascia and avoids damage to the underlying tissues (*Fig. 8.18*). Scissors are more likely to cause jagged edges and resultant imperfect approximation of the fascial edges at closure. This may predispose to inadequate healing, with a higher risk of dehiscence. Since the fascial layer is responsible for the tensile strength of the anterior abdominal wall, the adequacy of its closure must be kept in mind when the fascial incision is made. Small bleeding points are coagulated after the entire incision is completed.

MUSCLE

Depending on the location of the incision, the muscles may be separated (midline), split (gridiron, pararectal), or sectioned (Maylard). Separation of the rectus muscles offers no difficulty once the medial edges have been identified, and is best performed digitally (*Fig. 8.19*). In lower vertical midline incisions, the

midline is best found close to the umbilicus or at the level of the pyramidalis muscles.

Splitting the muscles requires attention to the direction of the fibers. With the help of a blunt instrument, such as a Kelly or Peon clamp, the fibers can be separated, preserving their integrity. This is helpful to prevent hematoma formation and muscle trauma, both of which may cause prolonged pain and delayed recovery.

The electrocautery (cut setting, blend 2) is useful for sectioning the rectus muscles (see *Fig. 8.47*). The Poly CS 57 (Autosuture Co.) stapling device may also be used for sectioning the rectus muscles while simultaneously achieving hemostasis (see *Fig. 8.47*).

PERITONEUM

With proper traction–countertraction and simultaneous elevation of the anterior abdominal wall, the peritoneum may be incised with the skin scalpel (*Fig. 8.20*). It is not necessary to "strip off" the preperitoneal fatty tissue. Elevation of the anterior abdominal wall separates the peritoneum from the underlying bowel.

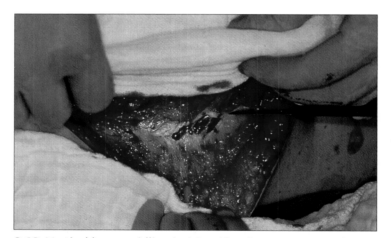

8.18 Vertical lower midline incision. Traction–countertraction and simultaneous elevation of the skin and subcutaneous tissue facilitate the exposure of the fascia.

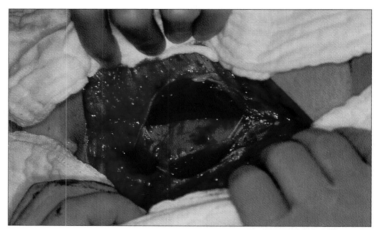

8.19 Vertical lower midline incision. The rectus muscles have been separated digitally at the midline.

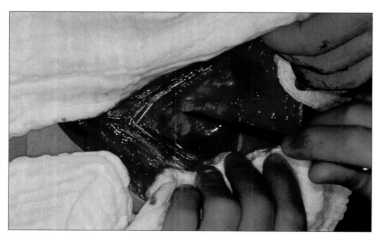

8.20 Vertical lower midline incision. Traction–countertraction and simultaneous elevation of the anterior abdominal wall result in separation of the peritoneum from the underlying bowel. The peritoneum is incised with the scalpel at a point away from the bladder.

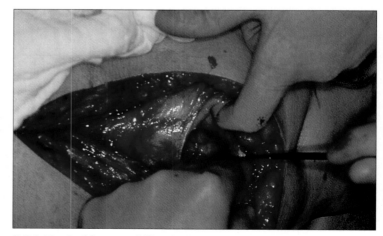

8.21 Vertical lower midline incision. Once peritoneal entry has been made, the fingers are used to check for adhesions.

Adjacent bowel will not be injured if a stroke of the scalpel is used. Tenting of the peritoneum between two clamps achieves the same result, with the exception that if the bowel is included in the clamps it will not then separate from the peritoneum and may be injured. Peritoneal entry is best performed as high as possible in the peritoneum, to prevent bladder injury. Once peritoneal entry has been made, two fingers are introduced to check for adhesions (*Fig. 8.21*). The remainder of the peritoneum is then incised using the scalpel, Metzenbaum scissors, or electrocautery (*Fig. 8.22*). The edges of the bladder can be identified by palpation or, preferably, by bringing a previously inserted Foley bulb upwards against the top of the bladder wall (*Fig. 8.23*).

REPEAT INCISIONS

Repeat or secondary incisions require special considerations. The old skin is preferably removed in a wedge fashion in conjunction with the subjacent scarred fibroadipose tissue (*Fig. 8.24*). The surgeon must be aware that the bowel may be attached immediately adjacent to the fascia and can be injured during the fascial incision. Elevation of the anterior abdominal wall and traction–countertraction are not helpful if the bowel is adhering to the anterior abdominal wall. Careful, light strokes of the scalpel can help to determine if the bowel is adhered, since the serosal layer of the bowel wall will become noticeable. Tenting the peritoneum carries the risk of incorporating the bowel; palpation may not be helpful owing to the presence of thickened, scarred peritoneum. Whenever possible it is preferable to enter the peritoneum in a fresh area away from the previous incision area. In repeat midline incisions with thick scar tissue or previous irradiation, it may be helpful to extend the incision superiorly to enter the peritoneal cavity through a fresh, previously nonoperated or irradiated area. In repeat paramedian incisions, dissection of the rectus muscle is usually not possible because of scarring[5]. A similar situation occurs with pararectal incisions. Repeat midline, Pfannenstiel, Maylard, or Cherney incisions are usually not a problem. In repeat Maylard incisions, the site of the previous muscle incision has been shown to have adequate healing[6].

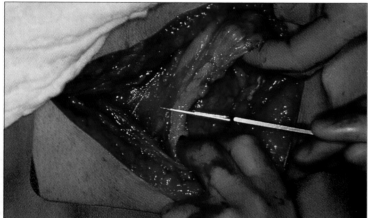

8.22 Vertical lower midline incision. The remaining peritoneum is incised with the scalpel.

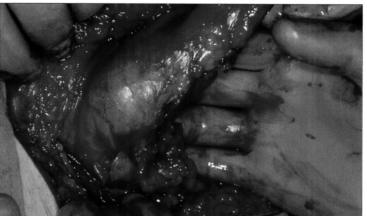

8.23 Vertical lower midline incision. The edge of the bladder can be easily identified by bringing the Foley bulb upwards against the top of the bladder wall.

8.24 Repeat incisions. Excision of old scar with subjacent scarred subcutaneous tissue.

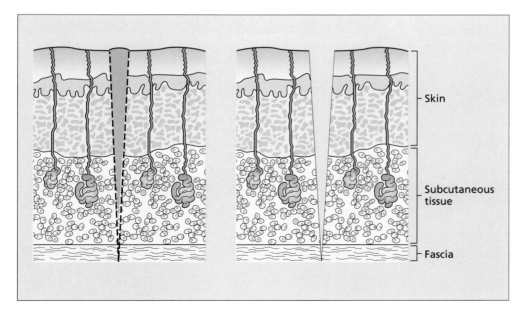

Skin

Subcutaneous tissue

Fascia

TYPE OF INCISION

The location and size of the incision must be such that they provide the necessary exposure to perform all aspects of the planned operation in an uncompromised fashion (*Fig. 8.25*). Unreasonable patient requests for a less-than-desirable type or size of incision for cosmetic purposes, can be dealt with by designing an alternative, acceptable, adequate incision or by offering cosmetic correction at a future date, but not by compromising the requisite exposure[7].

VERTICAL INCISIONS

Lower middle vertical

The lower midline incision is usually the reference for other types of incisions (see *Fig. 8.25*). It is quick, easy, relatively bloodless, and can be extended around the umbilicus for exposure to the upper abdomen. It is preferable to extend to the left of the umbilicus, since it is not then necessary to cut the falciform ligament, which is located to the right of the umbilicus (*Fig. 8.26*). Unfortunately, the lower midline incision is the weakest of all incisions, since it is performed through the weakest area in the anterior abdominal wall (where there is no posterior rectus fascia), through the relatively avascular linea alba (with decreased blood supply for healing), and is perpendicular to the lines of minimal tension of the skin (resulting in a wider scar than from incisions that follow these tension lines).

Under adequate traction–countertraction, the scalpel incises the skin and subcutaneous tissue with as few passes as possible (see *Fig. 8.14*). The superficial external pudendal vessels are sectioned in the lowermost part of the incision in the subcutaneous tissue (see *Figs 8.8, 8.17*). With elevation of the anterior abdominal wall, the fascial incision is facilitated (see *Fig. 8.18*). The midline is best found at the umbilicus, where the rectus muscles are slightly separated, or at the level of the pyramidalis muscles. The rectus muscles are digitally separated at the midline (see *Fig. 8.19*). With continued elevation of the edges of the incision, the peritoneum is incised with the scalpel at a point away from the bladder (see *Fig. 8.20*). Once peritoneal entry is made, two fingers are introduced to check for adhesions (see *Fig. 8.21*). The peritoneal incision is then extended (see *Fig. 8.22*). The upper limits of the bladder can be outlined by pulling upwards on the Foley bulb (see *Fig. 8.23*).

Paramedian

The skin incision is about 2 cm lateral to the midline incision (see *Fig. 8.25*). The fascia is incised over the lateral half of the rectus muscle and the muscle is retracted laterally (*Figs 8.27, 8.28*). The peritoneum is then entered.

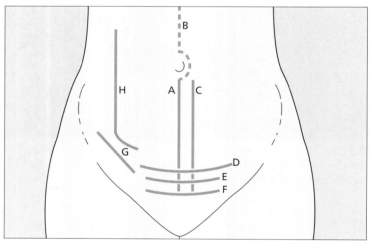

8.25 Gynecologic incisions. A: lower midline; B: extended lower midline; C: paramedian or pararectal; D: Maylard; E: Pfannenstiel; F: Cherney; G: gridiron; H: lateral vertical.

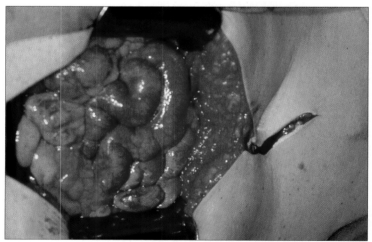

8.26 Vertical lower midline incision extended to the left and above the umbilicus to gain exposure to the upper abdomen.

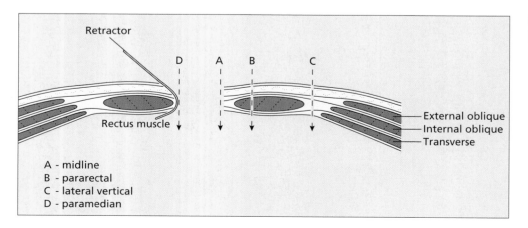

8.27 Gynecologic incisions. A: midline; B: pararectal; C: lateral vertical; D: paramedian.

The paramedian incision is not recommended in the presence of a midline incision whenever possible, because of the slight risk of necrosis of the tissues between close, parallel vertical incisions. It offers no significant advantages over the midline incision other than protecting the fascial incision with the belly of the muscle and thereby decreasing the risk of dehiscense or hernia. Repeat paramedial incisions are usually not possible because of the fixation of the rectus muscle[5]. In addition, they are associated with a high incidence of dehiscence[8].

The paramedian incision offers no significant advantages over the midline and is therefore not recommended. It is included for the sake of completeness.

Pararectal

The skin and subcutaneous tissue incision are about 2 cm lateral to the midline incision (see *Fig. 8.25*). The fascial incision is directly over the rectus muscle. The fibers of the rectus muscle are split vertically rather than retracted laterally as in a paramedian incision (*Fig. 8.29*; see also *Fig. 8.27*). It may be necessary to ligate the inferior epigastric vessels. The peritoneum is then incised vertically.

Because of the transverse orientation of the nerves of the anterior abdominal wall, splitting the rectus muscles results in some denervation of the medial half of the muscle, the collateral branches of the nerves of the anterior abdominal wall preventing total denervation. However, in long pararectal incisions, complete denervation of the medial half, and subsequent atrophy, may occur because of the limited reach of the collateral branches.

The pararectal incision is more time consuming and is associated with increased blood loss compared with a midline incision. It offers no significant advantages over a midline incision other than perhaps a decreased risk of dehiscence because of the shutter mechanism of the belly muscle under the fascial incision. The pararectal incision is not recommended for gynecologic operations. It is included for the sake of completeness.

Lateral vertical

The skin and subcutaneous tissue incisions are located following the linea semilunaris (see *Fig. 8.1*). A vertical fascial incision (see *Fig. 8.25*) is carried out immediately lateral to the rectus muscle and following the semilunaris line, in an area where no muscle tissue is found (*Fig. 8.30*; see also *Fig. 8.27*). The peritoneum, with the intraperitoneal contents, is reflected medially, allowing easy access to the aortic and common iliac nodal area (*Figs 8.31, 8.32*).

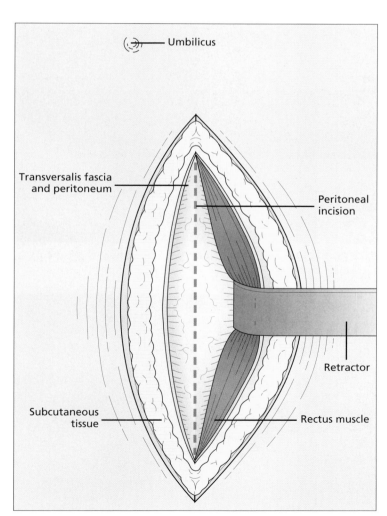

8.28 Left paramedian incision. The rectus fascia has been incised over the rectus muscle, which has been retracted laterally. The site of the peritoneal incision is shown.

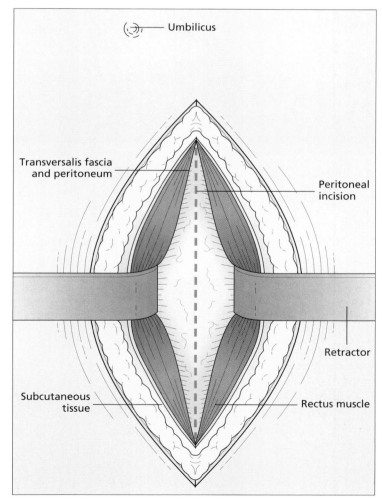

8.29 Left pararectal incision. The rectus muscle has been split and retracted medially and laterally. The site of the peritoneal incision is shown.

The incision can be extended downward and medially (J-shaped) as a gridiron incision to provide access to the pelvic nodes. Forward mobilization of the sigmoid mesentery from the presacral curvature allows access to the contralateral pelvic nodes.

Extraperitoneal aortic node dissection followed by external aortic irradiation is associated with a lower complication and mortality rate than with transperitoneal aortic lymphadenectomy[9]. The incision is outside of the lateral margins of the aortic irradiation field, allowing early initiation of the planned irradiation. Because of its location outside of the irradiation field and the presence of a continuous fascial layer in the incision, it appears more favorable than a midline incision for aortic node exploration.

TRANSVERSE INCISIONS
Pfannenstiel

This is the most common of all the low transverse incisions (see *Fig. 8.25*)[10]. It is cosmetic (the incision follows the direction of the lines of minimal tension of the skin) and is associated with a lower incidence of dehiscence than midline incisions. It is more time consuming, is associated with increased blood loss, offers limited exposure to the lateral pelvis, and provides no access to the mid- or upper abdomen.

Under adequate traction–countertraction, the skin and subcutaneous tissue are divided with the scalpel. The level of the incision is about two finger breadths above the pubis. The superficial epigastric vessels are encountered laterally and are coagulated or divided (*Fig. 8.33*). The fascial incision is made in a transverse fashion with the scalpel (*Fig. 8.34*). The lateral extensions of the fascial incision can be made digitally, thus protecting the external oblique muscle (*Fig. 8.35*). The upper edge of the rectus fascia is grasped with two straight Kocher clamps. With traction–countertraction, the rectus muscle is freed from the

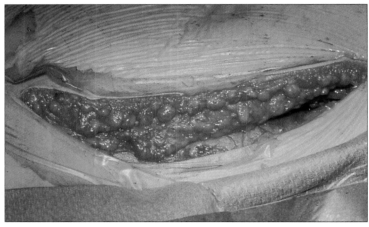

8.30 Left lateral vertical incision, performed following the linea semilunaris.

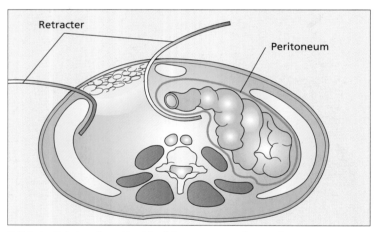

8.31 Left lateral vertical incision, retroperitoneal exposure.

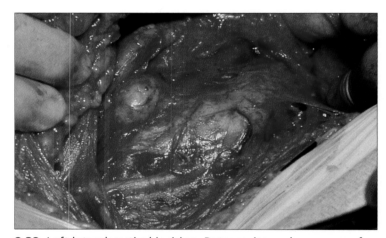

8.32 Left lateral vertical incision. Retroperitoneal exposure of the aortic nodal area.

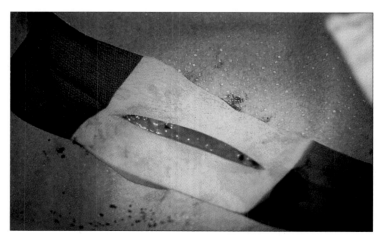

8.33 Low transverse incision. The superficial epigastric vessels have been coagulated at both ends of the incision.

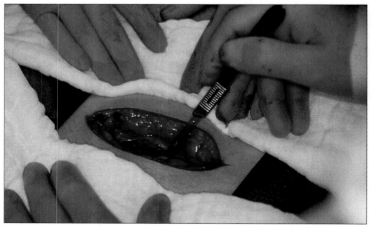

8.34 Low transverse incision. The fascial incision is made in a transverse fashion with the scalpel.

rectus fascia. The perforating branches of the inferior epigastric are coagulated or ligated as they are encountered (*Fig. 8.36*). The dissection is carried up to the level of the umbilicus, where the midline can usually be identified (*Fig. 8.37*). A similar dissection is performed in the lower portion of the fascial incision down to the pubic bone (*Fig. 8.38*). The rectus muscles are separated in the midline. The peritoneal incision is performed in a vertical fashion making the peritoneal entry in the upper portion of the peritoneum, away from the bladder (*Figs 8.39, 8.40*). On occasion, an additional transverse peritoneal incision is necessary to

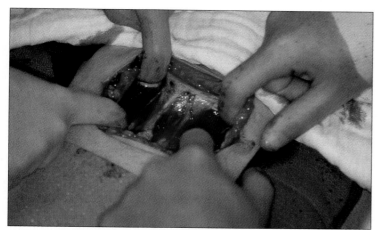

8.35 Low transverse incision. The lateral extensions of the fascial incision are made digitally to protect the external oblique muscle.

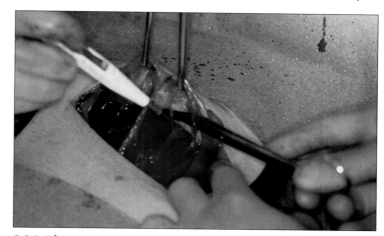

8.36 Pfannenstiel incision. Two Kocher clamps are holding the upper edge of the rectus fascia, which is freed from the rectus muscles. The perforating branches of the inferior epigastric have been isolated and are coagulated.

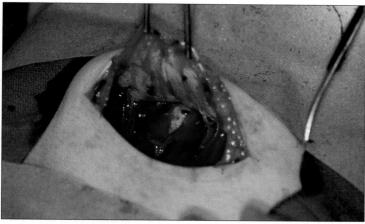

8.37 Pfannenstiel incision. The rectus fascia has been dissected from the rectus muscle to the level of the umbilicus. Some of the perforating branches of the inferior epigastric have been preserved.

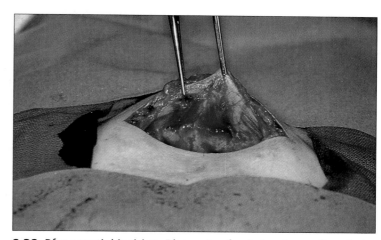

8.38 Pfannenstiel incision. The rectus fascia has been dissected from the rectus muscle to the pubic bone in the lower portion of the incision.

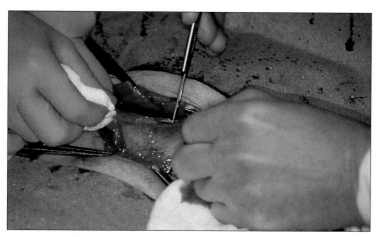

8.39 Pfannenstiel incision. With digital elevation of the peritoneum, the scalpel is used for peritoneal entry at a point away from the bladder.

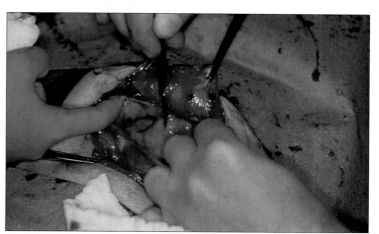

8.40 Pfannenstiel incision. The peritoneal incision is being extended vertically with the scalpel.

improve the exposure. With traction on the Foley bulb the limits of the bladder are easily identified (*Figs 8.41, 8.42*).

Modified Pfannenstiel

The skin and subcutaneous incisions are identical to a Pfannenstiel incision. The subcutaneous tissue is dissected from the rectus fascia at the umbilicus. Vertical fascial and peritoneal incisions are then performed (*Fig. 8.43*). These provide pelvic exposure similar to that with a midline incision but with improved cosmetic result. This procedure is time consuming, carries the risk of subcutaneous hematoma (unless meticulous hemostasis is obtained), and is weak (as with a midline incision). A combination of a modified Pfannenstiel with a transverse fascial and rectus muscle-cutting incision has been described as providing

adequate mid-abdomen exposure for staging purposes in thin patients who are opposed to a midline incision and who do not require an extensive operation.

Rectus muscle-cutting (Maylard)

The level of this skin incision is superior to a Pfannenstiel incision (see *Fig. 8.25*)[11]. The rectus fascia is not dissected off the rectus muscles (*Fig. 8.44*). After division of the rectus fascia transversely, the rectus muscles are digitally separated from their fascial sheath (*Fig. 8.45*). The muscle fibers are divided with the electrocautery (cut setting, blend 2) (*Fig. 8.46*). The inferior epigastric vessels are isolated and ligated when encountered, if necessary. An alternative to the electrocautery is to apply the Poly CS 57 stapling device (Autosuture Co.) to each belly of the rectus muscles

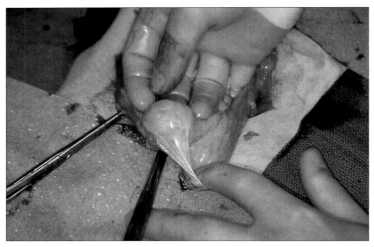

8.41 Pfannenstiel incision. The limits of the bladder are shown by upward traction of the Foley bulb intraperitoneally.

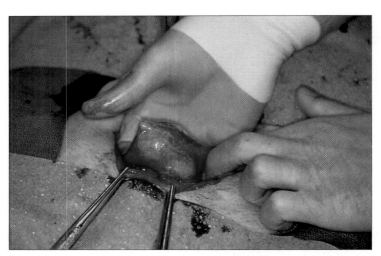

8.42 Pfannenstiel incision. The limits of the bladder are shown by upward traction of the Foley bulb retroperitoneally.

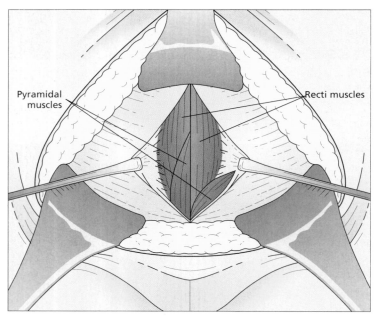

8.43 Skin and subcutaneous tissue. The subcutaneous tissue has been dissected from the rectal fascia, and vertical fascial and peritoneal incisions are then made.

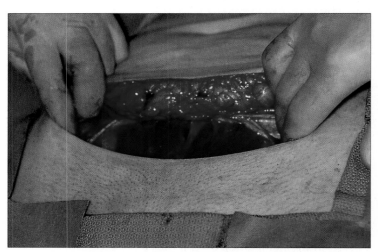

8.44 Maylard incision. The rectus fascia is incised transversely and is not dissected off the rectus muscles as in a Pfannenstiel.

(*Fig. 8.47*). The muscles are then cut between the two rows of absorbable staples (*Fig. 8.48*). The staples may fall off from the muscle edges by the end of the operation, but by then they have already provided their function of hemostasis. The peritoneum is incised transversely with the scalpel.

If additional lateral pelvic or mid-abdomen exposure is needed after a Pfannenstiel incision, division of the rectus muscles is helpful to solve the problem. Unilateral or bilateral division, including the entire or only the medial portion of the belly of the rectus muscle, can be performed, depending on the side and the degree of the requisite exposure.

At the time of closure, sutures are placed incorporating and approximating the rectus fascia and the divided rectus muscles.

Some authors prefer not to include the rectus muscle fibers in the fascial closure. The gap between the muscle ends will heal as a new linea transversa, resulting from fibroblastic proliferation between the muscle end and the rectus fascia. Subfascial drainage is used in instances where hemostasis is not adequate to prevent hematoma formation. A complication rate of 4–7% has been reported[12–14].

The Maylard incision is contraindicated in patients with impaired circulation of the lower extremities and reverse flow of the inferior epigastric vessels[15]. Ligation of the latter vessels may result in leg ischemia, caused by the interruption of the blood supply from the inferior epigastric vessels to the lower extremities in the presence of reverse flow.

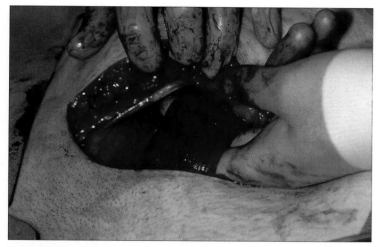

8.45 Maylard incision. The rectus muscles are isolated digitally, preserving the inferior epigastric vessels when possible. Note preservation of right inferior epigastric vessels.

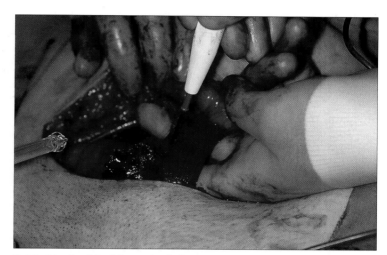

8.46 Maylard incision. The left rectus muscle is being divided with the electrocautery (cut setting, blend 2).

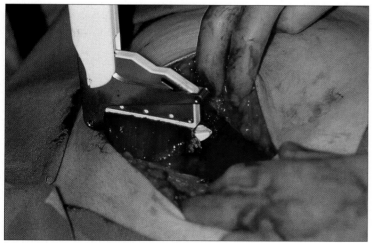

8.47 Maylard incision. The Poly CS 57 has been applied to the right rectus muscle after its isolation. The right inferior epigastric vessels have been preserved.

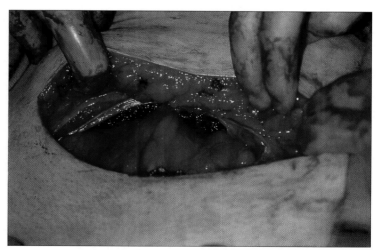

8.48 Maylard incision. The rectus muscles have been divided.

Rectus tendon-cutting (Cherney)

The skin incision is made inferior to a Pfannenstiel incision (see *Fig. 8.25*). The rectus fascia is not dissected off the rectus muscles[16]. After division of the rectus fascia, the tendinous insertion of the rectus and rectus pyramidalis muscles is sectioned instead of the muscle fibers (*Fig. 8.49*). The inferior epigastric vessels are preserved in most instances.

A poorly developed tendinous insertion is a contraindication for this incision, since a strong tendon approximation will not be possible at closure (*Fig. 8.50*). Postoperative tendon rupture occurs in 1–2% of patients if not repaired properly or if excessive tension exists[17].

Because the Cherney incision is a very low transverse incision, it provides excellent exposure of the retropubic and paravesical space, allowing the removal of high paravaginal masses extraperitoneally[18].

Gridiron

The skin and subcutaneous incisions are parallel and superior to the inguinal ligament, and lateral to the rectus muscles (see *Fig. 8.25*). The fascia encountered at that level is that of the external oblique muscle, since the rectus fascia ends at the lateral border of the rectus muscle. The external oblique fascia is split. The muscle fibers encountered are those of the internal oblique muscle. The fibers of the internal oblique and transverse muscles are split in the same direction, since their fibers are similarly orientated at this level (*Fig. 8.51*). The peritoneum is retracted or incised, depending on the operation planned.

This incision is most adequate for extraperitoneal pelvic procedures, e.g., lymph node biopsies or lymphadenectomy, hypogastric or uterine artery ligation, control of pelvic wall bleeding, drainage of lymphocysts, or transperitoneal pelvic operations (e.g., appendectomy, drainage of tubo-ovarian abscess). The incision can be extended upwards, i.e., vertically, allowing an extraperitoneal aortic node dissection (see *Figs 8.30, 8.32*) or transversally, in the case that additional pelvic pathology is found and added pelvic exposure becomes necessary.

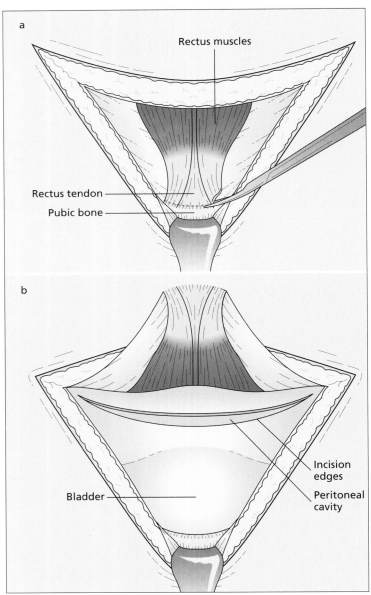

8.49 Cherney incision. **a**: The tendon of the rectus and pyramidalis muscles is cut at midlevel. **b**: The rectus muscles have been elevated; the peritoneal incision is performed transversely.

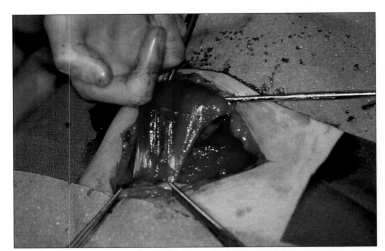

8.50 Cherney incision. Adequate length of the rectus tendon for Cherney incision to allow strong approximation. A short, poorly developed tendon is a contraindication for a Cherney incision since it will not allow a strong approximation and may result in postoperative tendon rupture.

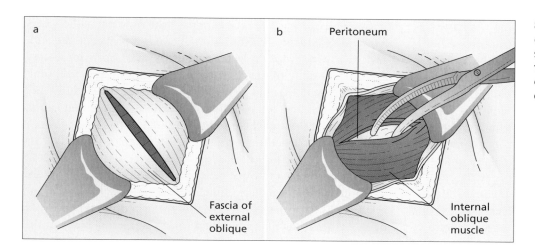

8.51 Gridiron incision. **a**: The fascia of the external oblique muscle is divided in the same direction as the skin and subcutaneous tissue incision. **b**: The fibers of the internal oblique muscle are separated in the direction of the orientation of its fibers.

EXPOSURE

The abdominal incision provides access to the desired anatomic area. Retraction of the intervening tissues provides exposure. This is usually achieved by the use of retracting blades and packing. Not uncommonly, these aspects of the operation are overlooked.

INCISION

Despite the generally held belief, it is not necessarily true that the smaller the incision, the better the surgeon. Surgical competency is based not only on the surgical act (including the incision) but on the application of proper indications, as well as excellence in postoperative management. The size of the incision bears no reflection of the adequacy of the internal operation. The incision must be of sufficient length to allow direct vision and manipulation of the tissues to be handled. Retraction will make this possible.

RETRACTION

Self-retaining retractors, such as the Balfour and O'Connor-Sullen, offer many advantages over hand-held retraction. The former is generally used for vertical incisions and the latter for low transverse incisions. Unfortunately, both of them carry the risk of femoral nerve injury[19,20] and have a fixed design and number of blades, thus preventing 'tailoring' of the retraction for each patient.

The Bookwalter retractor (Codman & Shurtleff Inc., Randolph, MA) allows tissue retraction with blades of different depth, size, and design to best fit the patient. By using shallow blades on thin patients or by placing the ring at different heights from the skin, femoral nerve injury can be prevented by retraction exclusively of the abdominal wall (and not of the psoas muscle) at both lateral aspects of the incision (*Fig. 8.52*).

The use of a fourth retracting blade increases exposure by keeping the bowel packed in the mid-abdomen (*Figs 8.53, 8.54*).

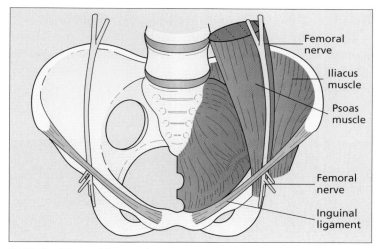

8.52 Position of femoral nerve.

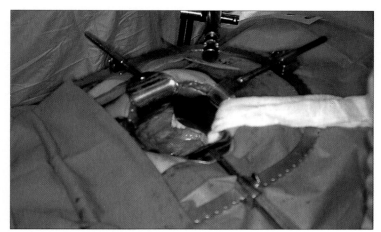

8.53 Fourth retracting blade used to increase exposure.

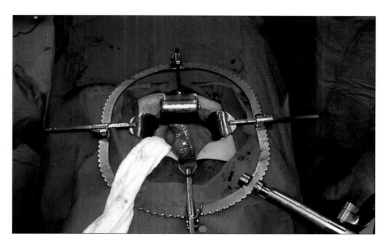

8.54 Bowel packing.

PACKING

For pelvic exposure, it is necessary to place the small bowel in the upper abdomen. This is usually accomplished by patient positioning, packing of the bowel, and retraction of the packed bowel.

Positioning the patient in the Trendelenburg position (20°) utilizes gravity to mobilize the stomach, omentum, and proximal small bowel to the uppermost portion of the abdominal cavity. The cecum, distal small bowel, and sigmoid are kept in the mid-abdomen by means of a gauze pack. To be effective, the pack must be properly placed. Use of a single, long and narrow (100 × 7.5") double layer gauze pack (Lintex Co, Minneapolis, MN) may be more efficient and safer than using multiple smaller gauze packs.

One end of the gauze is used to pack the right paracolic space, retracting the cecum. The distal small bowel is packed in the mid-abdomen with gauze by beginning at the root of its mesentery and piling it up until the inferior surface of the anterior abdominal wall is reached. The gauze is used to pack the sigmoid and its mesentery in the left paracolic area with the remaining gauze, if any, brought out of the incision (*Figs 8.55–8.57*).

The small bowel has a tendency to drop in the pelvis by escaping underneath the gauze pack. A properly placed pack at the root of the small bowel mesentery (against the pelvic brim) will prevent this from happening. In thin patients, packing alone is sufficient to keep the small bowel in the abdominal cavity. In other patients, the placement of a fourth retracting blade at the upper side of the incision will prevent this (see *Figs 8.53, 8.54*).

WOUND HEALING

The healing of a wound is an orderly process designed to provide function to the iatrogenically disrupted tissues. In the abdominal wall that function is regained, but only at about 50–70% of the original tissue strength[21].

The phases of wound healing can be arbitrarily divided into the inflammatory, fibroblastic, and maturation phases.

The inflammatory phase (days 1–4) consists of the normal inflammation of tissues in response to an injury. There is no wound strength other than that provided by the sutures.

The fibroblastic (repair) phase (days 5–20) consists of fibroblast proliferation and collagen synthesis. Collagen is responsible for wound strength and an increase of the wound strength is consequently noted during this phase. However, most of the wound strength still remains in the sutures.

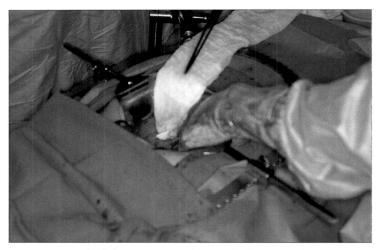

8.55 One end of the gauze used to pack the paracolic space.

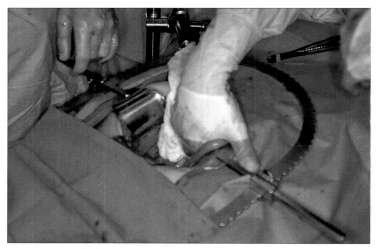

8.56 Packing of opposite paracolic gutter.

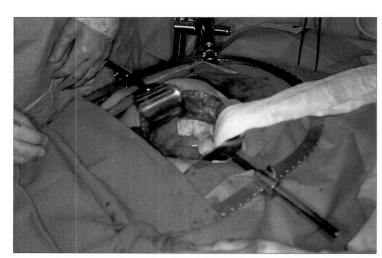

8.57 Packing of sigmoid colon and mesentery.

The maturation phase is characterized by organization and remodeling of the collagen until polymerized covalently bound collagen is formed. It can last from months to years. A continued increase of wound strength is noted during this phase. Collagen is extremely strong. To break a collagen fiber 1 mm in diameter a weight of 10–40 kg is required[22]. However, the process of collagen organization is delicate and can easily be disrupted by relatively mild nonphysiologic conditions[22], resulting in a weak wound with potential for incisional hernia. Minor changes, such as variations in pH and temperature, can affect collagen strength. These changes are difficult to appreciate clinically but may explain the subsequent development of an incisional hernia in a properly closed wound.

Wound contraction accompanies the last two phases of wound healing and begins about 5 days after wound closure. It is characterized by movement of the wound edges towards the center of the incision as a result of the contractile activity of the proliferating myofibroblasts.

WOUND STRENGTH

FASCIA
The postoperative fascial breaking strength as a percentage of normal is depicted in *Fig. 8.58*. At the time of hospital discharge (< 7 days), the fascial strength is about 5%. At 3 weeks (at the end of the collagen synthesis phase) it is about 25%. At 6–8 weeks it has increased to about 40%[23,24]. The final wound strength is about 50–70% of the original non-wounded fascial strength[21,23].

SKIN
The curve of the skin strength recovery follows a similar line to that of the fascia (see *Fig. 8.58*). At the time of hospital discharge (< 7 days) about 5% of the original skin strength is present[21]. This has implications for the skin closure technique.

SUTURES

The most important features in selecting a suture for abdominal fascial closure are its tensile strength and the type of material. The tensile strength of the suture needs to be great enough to hold the tissue for which it is being used and to remain at the same level until the tissues have regained their maximal strength. The suture material should be minimally reactive in order not to disrupt the synthesis and maturation of collagen.

Among the commonly available sutures, nylon (polyamide), Prolene (polyolefins), PDS (polydioxonone), and Maxon (polyglycolic acid copolymer) provide excellent tensile strength and have minimal reactivity. The tensile strength of these sutures is about half that of steel and they remain in the wound until the fascia has regained most or all of its tensile strength[25].

The tensile strength of Prolene remains almost unchanged at the end of one year. That of nylon decreases to just over 80% by the end of eight weeks, remaining at about that level during the remainder of the first year (*Fig. 8.59*).

Delayed absorbable sutures (PDS and Maxon) are reabsorbed by hydrolysis and have the advantage over permanent sutures that no foreign material remains in the wound. PDS maintains about 60% of its original strength at the end of 4 weeks; at 10 weeks this is decreased to 10%. Maxon maintains about 40% of its tensile strength at 6 weeks (see *Fig. 8.59*).

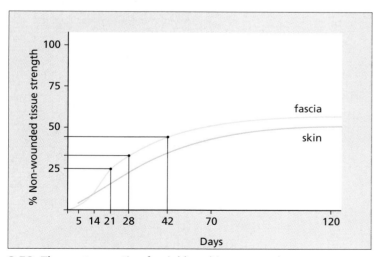

8.58 The postoperative fascial breaking strength.

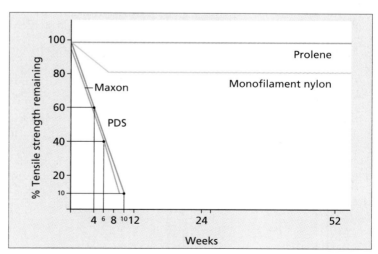

8.59 Comparative tensile strengths of commonly available suture materials.

#0 or #1 sutures sizes are preferred, not because of their increased tensile strength but because of their decreased tendency to cut through tissue compared with smaller-sized sutures. The tendency of a suture to cut through tissue, i.e., the pressure per unit area, is inversely proportional to the diameter of the suture material[26].

Prolene-closed wounds have been shown to have lower infection rates compared with multifilament nylon-closed wounds. Wounds closed with polyglycolic acid had the lowest infection rate (18%), a factor attributed to the bacteriostatic properties of this material's breakdown products. This could be an advantage for delayed absorbable polyglycolic acid sutures.

Nylon, Prolene, PDS, and Maxon sutures seem to perform in a similar fashion, and their selection appears to be based more on personal experience than on clinically significant advantages.

Early absorbable sutures, such as polyglycolic acid materials, provide a tensile strength of about 10% at 3 weeks, inadequate for fascial closure.

KNOTS

The tensile strength of a suture is as great as the efficiency of the knot with which it is tied. Slippage of knots has been found to be a cause of wound dehiscence[27,28], a preventable complication.

There is a direct relationship between the number of throws and knot stability[27,29]. For polyglycolic acid, a single throw provides a 5% knot efficiency, a square knot 58%, three throws 85%, and a square knot and three throws 100%[27].

For PDS, four throws provide maximal tensile strength[29]. Maxon requires six throws to achieve knot stability. Monofilament nylon and Prolene require four throws to achieve almost 100% knot efficiency.

As a rule of thumb, a surgeon's knot followed by five throws provides optimal knot efficiency for monofilament permanent or delayed absorbable sutures used for abdominal incision closure.

The results of seven series of gynecologic patients with mass closure and permanent or delayed absorbable sutures are shown in *Fig. 8.60*. The type of suture has not been shown to significantly influence outcome.

Outcome of Mass Closure Technique									
Author (ref.)	**No.**	**Incision[a]**	**Closure**	**Suture type**	**Size**	**Dehiscence**	**% Hernia**	**Infection**	**Sinus tract formation**
Wallace (32)	747	V	I	Nylon Prolene	0,1	0	N/A	14	N/A
Shepherd (33)	200	V,T	C	Surgilene	2	0	5	8.5	0.5
Gallup (34)	210	V	C	Surgilene	2	0	0.4	2.8	1
Gallup (35)	285	V	C	Maxon	1	0.3	0.3	2.4	N/A
Orr (25)	201	V,T	I	Maxon	1	0	2.4	1.6	N/A
	201	V,T	C	Maxon	1	0	3.9	4.1	N/A
Montz (36)	293	V,T	CSJ	Maxon	0	0	0	8[b]	N/A
Sorosky (37)	119	V,T	C	PDS	1	0	1.6	9.2	N/A
TOTAL	2,256					0.04	1.7[c]	6.3	

[a] V, vertical; T, transverse; I, interrupted Smead–Jones; C, continuous mass closure; CSJ, continuous Smead–Jones.

[b] Infection, seroma, cellulitis and/or breakdown.

[c] Based on 1,509 patients and 6 weeks – 24 months follow-up.

8.60 Outcome of mass closure technique in gynecological patients.

WOUND CLOSURE

Adequate closure of an abdominal incision consists of the approximation of the fascia and skin.

FASCIA

Experimental studies with vertical incisions have demonstrated that the security of wound closure doubles when the incisions are repaired with mass closure, taking fascial bites 1.5–2 cm away from the midline[29]. A bite taken more than 1 cm from the cut edge is twice as secure as a bite 0.5 cm from the cut edge[30]. The principle behind mass closure is that large bites avoid the problem of suture cutting through tissue, the most common cause of fascial dehiscence[30,31] The tendency to cut through a tissue is inversely proportional to the size of the tissue bite[26].

Mass closure has been shown to be associated with a decreased incidence of wound dehiscence compared with layer closure. The incidence of wound dehiscence among 2,256 gynecologic patients compiled from the literature from 1980 to 1991, with the use of mass closure and permanent or delayed absorbable sutures, was 1 in 2,500 patients (0.04%) (*Fig. 8.61*). The incidence of wound dehiscence was ten times higher, or 1 in 250 (0.4%, among 17,022 gynecologic patients from the literature (1954–1977) with layer closure and early absorbable sutures in the vast majority (*Fig. 8.62*).

The principle behind mass closure consists of incorporation of about 3–4 cm of fascia and muscle (1.5–2 cm from each side of the wound) in interrupted or continuous sutures placed 1.5–2 cm apart. The peritoneum is not necessarily included in the closure. The tissues are approximated in a loose fashion. Several techniques, offering similar results, are available:[32–37]

- **Smead–Jones** (far-far-near-near): With interrupted sutures (*Fig. 8.63*), the first bite is placed 2 cm away from the fascial edge through fascia and muscle. It is passed contralaterally to engage muscle and fascia and exits 2 cm away from the fascial edge. It then incorporates the ipsilateral fascial edge and finally the contralateral fascial edge.
- **Modified Smead–Jones** (far-near-near-far): With interrupted sutures (*Fig. 8.64*), the first bite is taken 2 cm away from the fascial edge through fascia and muscle. Next, the contralateral and ipsilateral fascial edges, respectively, are

Incidence of Wound Dehiscence		
Author (Ref.)	**No.**	**% Wound Dehiscence**
Wallace (32)	747	0
Shepherd (33)	200	0
Gallup (34)	210	0
Gallup (35)	285	0.3
Orr (25)	402	0
Montz (36)	293	0
Sorosky (37)	119	0
TOTAL	2,256	0.04

8.61 Incidence of wound dehiscence: patients in this series had mass closure, interrupted or continuous, and permanent or delayed-absorbable suture.

Incidence of Wound Dehiscence		
Author (Ref.)	**No.**	**% Wound Dehiscence**
Tweedie (38)	5,166	0.7
Hull (39)	1,810	0.2
Pratt (40)	2,500	0.3
Helmkamp (41)	7,546	0.6
TOTAL	17,022	0.4

8.62 Incidence of wound dehiscence: patients in this series had layer closure with catgut, wire, or silk sutures.

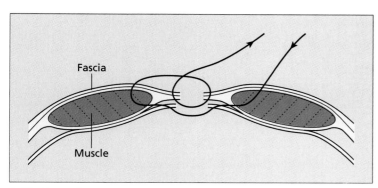

8.63 Smead–Jones suture.

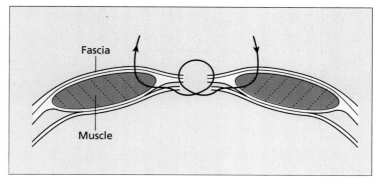

8.64 Modified Smead–Jones suture.

engaged. The suture is then passed contralaterally to engage muscle and fascia and exits 2 cm away from the fascial edge.

- **Continuous** (far-far): The suture is started at one end of the incision. It penetrates fascia and muscle 2 cm away from the fascial edge. It passes contralaterally, engaging muscle and fascia and exiting 2 cm away from the fascial edge. Bites are repeated in a similar fashion until the opposite end is reached, where the suture is tied (*Fig. 8.65*).
- **Continuous Smead–Jones** (far-far-near-near): The suture is started at one end of the incision (*Fig. 8.66*), incorporating the fascial edges, and is tied. A bite is taken 2 cm away from the fascial edge, engaging fascia and muscle, passing contralaterally to incorporate muscle and fascia, and exiting 2 cm away from the fascial edge. Next, the ipsilateral and contralateral fascial edges, respectively, are incorporated. The bites are repeated until the opposite end is reached, where the suture is tied.

In the continuous suture techniques, several points are worth mentioning. The total length of the suture must be approximately three to four times the length of the incision (suture : wound length ratio of 4:1). Tissues are approximated loosely, not tightly. A looped suture is advantageous; it allows a loop to be made at one end of the incision, reducing the number of knots to only at one end (*Fig. 8.67*). If the incision is too long, two continuous sutures are started at each end and tied at the midpoint. It is important to bury the knots as much as possible to prevent sinus tract formation.

In suturing the fascial ends of a low transverse incision, it is important to remember to incorporate only the fascial tissues into the suture and not the substance of the internal and external oblique muscle. The iliohypogastric and ilioinguinal nerves course within the internal and external oblique muscle and could therefore become entrapped.

The outcome of diverse mass closure techniques in 2,256 gynecologic patients is summarized in *Fig. 8.60*.

PERITONEUM

Closure of the peritoneum has not been shown to contribute to the prevention of wound complications, peritoneal adhesions, dehiscence, and hernia[5,38–48]. Mass closure of the wound, with or without including the peritoneum, is associated with a reduced incidence of wound dehiscence as compared to layer closure[39,49,50].

SUBCUTANEOUS TISSUE

Suture obliteration of the subcutaneous dead space should be abandoned, since it has not been substantiated by studies. Suture closure of the subcutaneous tissue impairs the wound's ability to resist infection and eliminates any benefits of dead space closure[51].

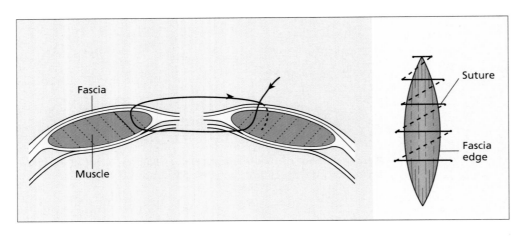

8.65 Continuous suture.

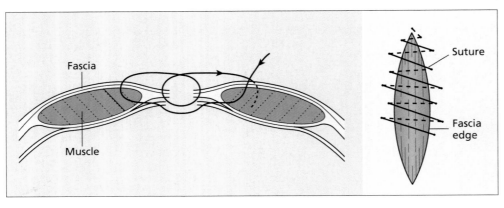

8.66 Continuous Smead–Jones suture.

SKIN

Skin closure is usually carried out by staples or a subcuticular continuous suture of early absorbable material. Staples are associated with a lower risk of infection than suture[52,53]. They provide a cosmetic result comparable to #3-0 Prolene closure in vertical incisions, but a less desirable result in transverse incisions when evaluated at 6 weeks[54]. Removal of skin staples within the first 5 postoperative days may result in skin dehiscence, a common occurrence in obese patients or those with other poor healing risk factors. Delaying the removal until 2 weeks postoperatively, however, has not been shown to offer additional protection and may result in epithelization of the staple tracts with poot cosmetic result. Staples are preferable in the absence of poor healing risk factors.

Subcuticular continuous closure offers additional protection relative to skin dehiscence compared with staple closure. It provides good cosmetic results and there is no need for suture removal, but it requires additional time under anesthesia. It is preferable to staples in the presence of poor health risk factors, such as in obese patients.

Although steri-strip closure has been associated with the lowest risk of infection compared with staples and suture[52,53] it has not gained popularity because of variability in adhesive properties. Cosmetic results with steri-strips at 6 months were superior to Dermalon (#3-0, #4-0) suture closure in abdominal incisions. However, late cosmetic results at 46 months were equal for both types of skin closure[55].

DELAYED SKIN CLOSURE

In the presence of risk factors for wound infection (e.g., obesity, bowel resection, contaminated wound, dirty wound), delayed primary skin closure has repeatedly been shown to be associated with a lower infection rate than primary closure at the time of operation[56–58].

Technique

A fascial mass closure is performed with a monofilament suture. The subcutaneous tissue is irrigated with saline. A gauze pack is placed in the subcutaneous space. A subcuticular continuous suture, vertical mattress sutures, or single stitches with a #4-0 Prolene are left untied in place (*Fig. 8.68*). After 4 days the pack is removed without disrupting the skin sutures and the wound is inspected. In the presence of a clean wound, the continuous suture is pulled or the interrupted sutures tied and the skin closed. The sutures are removed a few days later and steri-strips applied. Delayed primary skin closure is most useful in obese patients at risk of infection.

SUBCUTANEOUS DRAINS

The use of subcutaneous drains in clean wounds is not recommended, since this has been shown to increase the infection rate compared with undrained, clean wounds.

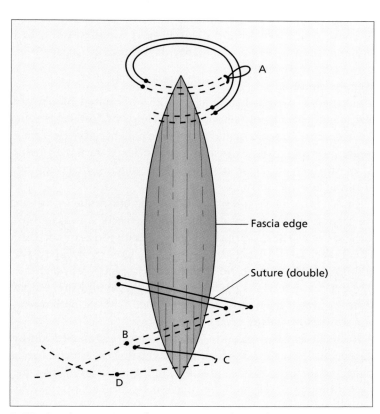

8.67 Continuous Smead–Jones suture: looped suture.

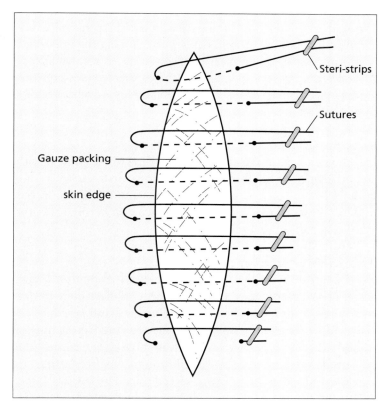

8.68 Delayed skin closure.

WOUND COMPLICATIONS
WOUND DEHISCENCE

The word *dehiscence* indicates any disruption of a suture line[59-61]. Wound dehiscence refers to the disruption of each of the suture lines of an abdominal wound and is synonymous with burst abdomen or wound disruption. The loops of small bowel may be in or out of the abdominal cavity. The latter case is known as evisceration.

Incidence

The incidence of wound dehiscence has decreased over the years owing to the use of mass closure techniques and permanent or delayed absorbable suture material. In a compiled series of 2,256 gynecologic patients (1980–1991) with the above closure technique and suture material, the incidence of wound dehiscence was 1 in 2,500 patients (0.04%) see *Fig. 8.61*. Compared with an earlier (1954–1977) compiled series of 17,022 patients with layer closure and catgut, wite, or silk sutures, the incidence of wound dehiscence was ten times higher, or 1 in 250 (0.4%) see *Fig. 8.62*.

Etiological factors

Factors that contribute to increased abdominal pressure, delayed wound healing, and/or faulty closure also predispose to wound dehiscence or incisional hernia. Usually they are found in combination. These factors may exist before the operation, result from the surgical technique, or develop postoperatively.

Preoperative factors

The general condition of the patient bears a strong influence relative to the risk of wound dehiscence. Among the important factors are obesity, pulmonary disease associated with coughing, advanced age, hypoproteinemia, diabetes, steroid use, previous irradiation, anemia, chronic medical conditions, advanced malignancy, and repeat incisions[33,42,62,63].

Intraoperative factors

The choice of closure technique has a direct relationship with the incidence of dehiscence. Low transverse incisions are commonly thought to be 'resistant' to wound dehiscence, but studies[64] have shown similar dehiscence and hernia rates for transverse and vertical incisions.

Postoperative factors

Wound infection or hematoma, abdominal distention (ileus, bowel obstruction), vomiting, coughing, and electrolyte imbalance[33,42,62,63] predispose to wound dehiscence and hernia.

The most common reason for dehiscence noted at the time of repair is that intact sutures are cutting through the tissues[31,32]. The length of an abdominal wall wound has been noted to increase by 30% in the presence of abdominal distension[31]. It is important not to approximate the tissues incorporated into the mass closure too tightly, and to leave reserve suture length to compensate for postoperative distension. A ratio of suture :

wound length of 4:1 is recommended for continuous sutures. Knot slipping has also been observed, as has protrusion of the bowel or omentum in between the sutures[31,32]. Suture breaking is rare with modern monofilament non-absorbable materials.

Clinical presentations and diagnosis

Serosanguineous fluid exuding from the incision is the most common presenting sign, being noted in 84% of patients[42]. A sudden tearing pain, "something giving way," in the incision is described by some patients at the time of coughing or straining and is suggestive of dehiscence. In 25% of patients with dehiscence, extrusion of the bowel (evisceration) is noted[65]. In about 15% of patients no signs other than abdominal distension and other predisposing factors exist, and the dehiscence is detected incidentally on routine inspection of the incision. When in doubt, CT scan of the abdomen is helpful to detect an occult wound dehiscence[66]. Small or incomplete fascial dehiscences usually are unnoticed postoperatively. With time, they present as incisional or ventral hernia.

In the presence of serosanguineous fluid, fascial dehiscence must be ruled out. A long, curved Kelly clamp is used to separated the skin edges over the area of exudation. A sudden gush of fluid may be noted, representing a collection of peritoneal fluid or a subcutaneous seroma. In the former, loops of bowel may be immediately apparent in the subcutaneous tissue but most commonly are not. After drainage of the fluid, probing the fascia with the Kelly clamp or with a sterile gloved finger will reveal the defect. Regardless of the defect size, inspection of the remainder of the fascia and closure are indicated in the operating room under satisfactory anesthesia.

The diagnosis of wound dehiscence is usually established within the first 5 to 10 postoperative days (range 2–22 days)[42,62].

Management

Moist packs, a tight bandage, and an abdominal binder are placed immediately for temporary prevention of bowel extrusion while preparations are made to carry the patient to the operating room. Insertion of a nasogastric tube is delayed until the patient is anesthetized because of the risk of gagging or coughing, resulting in evisceration.

Under general anesthesia, the skin and subcutaneous tissue are separated and the entire length of the fascia is explored for the size of the defect, seromas, infection, hematoma, or necrosis. The bowel is cleansed, if exteriorized, and returned to the abdominal cavity. Necrotic or infected tissues are debrided.

After the defect has been clearly identified and the wound cleaned, fascial mass closure is performed with monofilament, non-absorbable suture material (see above).

In the absence of infection, primary closure is carried out by stapling the skin edges together after irrigating the subcutaneous tissue. In the presence of infection, moist packs are left in the subcutaneous tissue and the incision is allowed to close by secondary intention.

Retention sutures are not used, since they have not been shown to be useful in the prevention of dehiscence[46,47,50,68-70].

Results

The possibility of a repeat dehiscence appears to be small; however, subsequent incisional hernia is noted in almost half of patients[69,71]. Most dehiscence patient are debilitated, and a second operation further aggravates their initial status. Prolonged hospital stay of over 8 days after dehiscence repair is customary because of potential secondary complications such as wound infection, pneumonia, pulmonary embolus, pelvic thrombophlebitis, tertiary operation, stress ulcers, and fistulae[42,62].

A recent report has shown a mortality rate of about 3% for gynecologic patients with dehiscence[42]. In most instances the mortality is related more to the general medical condition and the disease for which the patient underwent surgery than to the dehiscence itself. The mortality rate is similar for dehiscence patients with or without evisceration[65].

INCISIONAL HERNIA

Incidence

The incidence of incisional hernia is much greater than that of wound dehiscence[71-75]. In a compiled series of 1,509 gynecologic patients with mass closure and permanent or delayed absorbable suture techniques applied, the incidence of incisional hernia was 1.7% at a maximal follow-up of 2 years (*Fig. 8.69*). This incidence is probably a very low estimate, since the longest follow-up was only 2 years and a much longer follow-up has been shown to be required to determine the true incidence of incisional hernia.

Repeat incisions (re-incisions) appear to be associated with a higher incidence of incisional hernia compared with primary (fresh) incisions. It is unclear whether mass closure has reduced the incidence of incisional hernia among gynecologic patients, since the length of follow-up has been too short (see *Fig. 8.69*).

Etiology

The predisposing factors are similar to those for wound dehiscence. Among them, obesity (59%), malignancy (14%), chronic constipation (10%), and previous wound infection (10%) are most commonly noted[62]. Previous wound dehiscence has been noted in 5% of patients with incisional hernia. In 24% of patients no significant predisposing factors are noted.

An incisional hernia is the protrusion of the peritoneum and bowel into the subcutaneous tissue. Owing to repeated elevations of intra-abdominal pressure, the size of the peritoneal sac enlarges until the transmission of intra-abdominal pressure no longer exerts any effect on the hernia sac. When an incisional hernia is combined with progressive obesity, it may reach massive proportions (*Fig. 8.70*).

Diagnosis

The most common complaints are bulging of the lower abdomen and discomfort. On inspection and with the patient in the standing position, a protrusion is easily noticeable, since most incisional hernias are large. If not noticeable, it may become more apparent with a Valsalva maneuver. The fascial defect can be easily palpated and is usually smaller than the hernia contents. The protruding bowel may or may not be reducible, depending on the overall hernia size and the diameter of the hernia ring.

Incidence of Incisional Hernia

Author (ref.)	No.	% Incisional hernia	Length follow-up
Shepherd (33)	200	5	24 mos.
Gallup (34)	210	0.4	N/A
Gallup (35)	285	0.3	6 wks–12 mos.
Orr (25)	402	3.1	6 mos.
Montz (36)	293	0	6 wks
Sorosky (37)	119	1.6	6–12 mos.
TOTAL	1,509	1.7	

8.69 Incidence of incisional hernia: patients in this series had mass closure, interrupted or continuous, and permanent or delayed-absorbable suture.

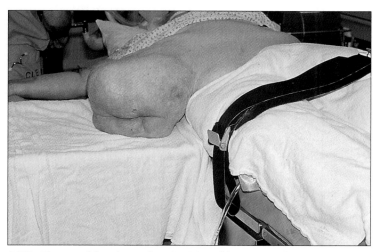

8.70 The combination of an incisional hernia and progressive obesity.

Management

Incisional hernias rarely become emergencies because of the large diameter of the ring. Correction is usually elective. Only about half of the patients with incisional hernia will require repair[76]. When diagnosed in the late postoperative period, repair is best postponed for at least 6 months until the inflammatory response has subsided. Temporary measures such as abdominal support, avoidance of abdominal strain, and weight reduction are indicated.

The principles of incisional hernia sac management focus on clear identification of the edges of the fascial defect (hernia ring) and closure. Because of improved results, in the majority of instances mesh (non-absorbable, monofilament) closure is performed. Primary mass closure is reserved for small hernia defects.

An elliptical incision is made in the skin directly over the hernia, encompassing the area of skin to be removed. The peritoneal sac is easily encountered immediately below the skin. It is dissected until the edge of the hernia ring (rectus fascia) is identifiable (*Fig. 8.71*). The sac is dissected in a 360° fashion until the entire circumference of the hernia ring is exposed (*Fig. 8.72*). The peritoneum of the hernia sac is incised if not previously opened, separated from the underlying adhered bowel, and excised. The hernia contents are reduced into the abdominal cavity.

Primary closure is performed only in the presence of a small fascial defect. In most cases, a non-absorbable mesh (usually Marlex or Mersilene) is used.

MESH CLOSURE

The mesh is fashioned to the sides of the defect, allowing a 3 cm margin. The margins of the mesh are placed preperitoneally, in a previously dissected space underneath the rectus muscle (*Fig. 8.73*). When this is not possible, they are placed intraperitoneally or immediately above the posterior or anterior rectus sheath. Once in place, and without undue tension, the fascial edge of the hernia ring is sutured to the mesh with a monofilament, non-absorbable suture #0 or #1 in a continuous fashion (*Fig. 8.74*). It is important to obtain a close fit with that suture, since recurrences are typically the result of partial separation of the mesh or bowel protrusion along the edges secondary to inadequate attachment[77]. The skin is closed as customary. No sutures are placed in the subcutaneous tissue. Antibiotic prophylaxis is routinely used.

In some situations, fascial closure over the mesh is possible. The mesh must be placed intra- or preperitoneally and sutured to the musculofascial layers. The fascia is then approximated

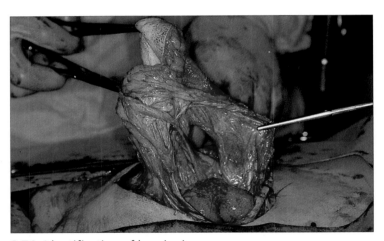

8.71 Identification of hernia ring.

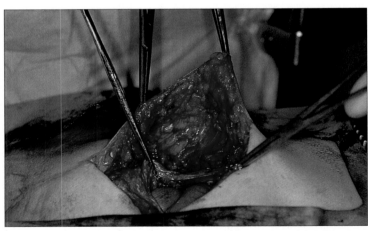

8.72 Exposure of hernia ring.

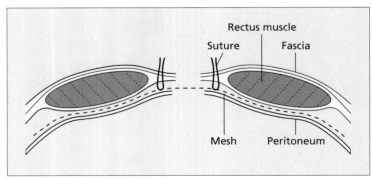

8.73 Placement of mesh graft.

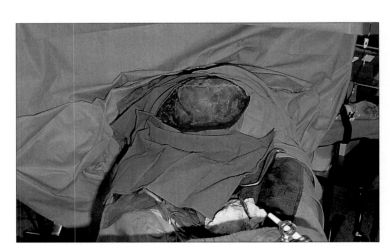

8.74 Mesh graft in-situ.

over the mesh in a mass closure fashion using monofilament, non-absorbable suture material (*Fig. 8.75*)[78–86].

PRIMARY CLOSURE

Primary closure consists of fascial mass closure using mono-filament, permanent #0 or #1 suture material (see above). The

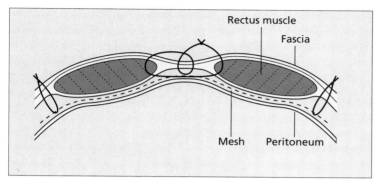

8.75 Mass closure using permanent suture material.

Incisional Hernia

Author	No.	Material	% Recurrence	Follow-up
Lewis (84)[78]	50	Marlex	6	2.6 yr
Validire (86)[79]	150	Toilinox*	9.5	4 yr
Adloff (87)[80]	130	Mersilene & Rectus Fascia	4.5	2 mo–3 yr
Bauer (87)[81]	28	EPTFE**	10.7	3.5 mo–3 yr
Wantz (91)[82]	30	Marsiline	3.4	N/A
Molloy (91)[77]	50	Marlex	8	4 yr
TOTAL	439		7	2 mo–4 yr

* metallic mesh
** expanded Polytetrafluoroethylene

8.76 Incisional hernia. Recurrence rates after repair with mesh closure.

bites extend 2 cm from the fascial edge and are placed 1.5–2 cm apart. The peritoneum is not necessarily included. No sutures are placed in the subcutaneous tissue. Any excess remaining skin is trimmed off and the skin closed.

Results

In a review of the literature, the recurrence rate after incisional hernia repair with mesh closure was much lower (7%) than after primary closure without mesh(36%) (*Figs 8.76, 8.77*). Failures typically result from the partial separation of the mesh from its attachment to the musculofascial tissues or from the protrusion of the bowel between the sutures along the edges.

Suprapubic incisional hernias

A special and different type of incisional hernia noted in gyne-cologic and urologic patients is the suprapubic incisional hernia. This hernia results from the dehiscence of the musculotendinous attachment of the abdominal wall muscles to the pubic bone (*Figs 8.78, 8.79*). Almost invariably it occurs in patients with multiple repeat incisions through the lower abdominal wall[87]. It may also occur after Cherney incisions.

Incisional Hernia

Author	No.	% Recurrence	Follow-up
Langer (85)[83]	154	31	5–10 yr
George (86)[84]	81	46	1 mo–13 yr
Lamont (88)[85]	36	44	1 yr
Read (89)[86]	206	25	1 yr
TOTAL	477	36	1 mo–13 yr

8.77 Incisional hernia. Recurrence rates after repair by primary closure (without mesh).

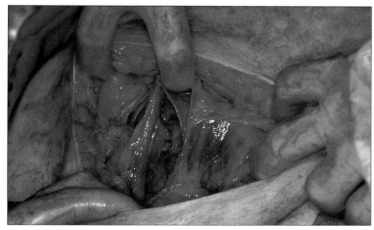

8.78 Suprapubic incisional hernia.

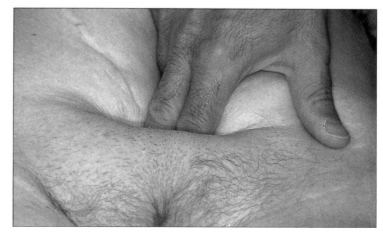

8.79 Physical examination showing suprapubic hernia.

Surgical correction is not possible without the use of a permanent mesh. Superiorly and laterally, the mesh is placed preperitoneally for a distance of 3 cm. The lower aspect is sutured directly to Cooper's ligament and the cartilage of the pubic symphysis (*Figs 8.80, 8.81*). This technique was successful in a series of seven patients[87] as well as in our own experience.

WOUND INFECTION

Incidence

In a compiled series of gynecological patients, the incidence of wound infection was 6.3% (range 1.6–14%) (see *Fig. 8.60*).

Predisposing factors

There are many factors related to wound infection. Among them are age, personal hygiene, socioeconomic group, skin preparation, disposable versus reusable drapes, type of operation, length of operation, medical condition, nutritional status, surgeon's experience, type of closure, suture material, and others.

Prevention

Disposable drapes are associated with a lower infection rate than reusable cotton drapes[88]. Chlorhexidine gluconate (Hibiclens) 4% in detergent solution has been shown to provide the fastest and most persistent reduction in hand flora compared with Betadine or Phisohex[89].

Prophylactic antibiotics given before the operation have been shown to reduce the infection rate significantly. Sutures in the subcutaneous tissue increase the risk of infection[50,66]. Hair removal should not be performed if possible, since not removing the hair is associated with the lowest infection rate; however, it may become necessary to allow identification of the wound edges and facilitate suturing. Hair clipping just before the operation is the second best method. Shaving is associated with the highest rate of infection and should not be done[90].

Diagnosis

Wound infections are usually not apparent until 5 days or more after the operation. Signs of deep subcutaneous infections may not surface until 10 days or more after surgery.

Erythema is the most common sign (*Fig. 8.82*). It should always evoke suspicion of wound infection, abscess, or lymphangitis. Slight temperature elevation is common in early infection; spiking fevers are common in the presence of an abscess.

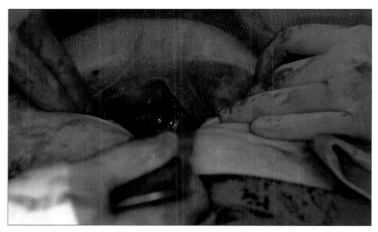

8.80 Placement of mesh with attachments.

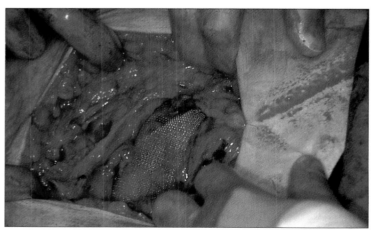

8.81 Permanent mesh placement.

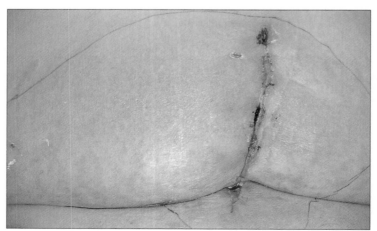

8.82 Erythema is the most common sign of wound infection.

Management

When a wound infection is suspected, probing with a Kelly clamp is indicated. If a seroma is drained, no further therapy is necessary, since the temperature will return to normal and the incisional pain will disappear. If an infection is demonstrated by the presence of purulent secretions, the wound is opened for the length of the infected area (probing with a Kelly clamp helps to determine the extent of the infected cavity) and cultures are taken.

The wound is cleaned with saline to identify necrotic tissues, which are debrided. The integrity of the fascia is demonstrated by probing with a Kelly clamp or a gloved finger. The wound is irrigated with Dakin's solution 25% concentration and packed with Marlex gauze. The gauze is changed four times daily. At every change it is irrigated with Dakin's solution. Debridement is performed once daily if necessary. Each change of the Marlex gauze results in automatic removal of further necrotic tissue, since the gauze becomes adhesed to the subcutaneous tissues. This gauze debridement is most helpful in the cleaning of the wound. As soon as healthy granulation tissue is noted, the Marlex gauze is replaced with fine mesh gauze and dressing changes are reduced to two or three times daily. The small size of the mesh openings does not allow penetration of the gauze by the budding capillaries of the granulation tissue. Consequently, when the gauze is changed no capillary damage occurs and the wound is allowed to granulate normally, without delay in healing. The number of daily changes decreases as soon as the wound becomes clean. Dakin's solution is used as an irrigant until no signs of infection are noted. Beefy red granulation tissue usually indicates the absence of infection. Secondary wound closure can be carried out if the patient is not obese, in which case there is a higher risk of reinfection[91].

Antibiotic therapy facilitates wound recovery. However, without proper wound care antibiotics will not be helpful. Most early wound infections can be satisfactorily managed with intensive local wound care without the need for systemic antibiotic therapy.

Early closure (between 4 and 6 days) of infected wounds has received some attention recently. Intensive systemic combination antibiotic therapy and local wound care, followed by closure after 4 days of therapy, have resulted in decreased morbidity and shorter hospitalization than closure by secondary intention[91]. Early closure should be considered when a prompt response to local and systemic therapy is noted. It should not be performed in the presence of unfavorable wound conditions.

NECROTIZING FASCIITIS

Necrotizing fasciitis is a rapidly progressing, aerobic and/or anaerobic necrosis of the fascia and subcutaneous tissue. It is described here because early recognition is associated with decreased morbidity and mortality.

A rapidly progressing wound erythema, or the development of ill-defined blue-gray skin patches in an erythematous area, or the development of anesthesia over an erythematous area that was initially very painful, should raise the suspicion of necrotizing fasciitis.

The involved area of the wound should be opened and the fascia inspected. Characteristically, the fascia and subcutaneous tissue appear dull gray. Necrosis of the fascia and subcutaneous tissue is obvious, and serosanguineous exudate is also noted. The skin appears undermined owing to subcutaneous tissue necrosis.

Management is based on repeated radical debridement of all the affected tissues and combination broad-spectrum antibiotic therapy. Saving the uninvolved healthy skin removed in the course of radical debridement can be helpful for later grafting. Reconstruction of the debrided area is accomplished by mesh prosthesis and skin grafting.

The mortality rate associated with necrotizing fasciitis is about 38%[92]. Factors affecting mortality include diabetes (mortality rate 63%), older age, general medical condition, malnutrition, and obesity[92].

REFERENCES

1. McCarthy JG. *Plastic Surgery, General Principles*, Vol 1. Philadelphia: WB Saunders, 1990: 42–3.

2. Hasselgren PO, Hagberg E, Malmer H, *et al*. One instead of two knives for surgical incision. *Arch Surg* 1984; 119:917.

3. Sowa DE, Masterson BJ, Nealon N, *et al*. Effects of thermal knives on wound healing. *Obstet Gynecol* 1985; 66:436–9.

4. Hambley R, Hebde PA, Abell E, *et al*. Wound healing of skin incisions produced by ultrasonically vibrating knife, scalpel, electrosurgery and carbon dioxide laser. *J Dermatol Surg Oncol* 1988; 14:1213.

5. Gilbert JM, Ellis H, Foweraker S. Peritoneal closure after lateral paramedian incision. *Br J Surg* 1987; 74:113.

6. Mouchel J. Transverse trans-rectus abdominis incision in gynecological and obstetrical surgery. 673 cases. *Nouv Presse Med* 1981; 10:413–15.

7. Barnes WA, Jr., Delgado G, Petrilli ES. An alternative approach to the vertical midline abdominal incision for staging in ovarian carcinoma. *Gynecol Oncol* 1987; 28:129.

8. Donaldson DR, Hegarty JH, Brennan TG, *et al*. The lateral paramedian incision. Experience with 850 cases. *Br J Surg* 1982; 69:630.

9. Weiser EB, Bundy BN, Hoskins WJ, *et al*. Extraperitoneal versus transperitoneal selective paraaortic lymphadenectomy in the pretreatment surgical staging of advanced cervical carcinoma (a gynecologic oncology group study). *Gynecol Oncol* 1989; 33:283.

10. Pfannenstiel HJ. Üeber die Vortheile des suprasymphysaren Fascienguer schnitt fur die gynnekologischen Koeliotomien. *Samml Klin Vortr Gynaekol (Leipzig)* 1900; 97:1735.

11. Maylard AE. Direction of abdominal incisions. *Br Med J* 1907; 2:895.

12. Helmkamp BF, Krebs HB. The Maylard incision in gynecologic surgery. *Am J Obstet Gynecol* 1990; 163:1554.

13. Mann WJ Jr, Orr JW Jr, Shingleton HM, *et al*. Perioperative influences on infectious morbidity in radical hysterectomy. *Gynecol Oncol* 1981; 11:207.

14. Tollefson DG, Russell KP. The transverse incision in pelvic surgery. *Am J Obstet Gynecol* 1954; 68:410.

15. Krupski WC, Sumchai A, Effeney DJ, *et al*. The importance of abdominal wall collateral blood vessels. *Arch Surg* 1984; 119:854.

16. Cherney LS. A modified transverse incision for low abdominal operations. *Surg Gynecol Obstet* 1941, 72:92.

17. Brand E. The Cherney incision for gynecologic cancer (letter). *Am J Obstet Gynecol* 1991, 165:235.

18. Cowles T, Schwartz PE. A suprapubic, retroperitoneal operative approach to solitary paravaginal tumors. *Obstet Gynecol* 1987; 69:420.

19. Georgy FM. Femoral neuropathy following abdominal operation. *Am J Obstet Gynecol* 1975; 123:819.

20. Sinclair RH, Pratt JH. Femoral neuropathy after pelvic operation. *Am J Obstet Gynecol* 1972; 112:406.

21. Masterson BJ. Wound healing in gynecologic surgery. In: Masterson BJ. ed. *Manual of Gynecologic Surgery,* 2nd ed. New York: Springer-Verlag, 1986: 71–9.

22. Grant ME, Prockop DJ. The biosynthesis of collagen. *N Engl J Med* 1972; 186:194.

23. Lichtenstein IL, Herzikoff, Shove JM, *et al*. The dynamics of wound healing. *Surg Gynecol Obstet* 1976; 130:685.

24. Pollack SV. Wound healing. A review. I. The biology of wound healing. *J Dermatol Surg Oncol* 1979; 5:389.

25. Orr, JW Jr. Incisions and closures. *Ala J Med Sc* 1986; 23:36.

26. Dudley HAF. Layered and mass closure of abdominal wall: a theoretical and experimental analysis. *Brit J Surg* 1970; 57:664.

27. Masterson BJ. Selection of incisions for gynecologic procedures. *Surg Clin North Am* 1991; 71:1041.

28. Tera H, Alberg C. Tissue strength of sutures involved in musculoaproneurotic layer sutures in laparotomy incisions. *Acta Chir Scand* 1976; 142:349.

29. Leaper DJ, Pollock AV, Evans N. Abdominal wound closure. A trial of nylon polyglycolic acid and steel sutures. *Brit J Surg* 1977; 64:603.

30. Jenkins TP. The burst abdominal wound: a mechanical approach. *Br J Surg* 1976; 163:873.

31. Stone IK, Von Frannhofer JA, Masterson BJ. The biomechanical effects of tight suture closure upon fascia. *Surg Gynecol Obstet* 1986; 163:448.

32. Wallace D, Hernandez W, Schlaerth JB, *et al*. Prevention of abdominal wound disruption utilizing the Smead-Jones closure technique. *Obstet Gynecol* 1980; 56:226.

33. Shepherd JH, Cavanagh D, Riggs D, *et al*. Abdominal wound closure using a non-absorbable single-layer technique. *Obstet Gynecol* 1983; 61:248.

34. Gallup DG, Talledo OE, King LA. Primary mass closure of midline incisions with a continuous running monofilament suture in gynecologic patients. *Obstet Gynecol* 1989; 73:675.

35. Gallup DG, Nolan TE, Smith RP. Primary mass closure of midline incisions with a continuous polyglyconate monofilament absorbable suture. *Obstet Gynecol* 1990; 76:872.

36. Montz FJ, Creasman WT, Eddy G, *et al*. Running mass closure of abdominal wounds using absorbable looped suture. *J Gynecol Surg* 1991; 7:107.

37. Sorosky JL, Hewett WJ, Kaminski PF, *et al*. Primary mass closure of fascial incisions using a continuous absorbable suture. *J Gynecol Surg* 1991; 7:41.

38. Tweedie FJ, Long RC. Abdominal wound disruptions. *Surg Gynecol Obstet* 1954; 99:41.

39. Hull HC, Hankins JR. Disruption of abdominal wounds. *Ann Surg* 1955; 21:223.

40. Pratt JH. Wound healing–evisceration. *Clin Obstet Gynecol* 1973; 16:126.

41. Helmkamp BF. Abdominal wound dehiscence. *Am J Obstet Gynecol* 1977; 128:803.

42. Jones TE, Newell ET, Brubaker RE. The use of alloy steel wire in the closure of abdominal wounds. *Surg Gynecol Obstet* 1941; 72:2056.

43. Hugh TB, Nankivell C, Meagher AP, *et al*. Is closure of the peritoneal layer necessary in the repair of midline surgical abdominal wounds? *World J Surg* 1990; 14:231.

44. McFadden PM, Peacock EE Jr. Preperitoneal abdominal wound repair: incidence of dehiscence. *Am J Surg* 1983; 145:213.

45. Karipineni RC, Wilk PJ, Danese CA. The role of the peritoneum in the healing of abdominal incisions. *Surg Gynecol Obstet* 1976; 142:729.

46. Tulandi T, Hum HS, Gelfand MM. Closure of laparotomy incisions with or without peritoneal suturing and second-look laparoscopy. *Am J Obstet Gynecol* 1988; 158:536.

47. Pietrantoni M, Parsons MT, O'Brien WF, *et al*. Peritoneal closure or non-closure at caesarean. *Obstet Gynecol* 1991; 77:293.

48. Baggish MS, Lee WK. Abdominal wound disruption. *Obstet Gynecol* 1975; 46:530.

49. Bucknall TE, Cox PJ, Ellis H. Burst abdomen and incisional hernia. a prospective study of 1129 major laparotomies. *Br Med J* 1982; 284:931.

50. deHoll D, Rodenheaver G, Edgerton MT, *et al*. Potentiation of infection by suture closure of dead space. *Am J Surg* 1974; 127:716.

51. Johnson A, Rodeheaver GT, Durand, *et al*. Automatic disposable stapling devices for wound closure. *Ann Emerg Med* 1981; 10:631.

52. Stillman RM, Marino CA, Seligman SJ. Skin staples in potentially contaminated wounds. *Arch Surg* 1984; 119:821.

53. Lubowski D, Hunt D. Abdominal wound closure comparing the proximate stapler with sutures. *Aust NZ J Surg* 1985; 55:405.

54. Pedersen VM, Struckman JR, Kjaergard HK, *et al*. Late cosmetic results of wound closure, strip versus suture. *Neth J Surg* 1987; 39:149.

55. Brown SE, Allen HH, Robins RN. The use of delayed primary wound closure in preventing wound infections. *Am J Obstet Gynecol* 1977; 127:713.

56. Hudspeth AS. Elimination of surgical wound infection by delayed primary wound closure. *South Med J* 1973; 66:934.

57. McLachlin AD, Wall W. Delayed primary closure of the skin and subcutaneous tissue in abdominal surgery. *Can J Surg* 1976; 19:37.

58. Cruse PJE. Some factors determining wound infection. A prospective study of 30,000 wounds; hospital-acquired infections in surgery. In: Polk HC Jr, Stone HH, eds. Baltimore: University Park Press, 1977:77–85.

59. Farnell MB, Worthington-Self S, Mucha, P Jr, *et al*. Closure of abdominal incisions with subcutaneous catheters. *Arch Surg* 1986; 121:641.

60. Magee C, Rodeheaver GT, Golden GT, *et al*. Potentiation of wound infection by surgical drains. *Am J Surg* 1976; 131:547.

61. Souders JC, Pratt JH. Wound dehiscence and incisional hernia after gynecologic operations. *Clin Obstet Gynecol* 1962; 5:522.

62. Funt MI. Abdominal incisions and closures. *Clin Obstet Gynecol* 1981; 24:1175.

63. Stone H, Heofling S, Strom P, *et al*. Abdominal incisions: transverse vs vertical placement and continuous vs interrupted closure. *South Med J* 1983; 76:1106.

64. Haddad V, Macon ML IV. Abdominal wound dehiscence and evisceration: contributing factors and improved mortality. *Am Surg* 1980; 4:508.

65. Smith-Behn J, Arnold M, Might J. Use of computerized tomography of the abdominal wall in the diagnosis of partial postoperative wound dehiscence. *Postgrad Med J* 1986; 62:947.

66. Ferguson DJ. Clinical application of experimental relations between technique and wound infection. *Surgery* 1968; 63:377.

67. Goligher JC, Irvin TT, Johnston D, *et al*. A controlled clinical trial of three methods of closure of laparotomy wounds. *Br J Surg* 1975; 62:823.

68. Daly JW. Dehiscence, evisceration and other complications. *Clin Obstet Gynecol* 1988; 31:754.

69. Tweedie FJ, Long RC. Abdominal wound disruptions. *Surg Gynecol Obstet* 1954; 99:41.

70. Grace RH, Cox S. Incidence of incisional hernia after dehiscence of the abdominal wound. *Am J Surg* 1976; 131:210.

71. Hull HC, Hankins JR. Distruption of abdominal wounds. *Am Surgeon* 1955; 21:223.

72. Mudge M, Hughes LE. Incisional hernia. a 10 year prospective study of incidence and attitudes. *Br J Surg* 1985; 72:70.

73. Regnard JF, Hay JM, Rea S, *et al*. Ventral incisional hernias: incidence date of recurrence, localization and risk factors. *Ital J Surg Sci* 1988; 18:259.

74. Lamont PM, Ellis H. Incisional hernia in re-opened abdominal incisions. an overlooked risk factor. *Br J Surg* 1988; 75:374.

75. Masterson BJ. Selection of incisions for gynecologic procedures. *Surg Clin North Am* 1991; 71:1041.

76. Molloy RG, Moran KT, Waldron RP, *et al*. Massive incisional hernia: abdominal wall replacement with Marlex mesh. *Br J Surg* 1991; 78:242.

77. Lewis RT. Knitted polypropylene (Marlex) mesh in the repair of incisional hernias. *Can J Surg* 1984; 27:155.

78. Validire J, Imband P, Dutet D, *et al*. Large abdominal incisional hernias: repair by fascial approximation reinforced with a stainless steel mesh. *Br J Surg* 1986; 73:8.

79. Adloff M, Arnaud JP. Surgical management of large incisional hernias by an intraperitoneal Mersilene mesh and an aponeurotic graft. *Surg Gynecol Obstet* 1987; 165:204.

80. Bauer JJ, Salky BA, Gelernt IM, *et al*. Repair of large abdominal wall defects with expanded polytetrafluoroethylene (EPTFE). *Ann Surg* 1987; 206:765.

81. Wantz GE. Incisional hernioplasty with Mersilene. *Surg Gynecol Obstet* 1991; 172:129.

82. Langer S, Christiansen J. Long-term results after incisional hernia repair. *Acta Chir Scand* 1985; 151:217.

83. George CD, Ellis H. The results of incisional hernia repair. a twelve year review. *Ann R Coll Surg Engl* 1986; 68:185.

84. Lamont PM, Ellis H. Incisional hernia in re-opened abdominal incisions: an overlooked risk factor. *Br J Surg* 1988; 75:374.

85. Read RC, Yoder G. Recent trends in the management of incisional herniation. *Arch Surg* 1989; 124:485.

86. Bendavid R. Incisional parapubic hernias. *Surgery* 1990; 108:898.

87. Moylan JA, Kennedy BV. The importance of gown and drape barriers in the prevention of wound infection. *Surg Gynecol Obstet* 1980; 151:465.

88. Peterson AF, Rosenberg A, Alatary SO. Comparative evaluation of surgical scrub preparations. *Surg Gynecol Obstet* 1978; 146:63.

89. Alexander JW, Fischer JE, Boyajian M, *et al*. The influence of hair-removal methods on wound infections. *Arch Surg* 1983; 118:347.

90. Walters MD, Dombroski RA, Davidson SA, *et al*. Reclosure of disrupted abdominal incisions. *Obstet Gynecol* 1990; 76:597.

91. Gottrup G, Gjode P, Lundhus F, *et al*. Management of severe incisional abscesses following laparotomy. *Arch Surg* 1989; 124:702.

92. Janevicius RV, Hahn SE, Butt MD. Necrotizing fasciitis. *Surg Gynecol Obstet* 1982; 154:97.

9

Gynecologic Surgery in Children and Adolescents

David Muram

Barbara R. Hostetler

Claudette E. Jones

Frederick J. Rau

LABIAL ADHESIONS

INTRODUCTION

Labial adhesion denotes the fusion of the labia minora in the midline (*Fig. 9.1*). Labial adhesion is quite common in the prepubertal period. The disorder is probably related to the low levels of estrogens in the prepubertal child. It has been suggested that the skin covering the labia is denuded by minor trauma (e.g., scratching), permitting the labia to adhere in the midline. Most children are asymptomatic. Many children respond to a short course of Premarin Vaginal Cream (Ayerst, New York, NY) applied twice daily for 7–10 days. In some children, gentle manual separation may be required after the estrogen therapy.

SURGICAL INDICATIONS

Separation of the labia is indicated when the labial fusion interferes with urination or with drainage of secretions from the vagina. However, medical therapy should be attempted first. Surgical division of the fused labia is reserved for patients in whom medical treatment has failed or when severe urinary symptoms preclude a trial of medical therapy.

SURGICAL PROCEDURE

Step 1

Locate a small fenestration between the fused labia. Such an opening is commonly found just above the external urethral meatus (*Fig. 9.1*).

Step 2

Insert a hemostat in a downward direction through that opening. Make sure that the hemostat is in front of the vestibule and not in the urethra or vagina. The hemostat is often visible through the thin labia. It serves to protect the vestibule and to apply traction on the fused labia to better delineate the line of fusion (*Fig. 9.2*).

Step 3

The line of fusion is incised with a scalpel blade. The incision is extended until the posterior fourchette is reached (*Fig. 9.3*).

Step 4

Only minimal bleeding is anticipated, and no sutures are required (*Fig. 9.4*).

Step 5

After the surgical separation, Premarin cream is applied to the area twice daily for 5 days to prevent immediate readhesion of the surgically separated labia.

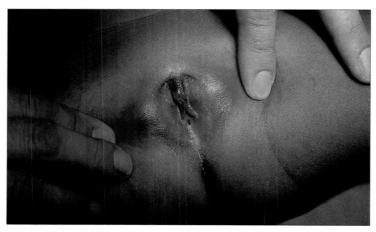

9.1 Labial adhesions. Note the line of fusion in the midline.

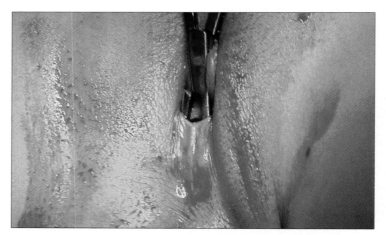

9.2 A hemostat is inserted behind the fused labia. It is used to protect the vestibule and to apply traction on the fused labia.

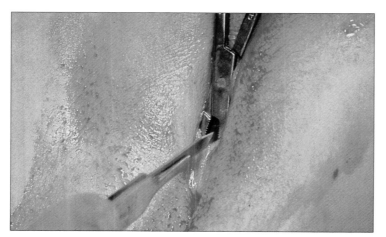

9.3 The labia are separated by sharp dissection along the line of fusion.

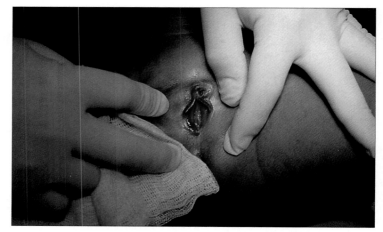

9.4 Normal anatomy is restored following surgical separation.

IMPERFORATE HYMEN

An imperforate hymen exists when the hymen consists of a solid membrane without an aperture. It is assumed that an imperforate hymen represents a persistent portion of the urogenital membrane and is caused by abnormal invasion by mesoderm of the primitive streak of the urogenital portion of the cloacal membrane. Demonstration of vaginal patency should be part of the examination of the genitalia of the newborn, and therefore an imperforate hymen should be diagnosed at birth. When the vagina is obstructed, it may become distended by accumulation of vaginal secretions, a condition called mucocolpos or hydrocolpos. When this occurs, the thin hymeneal membrane is stretched and forms a bulging, shiny, thin protuberance.

If the diagnosis of an imperforate hymen is not established during childhood, the condition is suspected when an adolescent girl presents with primary amenorrhea and recurrent lower abdominal pain. Menstrual flow fills the vagina (hematocolpos)

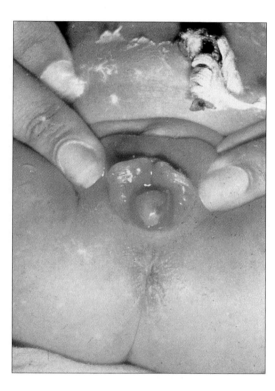

9.5 A 5-day-old patient with an imperforate hymen. Note the thin, bulging membrane filling the introitus.

and then the uterus (hematometra), and may spill through the tubes into the peritoneal cavity. Inspection of the vulva usually reveals a dome shaped, purplish–red hymeneal membrane bulging outward under pressure from the collection of menstrual fluid above it. On rectal examination, the distended vagina is palpable as a large cystic mass. Endometriosis and vaginal adenosis are known but not inevitable complications in such patients.

SURGICAL INDICATIONS

Hymeneal anomalies require surgical correction if they block the escape of vaginal secretions or menstrual fluid, interfere with intercourse, or prevent an indicated vaginoscopy and treatment of a vaginal disorder.

SURGICAL PROCEDURE

A 5-day-old patient with an imperforate hymen is shown in *Fig. 9.5*. Note the thin, bulging membrane at the introitus. The distension is caused by accumulation of vaginal secretions.

Step 1

The central portion of the membrane should be excised to provide a large aperture. If the hymen is only incised, the edges tend to coalesce and may again join to re-form an obstructing membrane.

Step 2

A careful examination of the external genitalia should be performed, including rectoabdominal palpation. This is particularly important in patients in whom the amount of vaginal fluid is small or the obstructing membrane is thick and fibrous. Under these circumstances, the imperforate hymen is similar in appearance to an absent vagina. In some instances a sonographic evaluation may be required to distinguish between these two conditions.

Step 3

The central portion of the hymen is grasped with a pair of forceps and, using scissors, is removed (*Fig. 9.6*).

Step 4

Bleeding is minimal and no sutures are required (*Fig. 9.7*). The procedure is identical in postmenarcheal girls.

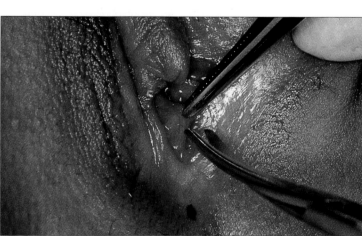

9.6 The central portion of the hymen is grasped with a pair of forceps and is excised with scissors.

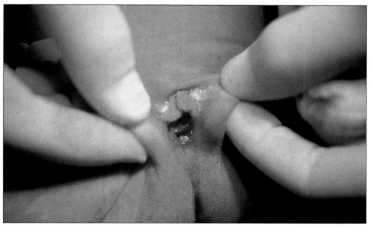

9.7 At the completion of the surgical procedure, an adequate aperture is created. No sutures are required.

Step 5

After a hymeneal aperture has been created, a large amount of old blood will be seen escaping from the vagina (*Fig. 9.8*).

Step 6

Evaluation of the vagina should be delayed for 4–6 weeks to reduce the risk of introducing infection. In addition, the significant distension of the uterus interferes with the examiner's ability to properly evaluate the pelvic organs.

TRANSVERSE SEPTUM

Transverse vaginal septa are the result of faulty canalization of the embryonic vagina. These septa may be without an opening (complete or obstructive) or may have a small central aperture (incomplete or non-obstructive). They are usually found in the midvagina but may occur at any level. When the septum is located in the upper vagina, it is more likely to be patent (incomplete), whereas those septa located in the lower part of the vagina are often complete (*Fig. 9.9*).

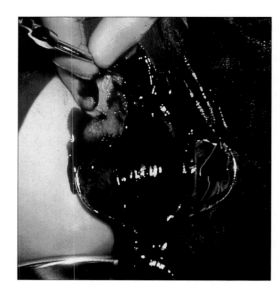

9.8 A hematocolpos is drained after excision of an imperforate hymen in a postmenarcheal girl.

SURGICAL INDICATIONS

An incomplete septum is usually asymptomatic and therefore does not require correction during childhood or early adolescence. The central aperture allows egress of vaginal secretions and menstrual flow. However, a complete septum will cause signs and symptoms similar to those of an imperforate hymen. Unfortunately, the diagnosis of a transverse vaginal septum is often delayed until after menarche, when menstrual fluid becomes trapped behind an obstructing membrane.

SURGICAL PROCEDURE

Step 1

Insert a speculum into the vagina until the septum comes into view (Fig. 9.9).

Step 2

Incise the central part of the septum using a No. 11 blade (*Fig. 9.10*). The aperture is dilated bluntly.

Step 3

A large amount of old, thick blood rapidly fills the vagina (*Fig. 9.11*).

Further evaluation should be delayed for 6–8 weeks.

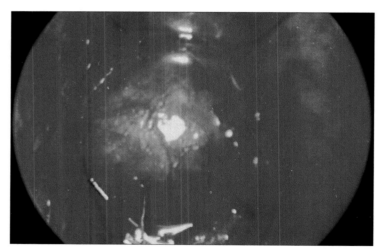

9.9 A bulging transverse septum is seen in the upper vagina.

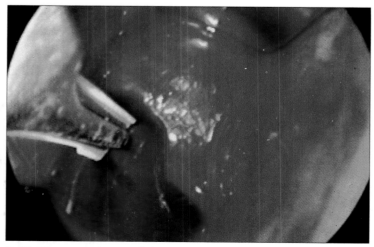

9.10 The central part of the septum is incised with a No. 11 blade.

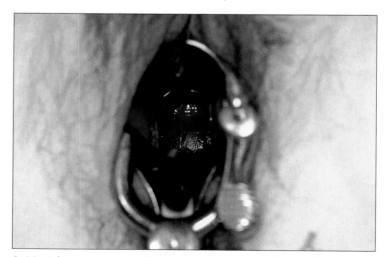

9.11 A large amount of old, thick blood rapidly fills the vagina.

DIVISION OF A LONGITUDINAL VAGINAL SEPTUM

These longitudinal septa occur when the distal ends of the Müllerian ducts fail to fuse properly (*Fig. 9.12*). Such failure results in a vagina divided by a longitudinal septum, with both parts encircled by the same muscle layer. Failure to fuse can be limited to the vagina only or can also affect the uterus, forming a bicornuate uterus or uterus didelphis.

SURGICAL INDICATIONS

Division of the septum is indicated when dyspareunia is present, when obstruction of drainage from one-half of the vagina is noted, or when the physician suspects that a septum would interfere with a vaginal delivery.

SURGICAL PROCEDURE

Step 1

Inspect the entire length of the vagina on both sides of the septum. The operator must determine whether the patient has one cervix or two (one on each side of the septum).

Step 2

Place the septum on tension by pushing the posterior vaginal wall downward (*Fig. 9.13*).

Step 3

Using scissors, cut the septum in the middle, at a point of equal distance from the anterior and the posterior vaginal walls (*Fig. 9.13*). Because the septum represents the line of fusion of two tubular structures, the septum is thinnest and least vascularized in midpoint (*Fig. 9.14*). In addition, if the septum is divided too close to the vaginal mucosa, a defect may form in the continuity of the vaginal mucosa as the divided septum retracts.

Step 4

Continue incising the septum until the cervix is reached (*Fig. 9.15*).

Step 5

Secure hemostasis by placing a continuous locking suture of #0-0 Vicril on each edge of the divided septum.

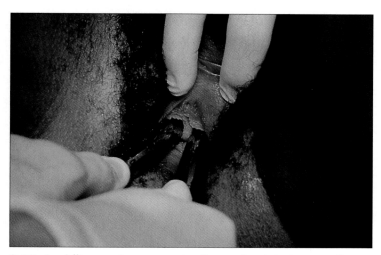

9.12 A midline septum separates the vagina into two smaller channels.

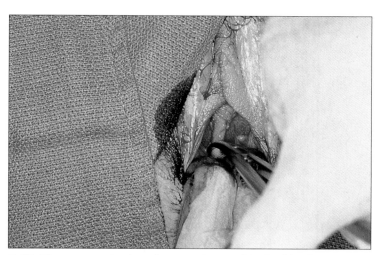

9.13 The septum is placed on tension and incised in the midline.

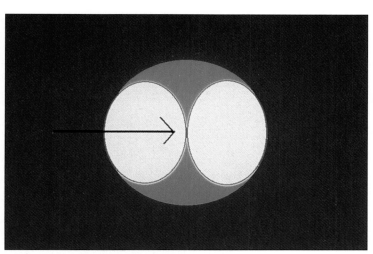

9.14 A schematic drawing for the division of the septum. The arrow indicates the thinnest and least vascularized portion of the septum.

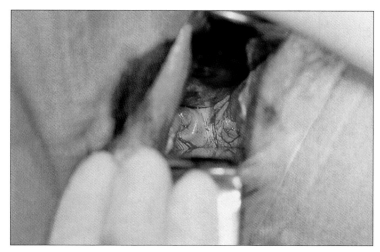

9.15 The septum is divided throughout its length. Two cervices are seen in the vaginal apex.

URETHRAL PROLAPSE

The urethral mucosa, an estrogen-dependent tissue, is thin and atrophic during childhood. Occasionally it prolapses through the urethral meatus (*Fig. 9.16*). Because of venous obstruction, the prolapsed tissue becomes swollen and sometimes undergoes necrosis. The diagnosis of urethral prolapse is relatively easy when a protruding tumor is found superior to the vagina, where the urethral meatus is located, and a central orifice is seen within that mass. When the lesion is small and urination is unimpaired, a short course of therapy utilizing a small amount of Premarin cream (applied twice daily for 5–7 days) is beneficial.

SURGICAL INDICATIONS

Surgical excision is indicated if urinary retention is present, if the lesion is large and necrotic, or if the child is being examined under anesthesia.

SURGICAL PROCEDURE

Step 1
Identify the urethral meatus and the vestibule. Identify the vestibule to determine the amount of tissue that needs to be resected (*Fig. 9.17*).

Step 2
Using scissors, excise the prolapsed urethral mucosa so that it is flush with the vestibule (*Fig. 9.18*).

Step 3
Using #3-0 Dexon suture, place three or four stay sutures, usually at the 12, 3, 6, and 9 o'clock positions, between the urethral mucosa and the vestibular mucosa (*Fig. 9.19*).

Step 4
An indwelling urinary catheter is left in place for 24 hours to prevent urine retention.

After the surgical resection, Premarin cream is applied to the area twice daily for 5 days to promote healing.

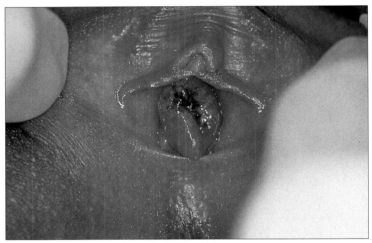

9.16 A 4-year-old girl presents with urethral prolapse. Despite application of Premarin cream, the urethral mucosa is still protruding and the patient remains symptomatic. Note the area of necrosis.

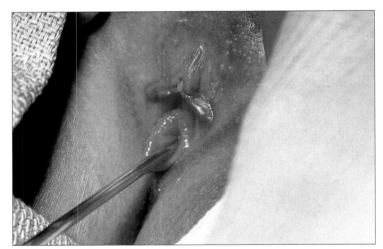

9.17 The urethral meatus is identified with a catheter.

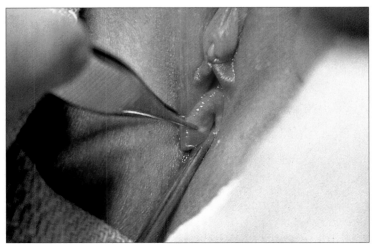

9.18 The prolapsed mucosa is excised.

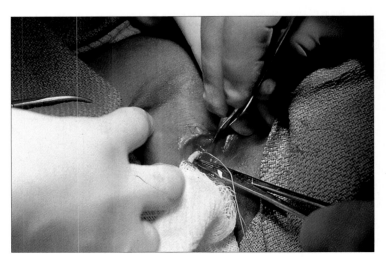

9.19 Stay sutures approximate the urethra to the vestibule.

VAGINOSCOPY

Instrumentation and vaginal inspection are not an integral part of the routine gynecologic examination in young girls. When required, the examination is usually performed under general anesthesia.

Many instruments have been used to separate the vaginal walls, e.g., nasal specula, otoscopes, and vaginoscopes. The vaginoscope is a modified otoscope consisting of a hollow cylinder with a removable obturator and a light source. It is available in a variety of diameters, permitting its use in various age groups (*Fig. 9.20*). Most recently, a small flexible endoscope has been used to visualize the vagina.

If the examination is to be performed in an office setting, the patient must be relaxed and cooperative. Lidocaine jelly is applied at the vaginal introitus and to the instrument.

Before insertion of the instrument, it must be shown to the girl in order to decrease apprehension. The child is allowed to touch the lubricated instrument and it is pointed out to her that it feels strange, slippery, and cool. Then the instrument is placed against the inner thigh and she is reminded that it feels cool, slippery, and unusual. Only then is the instrument passed through the hymeneal orifice.

If the aperture is too small for an instrument to be passed without discomfort, or if the child is uncooperative, vaginoscopy should not be attempted without general anesthesia. Indeed, persistent manipulation of the sensitive tissues without anesthesia will be traumatic and counterproductive. If the examination is performed under general anesthesia, the authors prefer to use a water cystoscope. The water distends the vagina, exposing the vaginal mucosa. At the same time, it irrigates secretions, blood, and debris.

SURGICAL INDICATIONS

Vaginoscopy may be required in patients with recurrent or persistent vaginitis. It is also performed when the upper third of the vagina requires evaluation, to determine the source of vaginal bleeding, to determine the extent of a penetrating injury, to remove foreign bodies and, sometimes, when the presence of a transverse septum is suspected.

SURGICAL PROCEDURE

Step 1

After inspection of the external genitalia, separate the labia to expose the hymeneal opening (*Fig. 9.21*).

Step 2

Insert the instrument (a cystoscope) through the hymeneal orifice (*Fig. 9.22*).

Step 3

Gently advance the instrument. The operator must exercise caution when the instrument is advanced, as the vaginal length varies with age.

Step 4

The labia minora are compressed together to retain the water in the vagina and maintain distension of the vaginal walls.

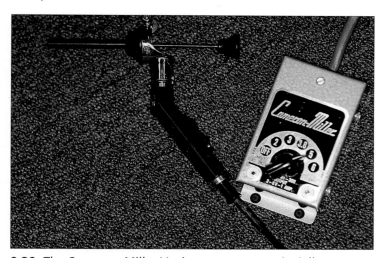

9.20 The Cameron–Miller Vaginoscope, a commercially available vaginoscope.

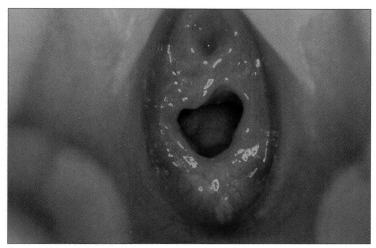

9.21 The labia are separated to expose the vaginal introitus.

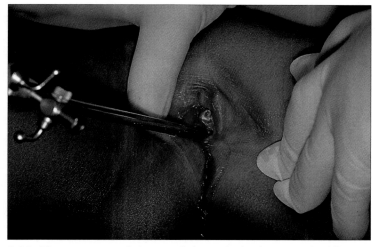

9.22 The cystoscope is inserted through the hymeneal orifice.

Step 5

Be sure to visualize the cervix and the entire length of the vagina. The cervix is seen in this picture flush with the vaginal vault (*Fig. 9.23*).

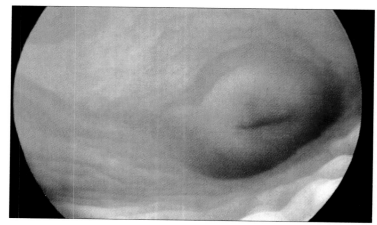

9.23 The cervix and vagina are inspected. The cervix can be seen at the vaginal apex.

CLITORAL REDUCTION

Androgens cause virilization of the external genitalia. The extent of such virilization depends on the timing, length of exposure, and the levels of androgens. In general, exposure to androgens after 12 weeks of gestation leads only to clitoral hypertrophy. Exposure at progressively earlier stages of embryologic development may also lead to retention of the urogenital sinus, fusion of the labioscrotal folds, and clitoral hypertrophy.

When significant ambiguity of the external genitalia is present, the true gender cannot be immediately determined. Surgical correction of ambiguous genitalia should be done only after completion of the medical and endocrine evaluation. Reconstruction of the female external genitalia is best accomplished in two stages. The first consists of clitoral reduction and should be performed before the infant's discharge from the hospital. The purpose of the surgical reduction is to achieve a female appearance of the external genitalia. When a reduction clitoroplasty is done, the surgeon should attempt to preserve the neurovascular connections to the glans. In this manner, a functional clitoris of normal size can be created. Removal of the entire clitoris is rarely indicated.

SURGICAL INDICATIONS

Surgical intervention is indicated in girls with clitoral enlargement sufficient to create conflict with the assigned sex of rearing.

SURGICAL PROCEDURE

Step 1

The skin overlying the clitoris is incised on both sides of the clitoris (*Fig. 9.24*). Dissection is then carried dorsally to isolate the neurovascular bundle.

Step 2

Once identified and dissected free from the phallus, the neurovascular bundle is displaced laterally. The corpora are transected just below the glans. The glans remains attached by the neurovascular bundle and the overlying dorsal skin (*Fig. 9.25*).

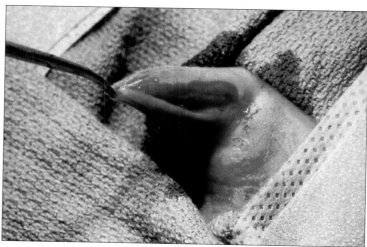

9.24 The skin of the phallus is incised.

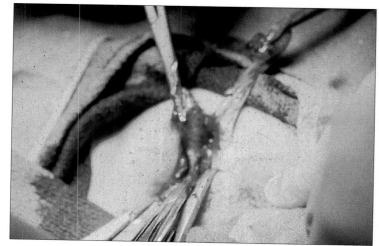

9.25 The glans is attached by the neurovascular bundle and the overlying dorsal skin.

Step 3

The corpora are transected at the base (*Fig. 9.26*). Two arteries are present at the base, and hemostasis is secured by proper placement of figure-of-eight sutures.

Step 4

The glans is trimmed and then is sutured to the base with interrupted absorbable sutures (*Fig. 9.27*).

Step 5

The skin is then closed over the new clitoris.

VAGINAL AGENESIS: THE McINDOE PROCEDURE

Individuals with vaginal agenesis are genetic females. They develop normally in adolescence and have all the usual feminine attributes. Unfortunately, because the Müllerian ducts fail to develop, the uterus and vagina are absent. A ruffled ridge of tissue represents the hymen, inside which there is an indentation marking the spot where the introitus would normally be found. In many patients other developmental defects are present as well, affecting the urinary tract (45–50%), the spine (10%) and, less frequently, the middle ear and other mesodermal structures. Therefore, at some time during childhood in any child with vaginal agenesis, there should be an evaluation of the urinary tract, the spine, and hearing. In addition, a chromosome analysis should be obtained on all patients with vaginal agenesis to rule out the rare instances in which vaginal agenesis represents the effects of testicular activity (testicular feminization syndrome). An exploratory laparotomy is not indicated in these patients, as the absence of the uterus can be confirmed by a pelvic sonogram.

SURGICAL INDICATIONS

The creation of a satisfactory vagina is the objective in treatment of vaginal agenesis, and this should be deferred until the girl is contemplating an active sex life.

SURGICAL PROCEDURE

Step 1

A Foley catheter is inserted into the bladder.

Step 2

The area which the vagina should occupy is a potential space filled with comparatively loose connective tissue which is capable of considerable indentation (*Fig. 9.28*).

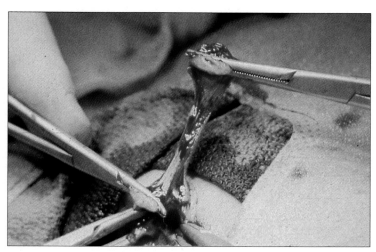

9.26 The phallus is transected at the base and just below the glans.

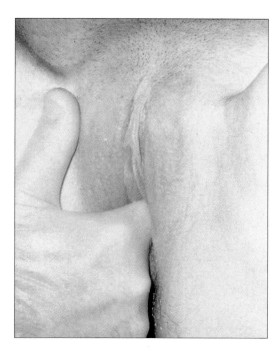

9.28 The vaginal dimple is very distensible.

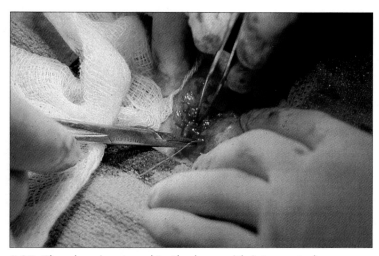

9.27 The glans is sutured to the base with interrupted absorbable sutures.

Step 3

Incise the mucosa overlying the introitus. Using a finger, bluntly dissect the space between the bladder and the rectum (*Fig. 9.29*). The operator may find dense tissue in the midline, which should be incised (*Fig. 9.30*).

Step 4

A mold is then covered with a split-thickness skin graft. Some surgeons prefer full-thickness grafts (*Fig. 9.31*).

Step 5

The mold is inserted into the newly created space and sutured into place (*Fig. 9.32*).

Step 6

The mold is removed a week later and the graft is inspected. Necrotic tissue is debrided (*Fig. 9.33*).

Step 7

The patient is then given a mold to maintain vaginal patency and to prevent contraction of the vagina (*Fig. 9.34*).

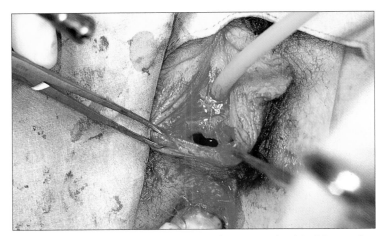

9.29 The surgeon dissects the space between the bladder and the rectum.

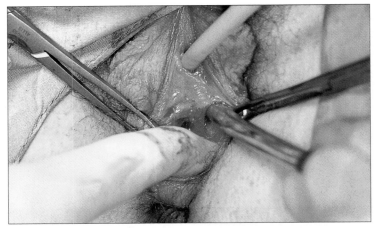

9.30 A midline structure separates a smaller cavity on either side.

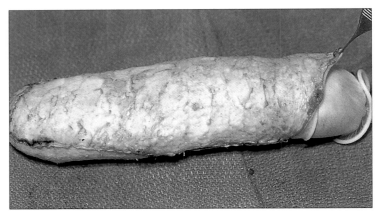

9.31 A mold is covered with a skin graft.

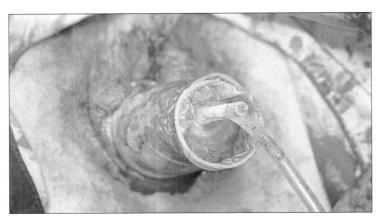

9.32 The mold is inserted into the newly created space and sutured into place.

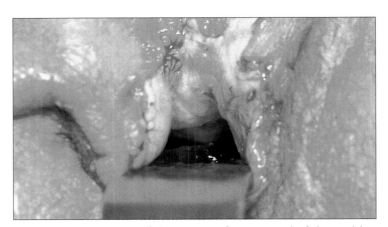

9.33 The appearance of the vagina after removal of the mold. Note the excellent take of the skin graft.

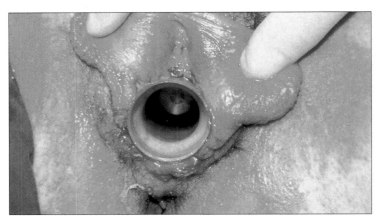

9.34 The patient is inserting a mold to maintain vaginal patency and to prevent contraction.

VAGINAL AGENESIS: THE WILLIAMS PROCEDURE

SURGICAL INDICATIONS

An alternative procedure is the Williams vulvovaginoplasty, which utilizes the labia majora to construct a coital pouch. The procedure is relatively simple and is not associated with skin grafts, scarring, or prolonged hospital stay. It can be done shortly before sexual activity is initiated. The axis of the coital pouch is different from that of the normal vagina. However, with continued use, it gradually changes to that of the anatomic vagina.

SURGICAL PROCEDURE

Step 1

A Foley catheter is inserted into the bladder.

Step 2

The labia are placed under tension. A U-shaped incision is carried down from the level of the urethra along the margins of the labia majora to the midpoint between the posterior fourchette and the anus (*Fig. 9.35*).

Step 3

The vulvar skin is dissected away from the subcutaneous fat to allow approximation without tension (*Fig. 9.36*).

Step 4

Closure is in three layers. First layer closure of the incision begins posteriorly and proceeds anteriorly, approximating the inner layer of skin (*Fig. 9.37*).

Step 5

Interrupted sutures are then used to approximate the subcutaneous tissues. The outer layer of skin is closed over the midline (*Fig. 9.38*).

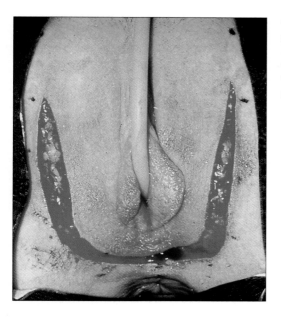

9.35 A U-shaped incision is made along the margins of the labia majora.

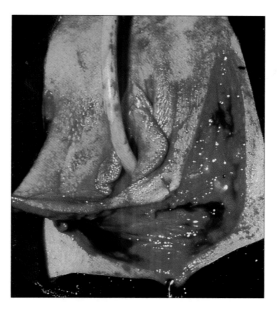

9.36 The vulvar skin is dissected away from the subcutaneous fat.

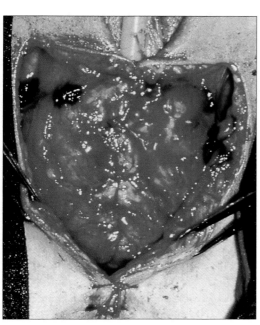

9.37 The inner layer closure begins posteriorly and proceeds anteriorly.

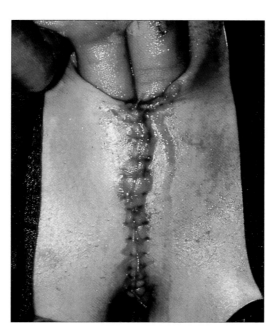

9.38 The skin is closed over the midline, creating a coital pouch.

REPAIR OF A UROGENITAL SINUS

The most prominent feature of congenital adrenal hyperplasia is virilization of the female fetus. An enzymatic deficiency, usually of 21-α-hydroxylase, causes increased production of adrenal androgens. Because adrenocortical function begins in the third month of gestation, the fetus is exposed to increased amounts of adrenal androgens at a critical time of sexual differentiation. Consequently, the infant exhibits signs of virilization of the external genitalia. Examination of the external genitalia of affected individuals reveals a single opening, the urogenital sinus, posterior fusion of the labioscrotal folds, and enlargement of the clitoris (*Fig. 9.39*).

The length of the urogenital sinus varies with the degree of virilization. In patients with severe virilization, the urogenital sinus is longer and the vagina enters into the proximal urethra. Therefore, urethroscopy is often performed to determine the urethral length and to identify the vaginal opening.

SURGICAL INDICATIONS

Repair of the urogenital sinus is required to create a vaginal introitus. The newly formed vaginal opening should be sufficiently large for intercourse and for vaginal instrumentation, e.g., insertion of a speculum.

SURGICAL PROCEDURE

Step 1

Inspect the external genitalia. In this particular instance (*Fig. 9.39*) there is a single opening, which represents a short urogenital sinus. Cystoscopy is performed to determine the relationship between the vaginal orifice and the bladder neck. The bladder, urethra, and sphincter function are evaluated as well. Although there is significant narrowing of the lower part of the vagina, vaginoscopy often shows a relatively normal upper vagina and cervix.

Step 2

An indwelling urinary catheter is then inserted into the bladder for drainage. It also identifies the urethra throughout the procedure.

Step 3

The future location of the vaginal orifice is marked on the perineum between the urethral opening and the anus. A semicircular incision is made and a skin flap is created, which will be used later to enlarge the newly created vaginal orifice (*Fig. 9.40*). To be viable, the width of the skin flap must be at least one and a half times greater than its height.

Step 4

A curved Kelley clamp is inserted through the vaginal orifice into the vagina and pushed downward and against the skin. It is used to estimate the distance between the vaginal wall and the perineal skin and to delineate the future vaginal orifice. The instrument, slightly open, is pushed against the perineum, which is incised in the midline. The vagina is thus being entered through its posterior wall (*Fig. 9.41*).

Step 5

A right-angled retractor is inserted into the vagina and the vaginal diameter is assessed (*Fig. 9.42*). If it is narrow, a midline incision through the posterior vaginal wall will increase the diameter of the vagina. Figure-of-eight hemostatic sutures are placed to control the bleeding from the perineal floor.

Step 6

The posterior vaginal mucosa is identified and is sutured to the apex of the previously prepared skin flap. Once these are approximated, the vaginal mucosa is advanced to the introitus (*Fig. 9.43*). The vaginal mucosa is then identified along its circumference and is sutured to the perineal skin. The operator must be certain that vaginal mucosa is closely attached to the perineal skin to prevent the formation of granulation tissue.

Step 7

After the vaginal mucosa has been sutured to the perineal skin, the small lateral V-shaped incisions are closed. A single suture at the apex will completely close the V-shaped incision (*Fig. 9.44*). A few interrupted sutures are used to approximate the remainder of the skin incisions. Meticulous approximation reduces scar formation and subsequent dyspareunia.

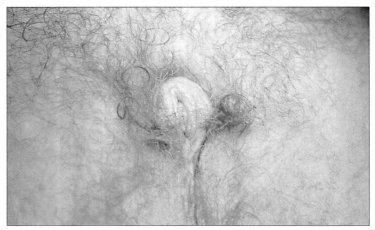

9.39 The external genitalia of a female patient with congenital adrenal hyperplasia. Note the small opening of the urogenital sinus beneath an enlarged clitoris.

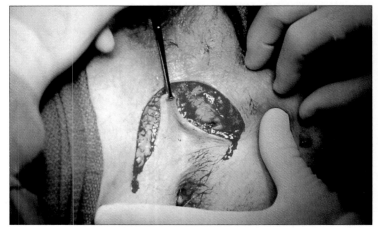

9.40 The future location of the vaginal orifice is marked on the perineum between the urethral opening and the anus. A semicircular incision is made to develop a skin flap.

Step 8

The size of the vaginal introitus is estimated by digital examination. An appropriately sized mold is inserted into the vagina and secured into position with a suture. The mold exerts local pressure to secure hemostasis (*Fig. 9.45*); it is removed 24 hours later. Intermittent use of vaginal dilators is required to prevent narrowing of the vaginal orifice. Although the appearance of the newly created vaginal introitus is not anatomically normal, it functions well (*Fig. 9.46*).

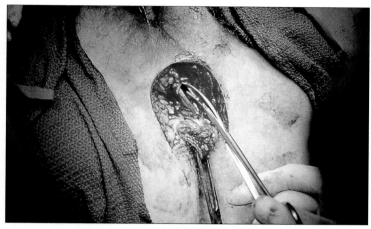

9.41 The thickness of the perineal floor is estimated with a curved Kelley. The perineum is then incised, and the vagina is entered through its posterior wall.

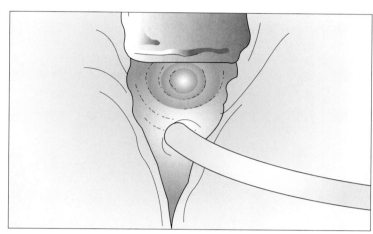

9.42 A right-angled retractor is inserted into the vagina and the vaginal diameter is assessed.

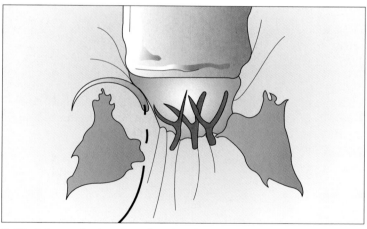

9.43 Schematic drawing showing how the previously prepared skin flap is sutured to the posterior vaginal mucosa.

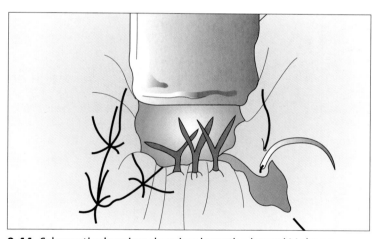

9.44 Schematic drawing showing how the lateral V-shape incisions are closed.

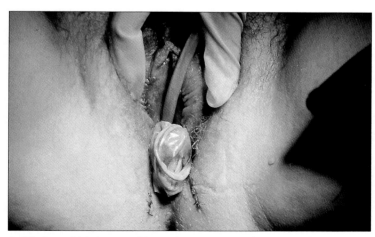

9.45 A mold is inserted into the vagina and is secured in position with a suture.

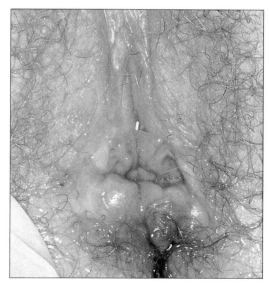

9.46 The appearance of the newly created introitus 6 weeks later. Note an adequate orifice. Sexual function was reported to be satisfactory.

LICHEN SCLEROSUS

Lichen sclerosus of the vulva is a hypotrophic dystrophy. The symptoms consist of vulvar irritation, dysuria, and pruritus. The lesions consist of flat, ivory papules which may coalesce into plaques. They tend to bruise easily, forming bloody blisters, and are susceptible to secondary infections. Scratching is common. Usually, these lesions do not extend laterally beyond the middle of the labia majora (*Fig. 9.47*). The clitoris is frequently involved as well as the posterior fourchette and the anorectal area. Histologically, typical findings include flattening of the rete pegs, homogenization of the dermis, and hyperkeratosis (*Fig. 9.48*).

SURGICAL INDICATIONS

In cases refractory to medical treatment, ablation of the skin lesions may result in symptomatic relief or even cure.

SURGICAL PROCEDURE

Step 1

Inspect the vulva and perianal region. All affected areas should be clearly delineated.

Step 2

Using the CO_2 laser, the affected areas of abnormal epithelium should be evaporated until the first surgical layer is reached (*Fig. 9.49*). Care should be taken not to cause thermal injury as this may cause disfigurement.

Postoperative care consists of meticulous perineal hygiene and the use of analgesics when required.

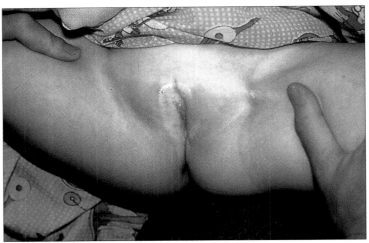

9.47 The typical appearance and distribution of pediatric lichen sclerosus. Note the white appearance of the vulva. The lesion does not extend beyond the midline of the labia majora.

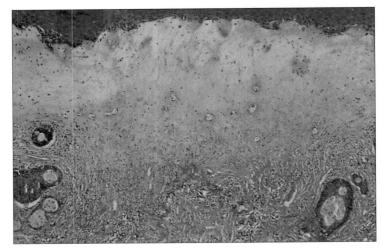

9.48 Histologic appearance of the lesion. Note the flattening of the rete pegs, homogenization of the dermis, and hyperkeratosis.

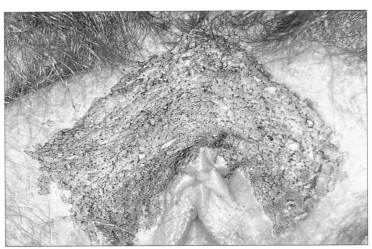

9.49 Ablation of the skin is accomplished using the CO_2 laser.

FURTHER READING

Ben-Ami T, Boichis H, Hertz M. Fused labia. Clinical and radiological findings. *Pediatr Radiol* 1978; 7: 33–5.

Capraro V, Capraro E. Creation of a neovagina. *Obstet Gynecol* 1972; 39: 545–9.

Carpraro VJ, Greenberg H. Adhesions of the labia minora. *Obstet Gynecol* 1972; 39: 65–9.

Cutler GB Jr, Laue L. Congenital adrenal hyperplasia due to 21-α-hydroxylase deficiency. *N Engl J Med* 1990; 323: 1806–13.

Davis AJ, Goldstein DP. Treatment of pediatric lichen sclerosus with CO_2 laser. *Adolesc Pediatr Gynecol* 1989; 2: 103–5.

Dewhurst CJ. Genital tract obstruction. *Pediatr Clin North Am* 1981; 28: 331–44.

Dewhurst CJ. Congenital malformations of the lower genital tract. *Clin Obstet Gynaecol* 1978; 5: 250.

Griffin JE, Edwards C, Madden JD, Harrod M J, Wilson J D. Congenital absence of the vagina. The Mayer-Rokitansky-Kuster-Hauser syndrome. *Ann Int Med* 1976; 85: 224–36.

Grumbach MM, Conte FA. Disorders of sexual differentiation. In: Wilson JD, Foster DW, eds. *Williams Textbook of Endocrinology*, 7th ed. Philadelphia: WB Saunders, pp 312–401 1985.

Huffman JW, Dewhurst CJ, Capraro VJ. *The Gynecology of Childhood and Adolescence*, 2nd ed. Philadelphia,WB Saunders,1981.

Ingram JM. The bicycle seat stool in the treatment of vaginal agenesis and stenosis: a preliminary report. *Am J Obstet Gynecol* 1981; 140: 867.

Jones HW Jr., Rock JA. *Reparative and Constructive Surgery of the Female Genital Tract*. Baltimore: Williams & Wilkins, 1983.

McIndoe AH, Banister JB. An operation for the cure of congenital absence of the vagina. *J Obstet Gynecol Br Emp* 1938; 45: 490–4.

Mercer LJ, Mueller CM, Hajj SN. Medical treatment of urethral prolapse. *Adolesc Pediatr Gynecol* 1988; 1: 182–4.

Monaghan JM. *Bonney's Gynecological Surgery*. 9th ed. London: Baillière Tindall, 1986.

Muram D. *Congenital Malformations. Textbook of Gynecology*. Copeland LJ, ed. Philadelphia: WB Saunders, Chapter 5, pp 121–41, 1993.

Muram D. *Pediatric and Adolescent Gynecology. Current Gynecologic and Obstetric Diagnosis and Treatment*. 7th ed. Pernol ML, ed. Norwalk, Appleton & Lange, Ch. 30, 629–56, 1991.

Muram D. *Pediatric and Adolescent Gynecology. Comprehensive Pediatrics*. Hughes JG, Summitt RL eds. St Louis: CV Mosby, 584–611, 1990.

Muram D. Vaginal bleeding in children and adolescents. *Obstet Gynecol Clin North Am* 1990; 17: 389–408.

Muram D, Elias S. The treatment of labial adhesions in prepubertal girls. *Surg Forum* 1988; 34: 464–6.

Muram D, Massouda D. Vaginal bleeding in children. *Contemp Obstet Gynecol* 1985; 27: 41–52.

Nowlin P, Adams JR, Nalle BC Jr. Vulvar fusion. *J Urol* 1949; 62: 75–9.

Reindollar RH, Tho SPT, McFonough PG. Abnormalities of sexual differentiation. *Clin Obstet Gynecol* 1987; 30: 697–713.

Rock JA, Azziz R. Genital anomalies in childhood. *Clin Obstet Gynecol* 1987; 30: 682–96.

Sanfilippo J, Muram D, Lee P, Dewhurst JC. *Pediatric and Adolescent Gynecology*. Philadelphia: WB Saunders, 1994.

Velcek FT, Kugaczewski JT, Klotz DH, Kottmeier PK. Surgical therapy for urethral propapse in young girls. *Adolesc Pediatr Gynecol* 1989; 2: 230–3.

Williams EA. Congenital absence of the vagina. A simple operation for its relief. *J Obstet Gynecol Br Commonw* 1964; 71: 511–16.

10

Fistulae

Thomas G. Stovall

Robert L. Summitt, Jr.

RECTOVAGINAL FISTULA REPAIR

Fistulae between the rectum and vagina are generally divided into anovaginal fistulae, those adjacent to or within 3 cm of the external anal sphincter, and rectovaginal fistulae, which are those > 3 cm above the external anal sphincter. Although most occur as a result of obstetric injury or after repair of a fourth-degree episiotomy, other predisposing factors have been reported (*Fig. 10.1*).

Rectovaginal Fistula
Fourth-degree episiotomy
Obstetric injury
Rectal injury during posterior colporrhaphy or other procedures involving the lower genital tract or anus
Perirectal abscess
Previous rectovaginal fistula repair
Inflammatory bowel disease
Systemic lupus erythematosus
Cul-de-sac obliteration (dissection during pelvic surgery)
Previous radiation therapy
Genital neoplasms
Idiopathic
Violence-induced
Foreign body
Congenital

10.1 Factors associated with the development of a rectovaginal fistula.

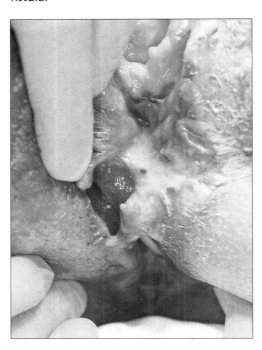

10.2 Characteristic findings in patients with Crohn's disease with vulvar manifestations include multiple fistulae, extensive excoriation, and multiple vulvar/rectal fissures.

Patients may present with complaints of gas or fecal loss but may also be asymptomatic. In young women who develop a spontaneous fistula, bloody diarrhea, weight loss, and vulvar lesions, or in patients with multiple fistulae, the possibility of Crohn's disease must be considered (*Fig. 10.2*). Patients with extensive disease such as demonstrated here require diverting colostomy with intensive local treatment before fistula repair.

SURGICAL INDICATIONS
The only indication for repair of a rectovaginal fistula is its presence in a symptomatic patient who requests repair. There is probably no need to repair an asymptomatic fistula. Whether or not a fistula should be repaired before a patient has completed her childbearing is controversial, but in our opinion this is not a contraindication to repair.

SURGICAL PROCEDURE
Preoperative preparation
The preoperative preparation of the patient may include a variety of bowel preparations including dietary restriction, mechanical preparation, or antibiotic prophylaxis. *Fig. 10.3* outlines several of these alternatives. There are no data demonstrating that these adjuncts increase the surgical success, nor are there data indicating that such preparation is detrimental.

Preoperative Adjuvants to Surgical Correction of a Rectovaginal Fistula
Laxatives
Magnesium citrate or Golytely
Enemas
Saline or soapsuds the day before and the morning of surgery
Antibiotics
Metronidazole 500 mg i.v. every 12 h the day before surgery and the day of surgery
Neomycin/Erythromycin: Neomycin 1 g by mouth at 10 AM, 2 PM, and 10 PM the day before surgery along with erythromycin 500 mg at the same time intervals
Diet
Low-residue 7 days before surgery
Full liquids 2 days before surgery
Clear liquids 1 day before surgery
Nothing by mouth after 6 PM on the evening before surgery

10.3 Regimens that can be used alone or in combination as preoperative adjuvants to surgical correction of a rectovaginal fistula.

Principles of repair

The surgical principles involved in the successful repair of a recto-vaginal fistula are similar to those for repair of other fistulae or hernias (*Fig. 10.4*).

Surgical Principles
Wide dissection of the surgical planes
Mobilization of tissue planes
Layered closure
Minimal tension on the repair
Treatment of the underlying condition
Small-caliber (#2-0, #3-0) synthetic absorbable suture material

10.4 Surgical principles involved in the repair of rectovaginal fistulae.

CONVERSION TO COMPLETE PERINEAL LACERATION WITH LAYERED CLOSURE

Step 1

Conversion to complete perineal laceration is used primarily when the rectal sphincter is disrupted (*Fig. 10.5*). The vaginal mucosa and rectal mucosa are cut sharply forming a complete perineotomy. This incision extends into the fistulous tract (*Fig. 10.6*).

Step 2

In a layered dissection, the vaginal mucosa is dissected from the rectal mucosa by sharp dissection. A 2- to 3-cm area should be mobilized around the fistulous tract. This allows layered closure without placing tension on the closure (*Fig. 10.7*).

Step 3

The fistulous tract is excised until the rectal and vaginal mucosa appear normal. This may require additional lateral dissection (*Fig. 10.8*).

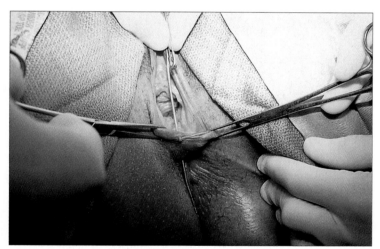

10.5 Identification of fistulous tract using a blunt probe.

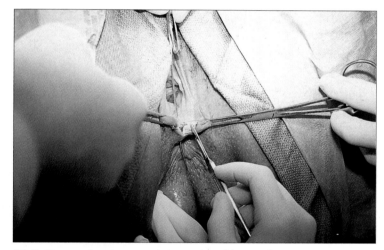

10.6 Conversion to complete perineal laceration.

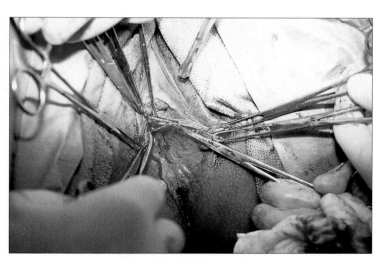

10.7 Mobilization of vaginal rectal mucosa.

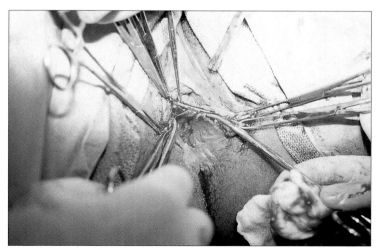

10.8 Completed dissection of rectovaginal fistula.

Step 4

The rectal mucosa is closed in two layers using a running suture of #3-0 delayed-absorbable suture material (*Fig. 10.9*). Our preference is to use a synthetic suture material such as polyglycolic acid. The puborectalis muscle is plicated to the midline as high as possible without constructing the vaginal orifice.

Step 5

The rectal sphincter is dissected so that the cut ends can be reapproximated. An attempt is made to preserve the capsule surrounding the muscle. The sphincter with its overlying capsule is grasped with an Allis clamp and brought to the midline. This step will, in effect, recreate the constricting function of the sphincter muscle. The sphincter ends are then reapproximated

with three or four interrupted sutures of a #2-0 delayed-absorbable suture material (*Fig. 10.10*). Some surgeons prefer a nonabsorbable suture for this step.

Step 6

The vaginal mucosa is closed with a #3-0 absorbable suture material using either a running continuous or an interlocking suture. The perineal body is reconstructed as the vaginal mucosa is approximated (*Fig. 10.11*).

TRANSVERSE TRANSPERINEAL APPROACH

The transverse transperineal approach is used if the fistulous tract is distal in the vagina in the presence of an intact sphincter (*Fig. 10.12*).

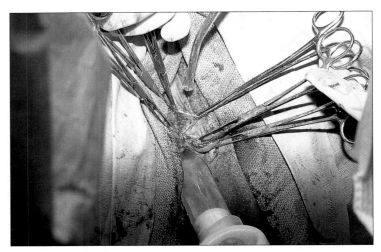

10.9 Rectal mucosa is closed in two layers and tested for complete closure.

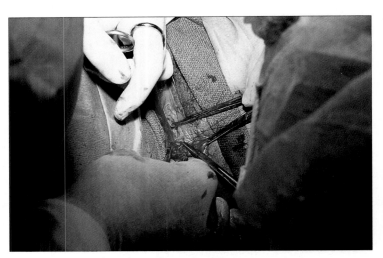

10.10 Reapproximation of rectal sphincter.

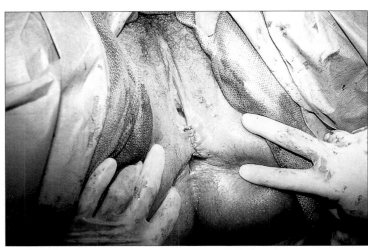

10.11 Completed closure of vaginal mucosa.

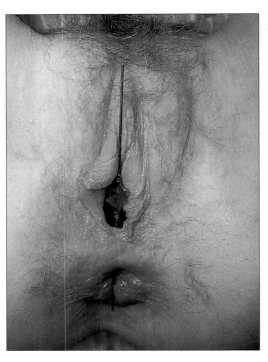

10.12 Demonstration of distal fistulous tract with intact sphincter.

Step 1
A transverse incision is made across the perineal body about 1 cm above the anus (*Figs 10.13, 10.14*). Both sharp and blunt dissection are used to dissect into the perirectal space.

Step 2
The vaginal mucosa is dissected away from the underlying connective tissue to a point above the vaginal opening of the fistulous tract, so that it is completely free (*Fig. 10.15*). The vaginal opening is then reapproximated using a #3-0 absorbable suture

material (*Fig. 10.16*). A second suture line is placed to incorporate additional connective tissue beneath the vaginal opening to reinforce the closure.

Step 3
The rectal opening of the fistulous tract is closed with either an interrupted or a continuous suture line so that the rectal mucosa is inverted (*Fig. 10.17*). A second suture line is placed to reapproximate the rectal muscularis and reinforce the initial suture line (*Fig. 10.18*).

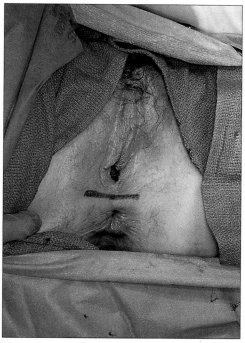

10.13 Marking demonstrates where transverse incision will be made.

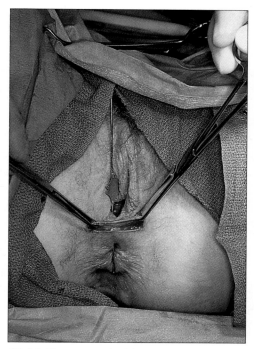

10.14 Transverse incision across perineal body.

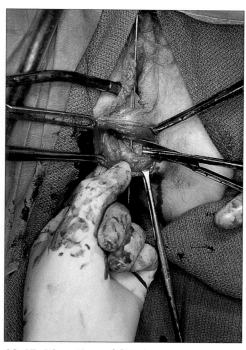

10.15 Dissection of fistulous tract.

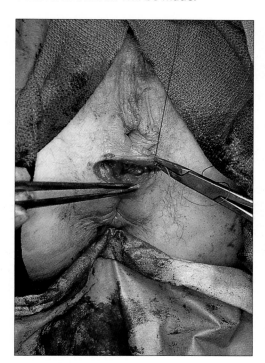

10.16 Closure of vaginal mucosa.

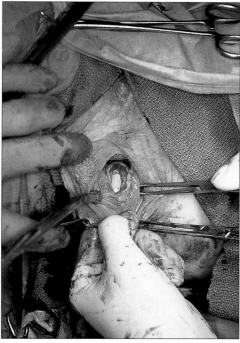

10.17 Demonstration of rectal opening of fistula.

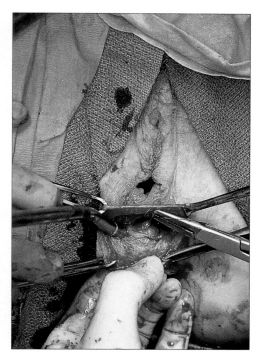

10.18 Closure of rectal mucosa.

Step 4

The perineal body is recreated and the perineal skin closed (*Fig. 10.19*).

TRANSPERINEAL ENDO-ANAL ADVANCEMENT

The transperineal endo-anal advancement is similar in approach to the transperineal approach and, in the same way, is best suited to the patient with a low rectovaginal fistula in association with an intact rectal sphincter.

Step 1

A semilunar incision is made just beneath the perineal body and just above the rectal orifice (*Fig. 10.20*). Both blunt and sharp dissection are used to extend the dissection into the rectovaginal space. This dissection mobilizes the rectal mucosa from the surrounding connective tissue (*Figs 10.21, 10.22*).

Step 2

The rectal mucosa is advanced until the fistulous tract is exteriorized and until sufficient length is obtained to ensure that there is no tension on the rectal mucosa (*Fig. 10.23*).

Step 3

The rectal mucosa is sutured to the capsule of the external anal sphincter with a series of interrupted #3-0 absorbable sutures (*Fig. 10.24*).

Step 4

The fistulous tract is then excised just distal to the suture line (*Fig. 10.25*). The remaining edge of the rectal mucosa is sutured to the perineal skin.

POSTOPERATIVE CARE

Much like the preoperative management of these patients, few scientific data exist to guide in their postoperative management. It is suggested that a patient is kept on a clear liquid diet for 24–72 hours, followed by a low-residue diet for about 2 weeks. A stool softener is used for 4 weeks and may be combined with mineral oil. An ice-pack can be used as an adjuvant to reduce swelling in the immediate postoperative period, and sitz baths are used to keep the area clean and to reduce postoperative pain.

EARLY REPAIR AFTER OBSTETRICAL INJURY

Early repair after breakdown of a fourth-degree obstetric laceration offers the advantage of avoidance of prolonged fecal and flatal incontinence. Hankins *et al.* reported 31 patients undergoing early repair with an excellent success rate. In this report, the average time from breakdown to repair was about 6 days. An outline for the management of these patients is presented in *Fig. 10.26*.

ALTERNATIVE PROCEDURES

Spontaneous closure of a fistulous tract has been reported and can be used for small openings. Once surgical repair has been selected, several procedures may be used. The selection of a particular procedure is dependent on the etiology, location, size, number of previous repairs, type of previous repairs, and the surgeon's experience.

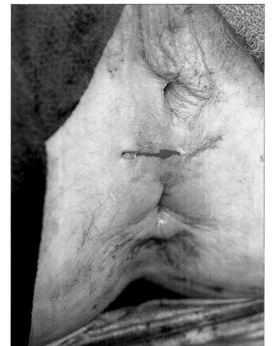

10.19 Perineal skin closure.

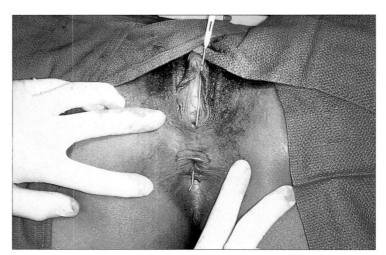

10.20 Demonstration of fistulous tract with marking for skin incision.

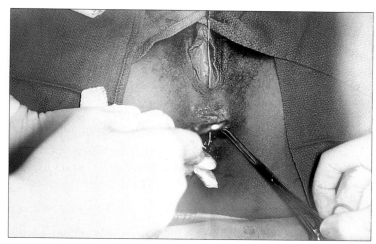

10.21 Dissection of fistulous tract.

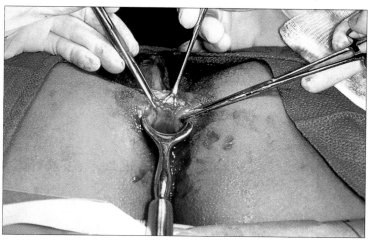

10.22 Mobilization of rectal mucosa.

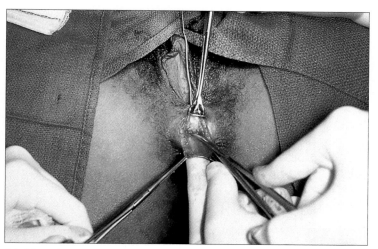

10.23 Advancement of rectal mucosa.

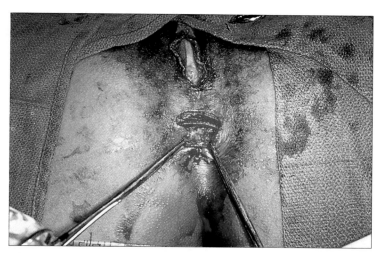

10.24 Attachment of rectal mucosa to external anal sphincter.

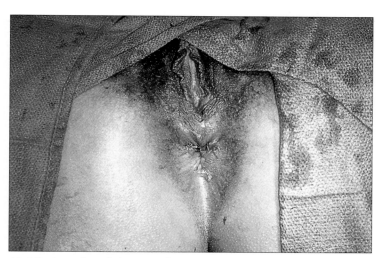

10.25 Completed closure of transverse incision.

Management Plan

Debridement of any infected tissue under intravenous sedation as soon as the breakdown is discovered

Wound is scrubbed and irrigated 2–3 times/day. The use of 1% lidocaine jelly applied topically helps to decrease the associated discomfort

Sitz baths or perineal irrigation are used after all bowel movements and after urination

A mechanical bowel prep using 1 l/h of Golytely until clear, colorless diarrhea

A single dose of preoperative antibiotics

Postoperatively, the patient remains NPO for 24–48 hours, followed by clear liquids for 48–72 hours. A low-residue diet is maintained for 2 weeks

A stool softener is used daily for up to 4 weeks so that there is no straining at the time of a bowel movement

10.26 Suggested management plan for the early repair of an episiotomy breakdown.

COMPLICATIONS

Potential intraoperative and postoperative complications of rectovaginal fistula repair are outlined in *Fig. 10.27*. The most common problem seen after rectovaginal fistual repair is breakdown of the repair or recurrence of the fistulous tract. This occurs most commonly in patients who have undergone previous repair or irradiation, or in those with inflammatory bowel disease.

VESICOVAGINAL FISTULA REPAIR: THE LATZKO TECHNIQUE

In the United States, benign gynecologic surgery is the most common etiology for development of a vesicovaginal fistula. Abdominal hysterectomy is the operation most likely to precede the formation of a fistula. Other procedures that may cause vesicovaginal fistula formation include vaginal hysterectomy, colporrhaphy, radical hysterectomy, and internal radiation therapy.

Vesicovaginal fistula formation after a hysterectomy most commonly occurs at the apex of the vagina or just anterior to the apex. The fistulous tract typically communicates with the bladder above the trigone and ureteral orifices. Because of this location, most vesicovaginal fistulae are amenable to a surgical approach through the vagina. An abdominal approach for repair can also be utilized but is usually reserved for recurrent or more complex fistulae.

The Latzko technique (or Latzko colpocleisis) is one of the most popular transvaginal methods for repair of vesicovaginal fistulae. Its simple approach leaves the fistulous tract in place and consists of a multilayer imbrication of the vaginal apex after denudation of the vaginal mucosa around the fistula. The success rate with this procedure exceeds 90%.

SURGICAL INDICATIONS

The surgical indications for the Latzko technique include primary vesicovaginal fistula and recurrent vesicovaginal fistula located at the vaginal apex.

SURGICAL PROCEDURE

Typically, the patient is placed in the dorsal lithotomy position before sterile preparation. However, some surgeons prefer to perform this operation with the patient in the jack-knife or prone lithotomy position, as they feel exposure is better. After draping of the patient, a transurethral Foley catheter can be placed for urine collection.

Step 1

After exposure with a weighted speculum and Deaver retractor, the position of the fistula in the vagina is noted (*Fig. 10.28*). As mentioned above, most vesicovaginal fistulae that develop after a hysterectomy are supratrigonal, and therefore the ureters are out of danger. The condition of the surrounding vaginal mucosa must also be inspected.

Potential Complications
Intraoperative
Bleeding
Rectal damage
Postoperative
Infection
Fecal/flatal incontinence
Fistula recurrence
Dyspareunia

10.27 Potential complications of rectovaginal fistula repair.

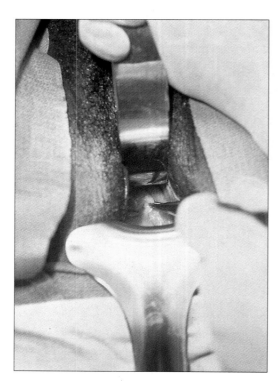

10.28 Demonstration of vesicovaginal fistulous tract.

Step 2

If exposure is still inadequate, the fistula can be drawn forward by placing one or more sutures through the vaginal mucosa around the tract. Once exposed, the vaginal mucosa is incised circumferentially around the fistula with a radius of 2–3 cm (*Fig.*

10.29). To facilitate removal of the mucosa, the circumscribed portion can be divided into quadrants (*Fig. 10.30*). The incised mucosa is then denuded by undermining, leaving the underlying vesical connective tissue and musculature undisturbed (*Figs 10.31, 10.32*). The fistulous tract can be left intact.

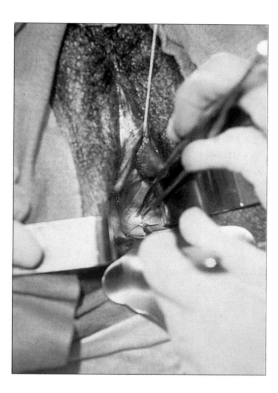

10.29 Excising the vaginal mucosa.

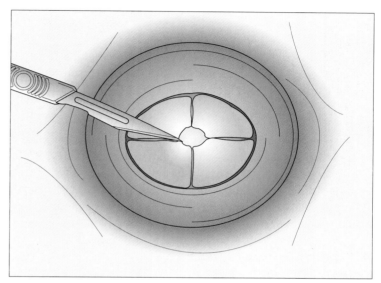

10.30 Demonstration of excision of vaginal mucosa.

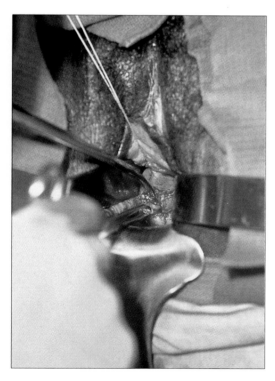

10.31 Removal of vaginal mucosa surrounding fistulous tract.

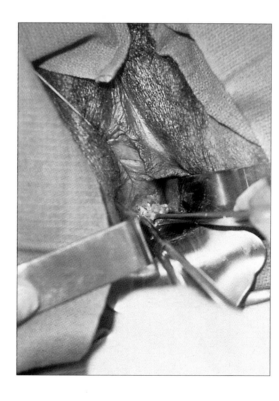

10.32 Completed dissection with mobilization of vaginal mucosa.

Step 3

An initial series of vertical mattress sutures is placed through the vesical tissue in a transverse axis, avoiding penetration into the vesical lumen (*Figs 10.33, 10.34*). We use a rapidly absorbed fine suture such as #3-0 chromic gut, but polyglycolic acid sutures can also be used. When the row of sutures is complete, they are all tied and cut, inverting the fistula (*Fig. 10.35*).

Step 4

A second layer of #3-0 polyglycolic acid mattress sutures is placed over the initial layer (*Figs 10.36, 10.37*), imbricating the first row of sutures when all are tied (*Fig. 10.38*).

Step 5

A final row of interrupted #3-0 polyglycolic acid sutures is placed to approximate the edges of the vaginal mucosa (*Fig. 10.39*). To reduce tension on the mucosal edges, the vaginal epithelium can be undermined and mobilized before the sutures are placed. When all sutures are tied, they are cut and the procedure is completed (*Fig. 10.40*).

ALTERNATIVE PROCEDURES
Catheter drainage

For small vesicovaginal fistulae, catheter drainage for 6–8 weeks may lead to spontaneous closure in 5–15% of cases.

Layered closure

Layered closures, with or without interposition of a bulbocavernosus fat pad, is an option for large vesicovaginal fistulae or for those that are located below the vaginal apex.

Transabdominal fistula repair

The transabdominal approach can be used for primary repair but is usually reserved for recurrent fistulae. The success rate approximates 100%.

COMPLICATIONS
Recurrence of fistulae

Fistula recurrence can usually be prevented by avoiding the placement of sutures that pass through both the bladder and vaginal mucosal layers. In addition, multiple layers of healthy tissue placed between the communicating organs prevents recurrence.

Ureteral obstruction

Obstruction of either or both ureters can occur as a result of excessively wide denudation of the vaginal mucosa combined with suture penetration into the bladder.

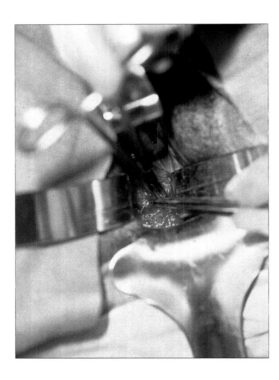

10.33 Placement of sutures to close vaginal mucosa.

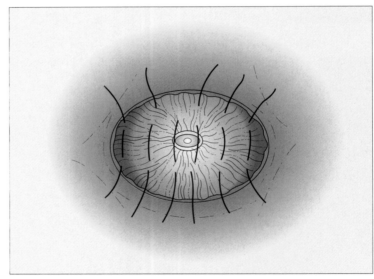

10.34 Demonstration of initial series of vertical mattress sutures.

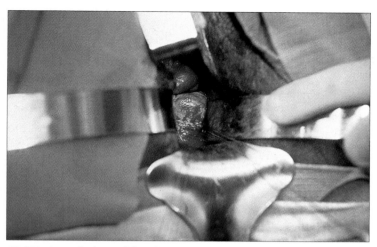

10.35 Completion of first layer closure.

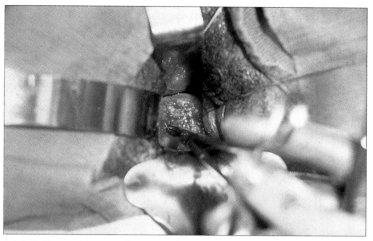

10.36 Second layer of suture closure.

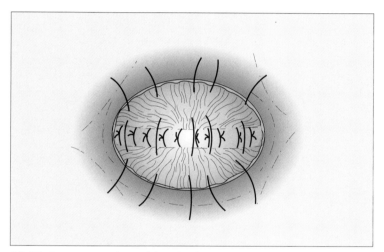

10.37 Demonstration of fistula closure.

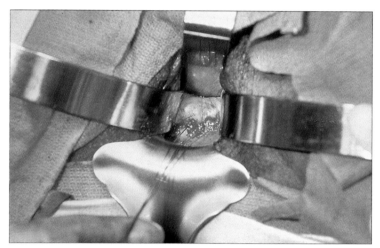

10.38 Completion of second layer of closure.

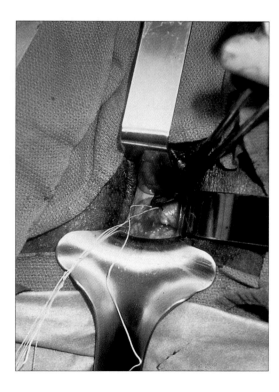

10.39 A third row of sutures can be place but is not necessary.

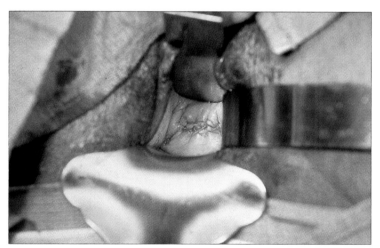

10.40 Completed closure of vesicovaginal fistula.

FURTHER READING

Hankins GDV, Hauth JVC, Gilstrap LC, *et al*. Early repair of episiotomy dehiscence. *Obstet Gynecol* 1990;75:48.

Hauth JC, Gilstrap LC, Ward SC, Hankins GDV. Early repair of an external sphincter ani muscle and rectal mucosal dehiscence. *Obstet Gynecol* 1986;67:806.

Hibbard LT. Surgical management of rectovaginal fistulas and complete perineal tears. *Am J Obstet Gynecol* 1978;130:139.

Lee RA, Symmonds RE, Williams TJ. Current status of genitourinary fistula. *Obstet Gynecol* 1988;72:313–19.

Mengert WF, Fish SA. Anterior rectal wall advancement. *Obstet Gynecol* 1955;5:262.

Nichols DH, Randal CL. *Vaginal Surgery*. 3rd ed. Baltimore: Williams & Wilkins, 1989:369–87.

Pepe F, Panella M, Arihian S, Panella P, Pepe G. Low rectovaginal fistulas. *Aust NZ J Obstet Gynecol* 1987;27:61.

Rothenberger DA. Christenson CE, Balcos EG, *et al*. Endorectal advancement flap for treatment of simple rectovaginal fistulae. *Dis Colon Rectum* 1982;25:297.

Thompson JD. Vesicovaginal fistulas. In: Thompson JD, Rock JA, eds. *TeLinde's Operative Gynecology*. 7th ed. Philadelphia: JB Lippincott, 1992:785–818.

11

Obstetrical Surgical Procedures

David Shaver

EPISIOTOMY

Routine episiotomy has long been recommended to reduce the incidence of perineal lacerations and to preserve the integrity of the pelvis during labor and childbirth. That disruption of the pelvic floor occurs as a natural consequence of vaginal delivery is not disputed. What has long been debated is the role of episiotomy in preventing this injury. More recently, much has been written about the role of episiotomy in actually increasing extension of perineal lacerations into the anal sphincter and rectum.

DeLee was one of the first obstetricians to recommend routine episiotomy to prevent injury to the fetal head and to hasten delivery. Pomeroy, in 1918, suggested that episiotomy should be practiced routinely in all primiparae.

It is clear that episiotomy results in a cleaner incision of the perineum than that resulting from a spontaneous tear. It is also apparent that extension into the rectum is more common in patients who undergo episiotomy than in those who do not. What is less clear and is still debated is whether episiotomy has any role in decreasing injury to the pelvic floor.

SURGICAL INDICATIONS

Most episiotomies are performed prophylactically. The alternative is to allow slow stretching of the perineum, coupled with careful control of delivery of the head and the aftercoming shoulders. Performance of an episiotomy is indicated if lacerations are felt to be inevitable or if a difficult vaginal delivery is encountered, such as with breech or occiput posterior delivery.

SURGICAL PROCEDURE

Two types of episiotomy are commonly performed (*Fig. 11.1*). The midline episiotomy involves an incision to the median raphe of the perineum and is the procedure most commonly employed in this country. Mediolateral episiotomies (either right or left) offer the advantage of a lower incidence of extension into a third- or fourth-degree tear but usually are associated with greater blood loss and greater discomfort during the puerperium.

MIDLINE EPISIOTOMY
Step 1

Blunt or rounded scissors are introduced along the midline of the perineum, and the incision is carried down to, but should not include, fibers of the external anal sphincter. The use of blunt scissors prevents lacerations and damage to the fetal scalp. Performance of the procedure after distension of the perineum is easier and is associated with less blood loss (*Fig. 11.2*).

Step 2

After delivery, a #3-0 absorbable suture is used to close the vaginal mucosa (*Fig. 11.3*). Care is taken that the suture is placed above the apex of the vaginal incision, and a running interlocking closure is performed down to the level of the hymenal ring (*Fig. 11.4*). At this point, the suture is passed through the vaginal mucosa and is brought out through the perineum underneath the hymenal ring (*Fig. 11.5*).

11.1 Demonstration of the two types of episiotomy commonly performed.

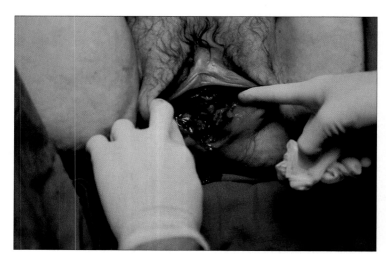

11.2 Prior to cutting the episiotomy, there is distension of the perineum.

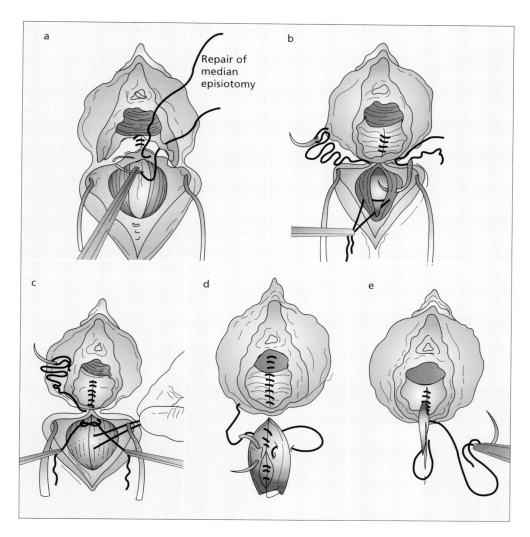

Repair of median episiotomy

11.3 Closure of midline episiotomy: **a** closure of vaginal mucosa; **b** approximation of perineal musculature; **c** perineal muscles closed; **d** closure of fascia over muscles; **e** approximation of skin with subcuticular continuous suture.

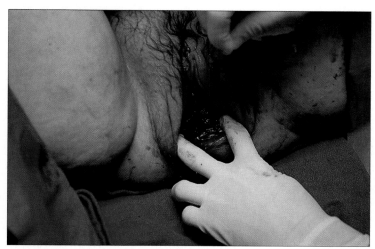

11.4 Placement of the suture above the apex.

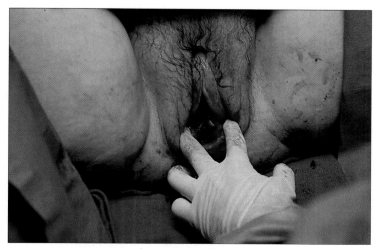

11.5 Suture placement at hymenal ring.

Step 3

This continuous suture is then utilized to incorporate the bulbo-cavernosus muscles at the upper margin of the incision, utilizing deep bites at right angles to the perineal incision (*Fig. 11.6*).

Step 4

Deep interrupted #3-0 absorbable sutures are then placed along the length of the perineal incisions to reapproximate the muscles of the perineum (*Fig. 11.7*).

Step 5

The original continuous suture is then run in a non-interlocking fashion to reapproximate the subcutaneous tissue down to the apex of the perineal incision (*Fig. 11.8*).

Step 6

The same suture is then run in a subcuticular fashion back towards the hymenal ring to close the skin. The suture is then tied at the level of the fourchette (*Fig. 11.9*).

MEDIOLATERAL EPISIOTOMY AND REPAIR

The technique of right mediolateral episiotomy is described.

Step 1

As with the midline episiotomy, performance of a mediolateral episiotomy after distension of the perineum by the fetal head eases performance of the procedure and is associated with less bleeding. The incision should start on the posterior fourchette at the 6 o'clock position and should be placed at an angle of about 30 degrees from the midline.

Step 2

After delivery, to reapproximate the vaginal mucosa a running interlocking suture of #3-0 absorbable material is again utilized, with care taken to begin above the apex of the vaginal incision (*Fig. 11.10*). Care must also be taken to place the sutures at longer intervals on the lateral margin of the incision to prevent an asymmetric repair.

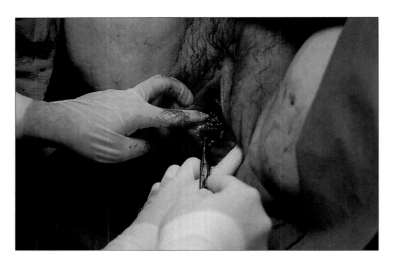

11.6 Reapproximation of bulbocavernosus muscle.

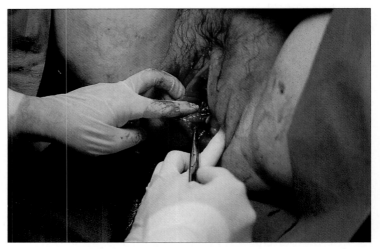

11.7 Reapproximation of perineum.

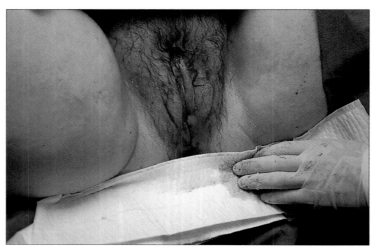

11.8 Closure of subcutaneous tissue.

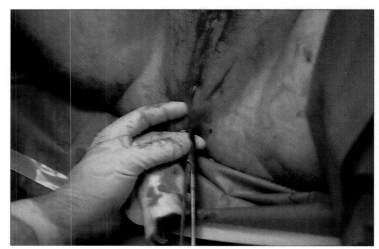

11.9 Closure of perineal skin.

Step 3

After closure to the level of the hymen, the suture is placed through the vaginal mucosa and is brought out through the perineum, and a deep crown stitch is again taken.

Step 4

Deep interrupted absorbable sutures are then placed at right angles to the perineal incision to incorporate the muscles of the perineum.

Step 5

The continuous suture is then carried down to the apex of the perineal incision to reapproximate the subcutaneous tissues.

Step 6

The same suture is then used to reapproximate the skin in a running subcuticular fashion. The suture is tied at the level of the hymenal ring.

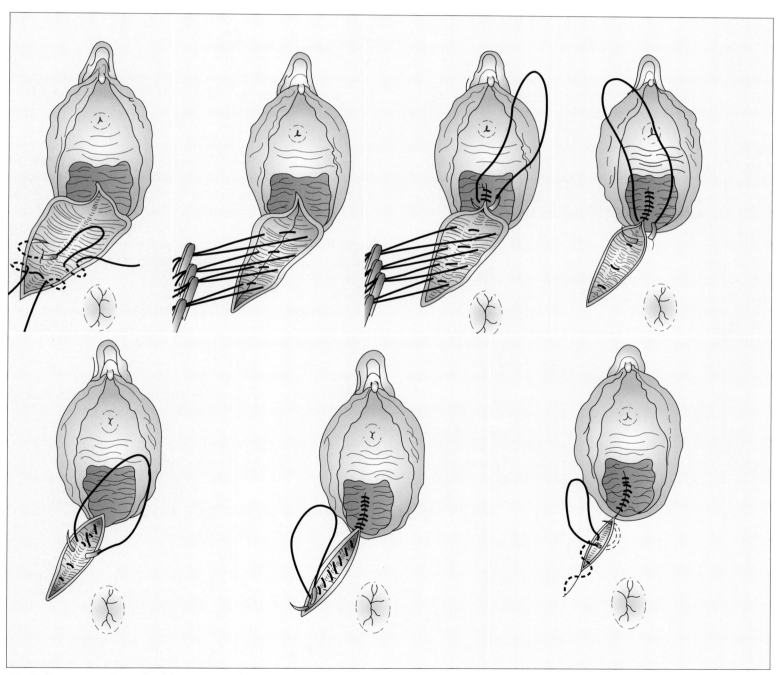

11.10 Demonstration of episiotomy repair.

OPERATIVE PROCEDURES FOR INCOMPETENT CERVIX

The term "incompetent cervical os" is used to describe a defect of the uterine cervix that allows painless dilatation and effacement of the cervix with loss of the pregnancy, usually during the second trimester. Although the etiology is poorly understood in most cases, the condition is thought to occasionally result from injury to the cervix by previous obstetric or gynecologic procedures. There is also an increased incidence of incompetent cervix in patients exposed to diethylstilbestrol *in utero* and in patients with coexistent uterine anomalies.

The concept of an incompetent cervix has been recognized since the seventeenth century, but only in the last 40 to 50 years have operative procedures for correction of the incompetent cervix been developed. Initially, preconceptional procedures were used. However, these soon fell into disfavor after procedures were introduced that could be performed during early gestation.

Most cerclage procedures are performed electively late in the first trimester or early in the second trimester in patients with a history consistent with an incompetent cervix. This timing enables the cerclage to be placed after the greatest risk of spontaneous abortion has passed and before the dilatation and effacement associated with the natural course of the cervical incompetence. Cerclage may occasionally be performed emergently when painless dilatation and effacement are discovered during the course of the pregnancy.

INDICATIONS

The procedure should be reserved for patients whose history is suggestive of an incompetent cervical os. Success rates of 75–85% are frequently quoted.

Emergent cerclage may be performed when a patient presents with painless dilatation and effacement, usually between 18 and 26 weeks' gestation. Procedures performed at this time are technically more difficult and are generally associated with a much lower chance of success.

It should be emphasized that cerclage does not appear to be of benefit in patients who are considered to be at increased risk of premature labor. Many studies performed on patients with multiple gestation or with a previous history of preterm delivery have shown no advantage with elective cerclage placement.

THE SHIRODKAR CERCLAGE PROCEDURE

Shirodkar was the first to describe a surgical treatment for incompetent cervical os performed after conception. The operation is designed to place a suture near the level of the internal cervical os to prevent dilatation of the cervix. Shirodkar originally described the use of fascia lata, but the procedure is most commonly performed now with the use of synthetic suture. The technique is more difficult than the McDonald procedure, and many modifications have been suggested to simplify it. The original report described the knot being tied anteriorly on the cervix, but there does not seem to be an advantage with either anterior or posterior knot placement.

SURGICAL PROCEDURE
Step 1
The posterior lip of the cervix is grasped with an atraumatic forceps (ring forceps or Allis clamp) and is pulled anteriorly to expose the posterior fornix.

Step 2
A short vertical incision is then made at the cervical vaginal junction, and blunt dissection is used to separate the mucosa from the underlying cervix. The cervix is pulled posteriorly and downwards, and a transverse incision is made at the cervicovaginal junction anteriorly. Again, blunt dissection is carried out to the level of the internal cervical os, which can be identified as the lowermost attachment of the bladder pillars.

Step 3
An Allis clamp is then used to bridge the tissue between the two incisions. The blade of the clamp is placed under the edges of both the anterior and the posterior incision.

Step 4
A Mersilene strip on an attached needle is then passed through the incision from anterior to posterior on both sides.

Step 5
The band is then pulled taut and tied posteriorly.

Step 6
The vaginal incisions are closed in a running fashion with fine absorbable sutures.

THE McDONALD CERCLAGE PROCEDURE

McDonald was the first to popularize a simple purse-string suture of the cervix for treatment of the incompetent cervical os. The advantages of the McDonald procedure were that it could also be carried out in early pregnancy and was extremely simple to perform. In addition, it was better suited for emergent procedures than was the Shirodkar procedure.

McDonald's original report described the use of #4 suture, which was tied anteriorly. Subsequent reports have described various permanent sutures and tying the knot either anteriorly or posteriorly. There appear to be no advantages with either technique, and operator preference is most important.

SURGICAL PROCEDURE
Step 1
The cervix is grasped on the anterior and posterior lips with an atraumatic clamp (ring forceps or Allis clamp). The cervix is pulled anteriorly and downwards, and a purse-string suture is placed around the circumference of the cervix at the cervicovaginal junction. Four to six bites are usually required. Re-entry of the needle with each successive bite is placed next to the exit of the previous bite to minimize the amount of suture exposed.

Step 2
The suture is tied anteriorly and the ends are left long to aid in identification for suture removal.

TRANSABDOMINAL CERCLAGE

Transabdominal cerclage was first described by Benson and Durfey in 1965. The procedure was introduced to allow treatment of those patients who were not candidates for the transvaginal procedure or in whom transvaginal procedures had failed in the past. Many reports have appeared since the original description; however, it still is a very selectively used operation, and there are no large series from any single institution.

SURGICAL INDICATIONS
As with any cerclage procedure, transabdominal cerclage is indicated only in patients whose history or examination is consistent with an incompetent cervical os. The transabdominal approach is usually reserved for patients in whom a transvaginal approach is considered impossible or likely to be associated with a very low success rate. Indications include:
- Patients with a very short or amputated cervix.
- Marked scarring of the cervix.
- Deeply notched or penetrating cervical or forniceal lacerations.
- Previous failed vaginal procedures.

SURGICAL PROCEDURE
Access to the abdominal cavity can be gained through either a midline or a transverse abdominal incision (*Figs 11.11, 11.12*).

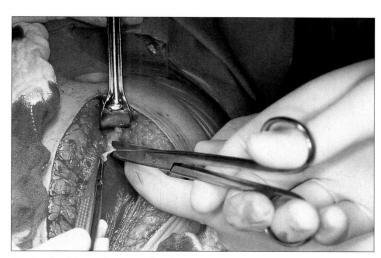

11.11 Midline abdominal incision.

11.12 Incision of rectus fascia.

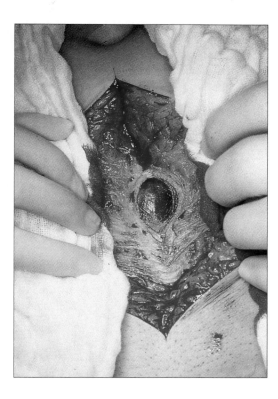

Step 1

The uterus is gently retracted superiorly (*Fig. 11.13*), and the loose visceral peritoneum is picked up over the lower uterus and dissected sharply laterally (*Fig. 11.14*). The bladder is gently dissected off the lower uterus in the midline (*Fig. 11.15*). Great care is taken to avoid dissecting too far laterally owing to the marked vascularity present in the pregnant state.

Step 2

An avascular plane (*Fig. 11.16*) is identified between the uterine vessels and the cervix at the level of the internal cervical os, which corresponds to the lower edge of the uterine isthmus (*Fig. 11.17*). The space is carefully dissected with right-angled forceps, and the posterior sheath of the broad ligament is perforated (*Fig. 11.18*).

Step 3

A 5-mm Mersilene strip on an atraumatic needle is then passed through this space and is brought around the uterus posteriorly.

Step 4

A similar procedure is carried out on the left side, and the Mersilene strip is brought anteriorly through this avascular space (*Fig. 11.19*).

Step 5

The suture is tied snugly anteriorly (*Fig. 11.20*).

Step 6

The cut ends of the Mersilene strip are then sutured to the uterus with #3-0 silk sutures (*Fig. 11.21*).

Step 7

The vesicouterine fold is then closed with a running suture of a #3-0 absorbable type (*Fig. 11.22*).

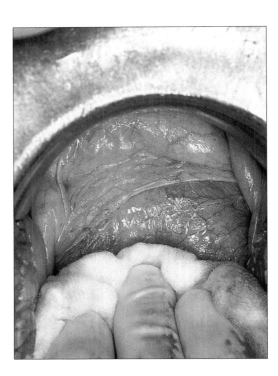

11.13 Retraction of uterus superiorly.

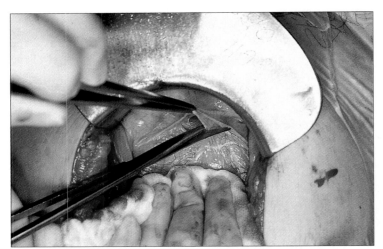

11.14 Peritoneal incision.

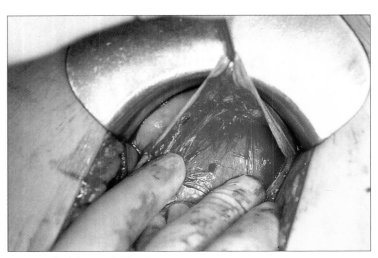

11.15 Bladder mobilization.

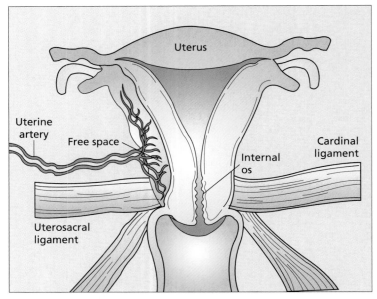

11.16 Demonstration of avascular plane between the uterine vessels and cervix.

COMPLICATIONS

The potential for complications with the transabdominal approach for cerclage is much greater than with the transvaginal approach. First, because of the marked vascularity in the area of the broad ligament, the potential for hemorrhage is markedly increased, as is the need for blood transfusion. Second, immediate abortion may

be more common, owing to increased manipulation of the uterus. Finally, because of the difficulty of cerclage removal, a cesarean section is necessary for delivery. More importantly, delivery of a nonviable fetus after cerclage placement may also require abdominal delivery or posterior colpotomy and division of the cerclage over the posterior aspect of the uterus.

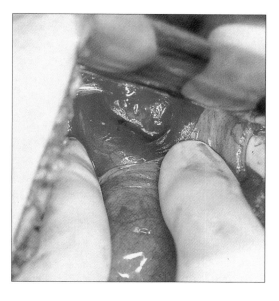

11.17 Avascular plane at the level of the internal cervical os.

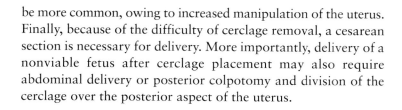
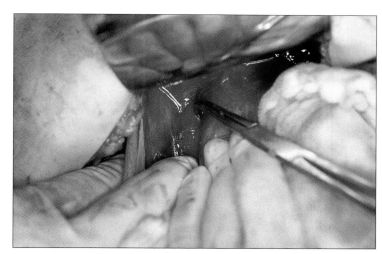

11.18 Perforation of posterior broad ligament.

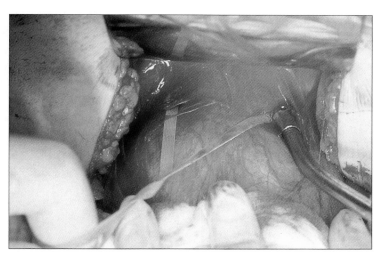

11.19 Placement of Mersiline strip.

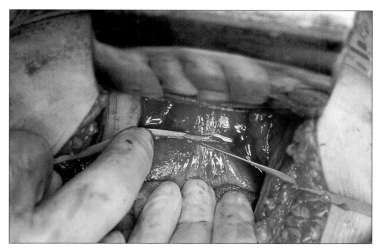

11.20 Tying of Mersiline strip.

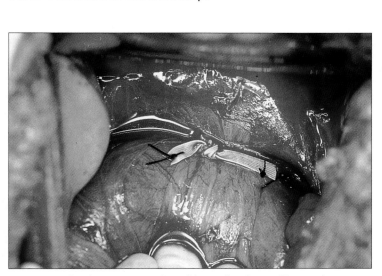

11.21 Anchoring sutures placed in ends of Mersiline strip.

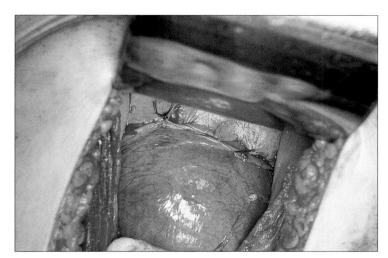

11.22 Closure of vesicouterine fold.

CESAREAN SECTION

There has been a tremendous increase in the use of cesarean section for delivery over the last 20 to 30 years. Although there is general agreement that the incidence of cesarean section is probably higher than necessary, this procedure continues to be utilized in a high percentage of cases. Most of the increase has been due to a perceived decrease in fetal morbidity and mortality when delivery is accomplished by abdominal delivery.

INDICATIONS

The indications for cesarean section are quite varied. They are frequently classified into fetal versus maternal indications, although this is arbitrary and indications often overlap.

Dystocia can be the result of dysfunctional labor such as arrest disorder. It can also be classified as mechanical dystocia, such as that caused by fetal macrosomia, or obstructive dystocia, such as that resulting from pelvic tumors.

Other indications for cesarean section include previous uterine surgery such as cesarean section or myomectomy; abnormal fetal presentation such as a breech presentation or a transverse lie; and fetal distress. Still other reasons include hemorrhage, such as with placenta previa or abruptio placentae; planned or indicated preterm delivery with an unfavorable cervix; active genital herpes; and cervical cancer.

SURGICAL PROCEDURE

Access to the abdominal cavity is usually carried out through either a Pfannenstiel or a low midline incision. Although advantages and disadvantages of both are widely quoted, both provide adequate access for performance of abdominal delivery in most cases.

Step 1

After entry into the abdominal cavity, the area over the lower part of the uterus is exposed. The non-adherent peritoneum of the vesicouterine fold is elevated and is incised transversely (*Fig. 11.23*).

Step 2

The bladder is bluntly dissected off the lower uterine segment.

Step 3

The uterus is then entered sharply (*Fig. 11.24*) with the scalpel in the midline. At this point, the uterine incision can be extended laterally using several different methods:

- By inserting the forefinger of each hand into the lateral margins of the uterine incision and forcibly splitting the muscles upwards and outwards.
- By cutting the uterine incision with scissors in a crescentic manner.
- By utilizing a stapling device.

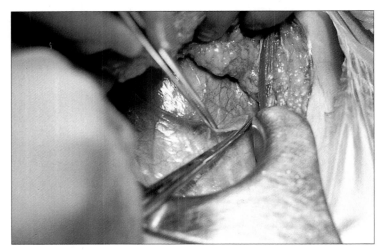

11.23 Incision of vesicouterine fold.

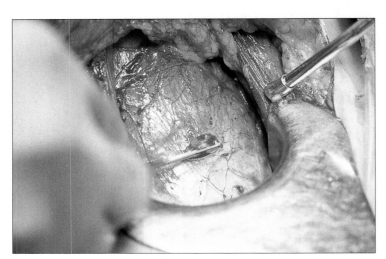

11.24 Initial uterine incision.

Step 4

After the incision has been made in the midline, the area to be incorporated into the stapling device is explored manually to ensure that no small parts or umbilical cord could be occluded by the device (*Fig. 11.25*). The instrument is then inserted into the incision and directed cephalad to form a V-shaped incision (*Figs 11.26–11.29*).

Step 5

The fetus and placenta are then delivered.

Step 6

After delivery, the uterus is exteriorized, and the uterine incision is adequately exposed (*Fig. 11.30*).

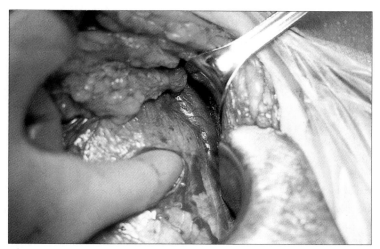

11.25 Exploration of lower uterine segment.

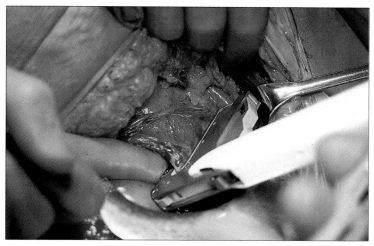

11.26 Insertion of stapling device over a finger for protection of the infant.

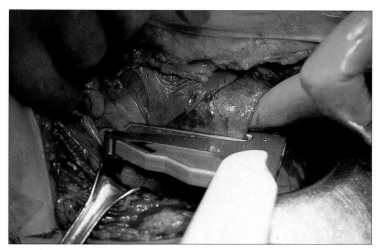

11.27 Recheck of stapler position.

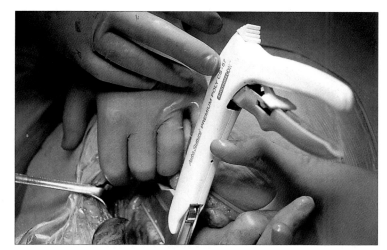

11.28 Repeat of procedure on opposite side.

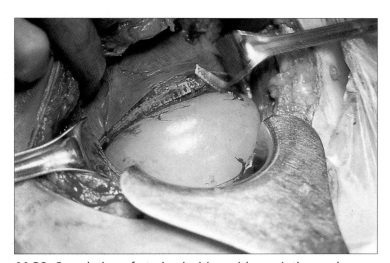

11.29 Completion of uterine incision with amniotic membrane bulging.

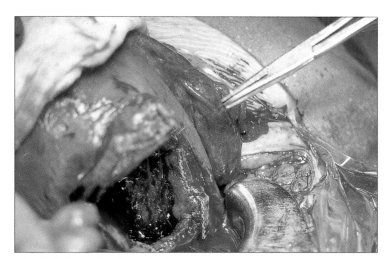

11.30 Exteriorization of uterus.

Step 7

The uterine incision is closed in a running manner with absorbable #0 suture in a single layer (*Figs 11.31–11.33*).

Step 8

The uterus is then placed back inside the abdominal cavity (*Fig. 11.34*).

Step 9

The fascia and skin are closed (*Fig. 11.35*).

COMPLICATIONS

Bleeding is more common with abdominal delivery compared with vaginal delivery. Typically, blood loss associated with a normal vaginal delivery is about 500 ml, whereas that associated with cesarean section is 1000 ml. Clearly, the potential for massive hemorrhage is increased with cesarean section.

The incidence of postpartum endometritis is also increased by abdominal delivery. Routine use of prophylactic antibiotics significantly decreases the incidence of this complication. Typically, a broad-spectrum antibiotic is administered after clamping of the umbilical cord. Unless overt infection is present, only 1–3 doses of antibiotics are necessary.

Occasionally, laceration of the uterine artery may occur, either as a result of incision across the uterine artery during development of the uterine incision or by extension of the uterine incision during delivery of the fetus. This can often be prevented if care is taken to be sure that the uterine incision is made in a U- or V-shaped manner. If laceration does occur, ligation of the uterine vessels is necessary to control bleeding.

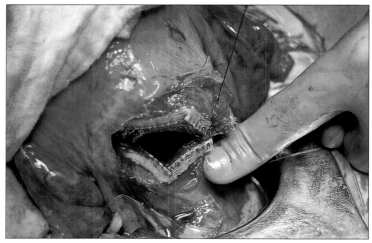

11.31 Closure of uterine incision.

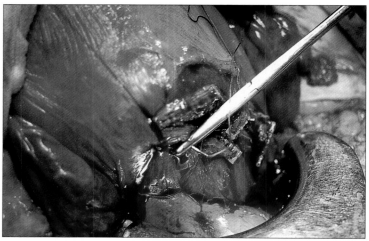

11.32 Closure of uterine incision.

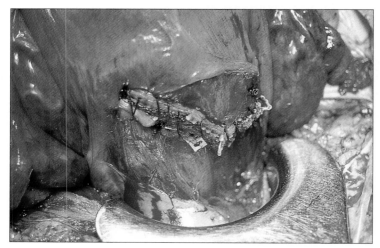

11.33 Completed closure of uterine incision.

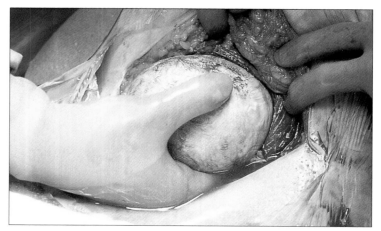

11.34 Intra-abdominal placement of uterus.

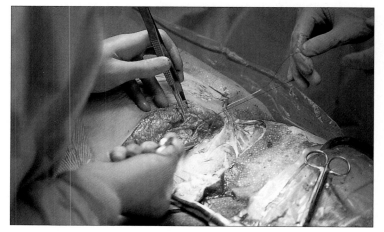

11.35 Rectus fascia closure.

Injury to other pelvic structures, especially the bladder, may occur. Bladder injury frequently takes place during entry into the abdominal cavity, especially in women who have undergone previous abdominal surgery, after which the bladder may be adherent to the anterior abdominal wall. Less commonly, injury occurs during dissection of the bladder off the lower uterine segment. If injury is recognized, immediate repair seldom results in any long-term complications. However, unrecognized injury to the bladder may lead to eventual fistula formation.

TECHNIQUE FOR REPLACEMENT OF INVERTED UTERUS

Uterine inversion is a rare complication in the immediate puerperium (*Fig. 11.36*). It is an obstetric emergency associated with a high incidence of hemorrhage and maternal mortality if not properly managed. The incidence is variously quoted as being from 1:500 to 1:20,000 but probably occurs in 1 out of every 2–3000 deliveries.

Many reports have suggested predisposing factors to development of uterine inversion. These include primiparity, short umbilical cord, fundal implantation, adherent placenta, and improper management of the third stage of labor. Indeed, undue traction on the umbilical cord is thought by many to be the primary risk factor for uterine inversion, although the rarity of the event does not enable this to be easily confirmed.

Prompt recognition and treatment of blood loss is an integral part of therapy, although shock out of proportion to the degree of blood loss is often mentioned in the literature. It is also probable that the amount of blood loss is frequently underestimated.

Manual replacement of the uterus should be attempted initially when uterine inversion is recognized. This method is successful in most cases of uterine inversion. It is important that any uterotonic agents are discontinued before attempted replacement of the uterus. The use of general anesthesia, beta-mimetics, or tocolytic agents such as magnesium sulfate may be helpful in relaxing the cervical ring and enabling the uterus to be replaced more easily. Debate exists as to whether or not the placenta should be manually detached before replacement of the uterus.

HYDROSTATIC TECHNIQUE OF O'SULLIVAN

Although often discounted by various authors as being of historical interest only, the hydrostatic technique is frequently successful in replacing a uterus that cannot be manually replaced. Conceptually, it appears to be successful because of the equal pressure that it places on the lateral fornices of the vagina, which creates distension of the cervical ring while at the same time placing pressure on the fundus of the uterus, thus allowing slow return to its original position (*Fig. 11.37*).

TECHNIQUE
Step 1
A receptacle with a large-bore tubing, such as an enema bag, is used for the procedure. The bag and tubing are filled with saline.

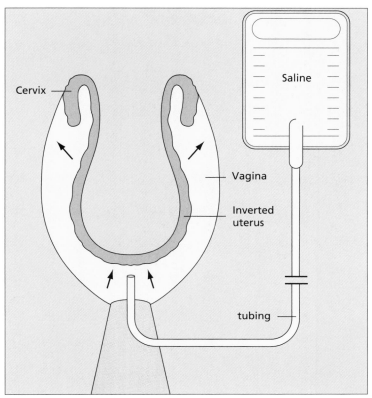

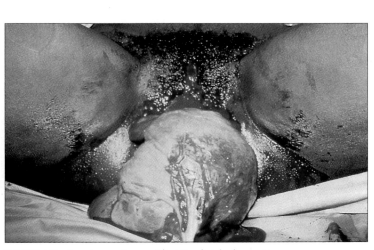

11.36 Uterine inversion with attached placenta.

11.37 Hydrostatic technique of O'Sullivan.

Step 2
The uterus is replaced in the vagina (*Fig. 11.38*).

Step 3
The tubing is then introduced into the vagina, and the introitus is manually occluded (*Fig. 11.39*). Saline is continuously added to the receptacle, which is held several feet above the level of the patient's introitus (*Fig. 11.40*).

Step 4
The uterus is slowly returned to its original position. The fundus can be visualized as it returns to its abdominal position. Tocolytic agents may be helpful in allowing relaxation of the cervical ring.

Step 5
After replacement of the uterus (*Fig. 11.41*), uterotonic agents are given to cause contraction of the uterus.

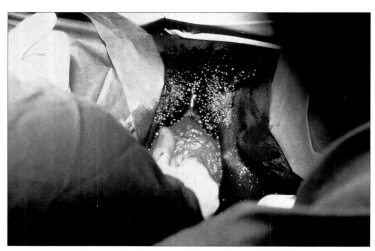

11.38 Placement of uterus in vagina.

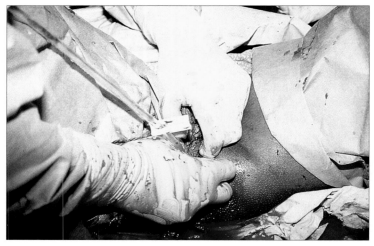

11.39 Insertion of tubing into vagina.

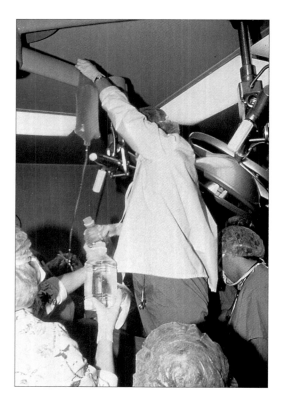

11.40 Saline infusion.

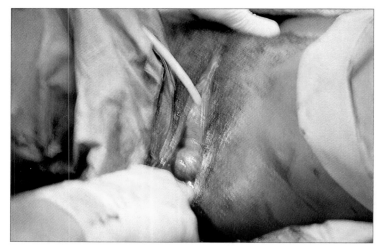

11.41 Uterus in proper anatomic position.

FURTHER READING

Combs CA, Robertson PA, Laros RK. Risk factors for third and fourth degree lacerations in forceps and vacuum deliveries. *Am J Obstet Gynecol* 1990;163:100.

Druzin ML, Berkley AS. A simplified approach to Shirodkar cerclage procedure. *Surg Gynecol Obstet* 1986;162:375.

Harger JH. Comparison of success and morbidity in cervical cerclage procedures. *Obstet Gynecol* 1980;56:543.

Kerr JMM. The technic of Cesarean section, with special reference to the lower uterine segment incision. *Am J Obstet Gynecol* 1926;12:729.

Novy MJ. Transabdominal cervicoisthmic cerclage for the management of repetitive abortion and premature delivery. *Am J Obstet Gynecol* 1982;143:44.

Phelan JP, Clark SL. Cesarean delivery – the transperitoneal approach. In: Phelan JP, Clark SL (eds.) *Cesarean Delivery* New York: Elsevier, 1988;201–214.

Thorp JM, Bowes WA, Brame RG Cefalo R. Selected use of midline episiotomy: effect on perineal trauma. *Obstet Gynecol* 1987;70:260.

Treadwell MC, Bronsteen RA, Bottoms SF. Prognostic factors and complication rates for cervical cerclage: a review of 482 cases. *Am J Obstet Gynecol* 1991;165:555.

Wilcox LS, Strobino DM, Baruffi G, Dellinger NS. Episiotomy and its role in the incidence of perineal lacerations in a maternity center and a tertiary hospital obstetric service. *Am J Obstet Gynecol* 1989;160:1047.

12

Pregnancy Termination

Lee P. Shulman

Frank W. Ling

PREGNANCY TERMINATION

Since the legalization of abortion throughout the USA in the early 1970s, obstetrician/gynecologists, family practitioners, and surgeons have made available such procedures to women during the first and second trimesters of pregnancy. Pregnancy termination can be divided into three categories, based on the indication for the abortion: elective, fetal (e.g., diagnosis of fetal abnormalities), or maternal (e.g., maternal Eisenmenger syndrome). Although the vast majority of pregnancy terminations performed in the USA are for elective indications, the techniques used for all pregnancy terminations are fundamentally the same

Even obstetrician/gynecologists who do not perform elective pregnancy terminations are frequently called on to carry out uterine evacuation procedures on women who present with nonviable fetuses or hydatidiform moles. This chapter reviews uterine evacuation techniques for first-trimester pregnancies, second-trimester pregnancies, nonviable pregnancies, and the management of complications resulting from uterine evacuation procedures.

FIRST-TRIMESTER PREGNANCY TERMINATION

Physicians who perform first-trimester pregnancy terminations should obtain a comprehensive history from all patients desiring first-trimester termination (i.e., pregnancy termination performed at or before 13 weeks of gestation), regardless of the indication for the procedure. *Fig. 12.1* outlines the information that should be obtained before pregnancy termination is undertaken.

All patients who present for first-trimester pregnancy termination, irrespective of the indication for the procedure, should be informed of the procedure's risks; a signed informed consent should therefore be obtained from all patients. The physician should also perform a physical examination before the procedure, with particular attention to uterine size and position. A complete blood count, blood type and Rh, and indirect Coombs' test should also be performed. Other laboratory tests may be necessary on the basis of the individual patient's past medical or surgical history. Local anesthesia, such as a paracervical block, is usually sufficient for most procedures; spinal, epidural, or general anesthesia can also be used according to patient wishes and the indications for the procedure. The risks and benefits of regional or general anesthesia should be reviewed with all patients who request either of these.

SURGICAL PROCEDURE
Step 1
After the patient empties her bladder, a bimanual pelvic examination is performed. If the uterine size is more than 3 weeks different from that for the gestational age based on menstrual history, an ultrasonographic examination should be obtained to confirm gestational age (*Fig. 12.2*).

Step 2
A Graves'-type vaginal speculum is inserted into the vagina and the cervix is visualized (*Fig. 12.3*).

Step 3
The vagina is cleansed with an iodine-based solution, using cotton swabs (*Fig. 12.4*).

Step 4
A single-toothed tenaculum is placed at the 12 o'clock position on the anterior cervical lip (*Figs 12.5–12.8*). A clear and unimpeded view of the cervix is required for safe performance of procedures that involve instrumentation of the cervix or the intrauterine cavity.

Historical Parameters

Age, gravidity, parity

Last menstrual period or other indications of gestational age

Indication for procedure

Any problems with current pregnancy

Past medical and surgical history

Past gynecologic history

Outcome and problems in all previous pregnancies

Allergies

Drug/medication use

12.1 Historical parameters of importance on patients undergoing uterine evacuation.

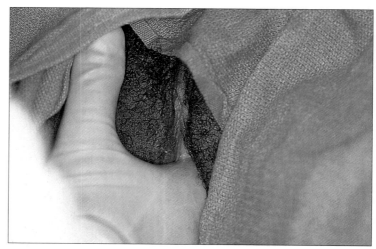

12.2 Bimanual examination to determine uterine size.

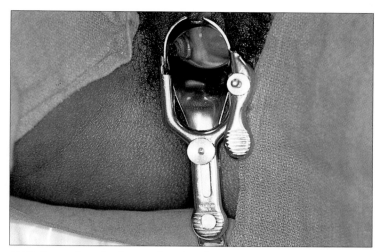

12.3 Graves' vaginal speculum in place.

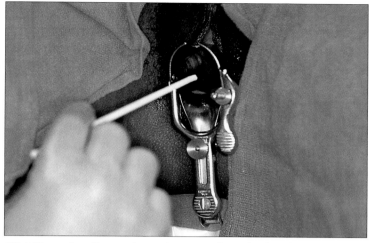

12.4 Cleansing the vagina using a swab soaked with iodine-based solution.

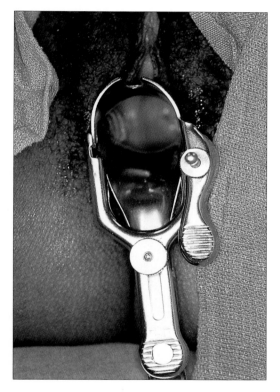

12.5 Visualizing the cervix following application of betadine solution.

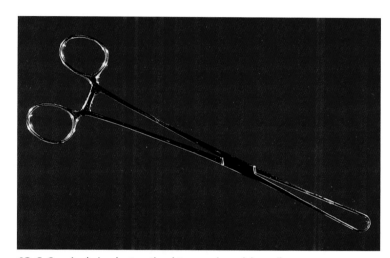

12.6 Cervical single-toothed tenaculum (closed).

12.8 Cervical tenaculum applied to anterior lip (12 o'clock) of cervix.

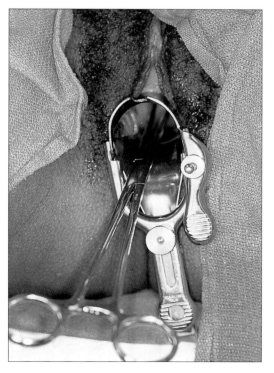

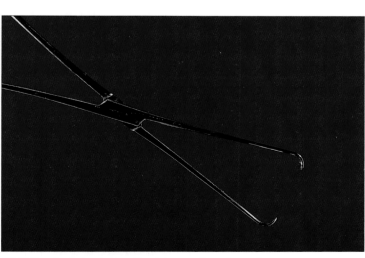

12.7 Cervical single-toothed tenaculum (open).

Step 5

A paracervical block is placed, using 10 ml of 1% lidocaine with epinephrine. A 20-gauge spinal needle is inserted at the 4 o'clock and 8 o'clock positions of the cervix (5 ml at each injection site) (*Figs 12.9, 12.10*). Before injection of lidocaine, 3–5 ml of negative pressure is applied to prevent intravascular injection.

Some authors suggest that a uterine sound be inserted through the cervical os to further assess uterine and cervical orientation and uterine size. The concern with such instrumentation, however, is the added risk of uterine perforation caused by the narrow-caliber sound.

Step 6

The os is gently dilated with manual dilators (*Fig. 12.11*). If Hegar dilators are used, dilation is sequentially performed to the dilator number that is equal to the weeks of gestation (e.g., No.

9 dilator if the patient is at 9 weeks' gestation). If French/Pratt dilators are used (*Fig. 12.12*), the dilator number is divided by 3 and dilation is done using the number closest to or slightly greater than the weeks' gestation (e.g., a No. 31 dilator if the patient is at 10 weeks' gestation. This set of Pratt dilators ranges from No. 13 (4.33 mm diameter) to 43 (14.33 mm diameter). Each individual dilator has two different diameters on each end, with one being two sizes larger than the other (e.g., one dilator has a No. 13 and a No. 15 end). In addition, each larger dilator increases by two sizes (e.g., the next larger dilator after the 13/15 dilator is a 17/19 dilator) over the previous dilator. Extreme force is never used to dilate the cervix; if smooth dilation is not initially achieved, uterine and cervical orientation should be reassessed and the dilator rotated along its axis during dilation. If the dilation does not progress smoothly, consideration of ultrasonographic guidance is warranted.

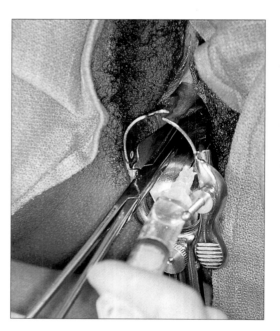

12.9 Negative pressure aspiration prior to injection of paracervical block; this step is performed to ensure that the injection will not be intravascular.

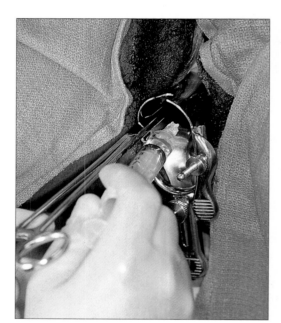

12.10 Injection of lidocaine for paracervical block.

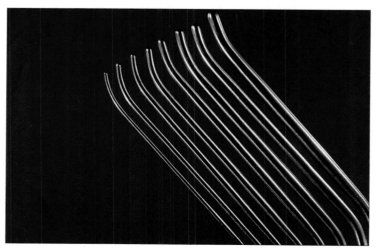

12.11 A set of Pratt dilators used for first-trimester procedures.

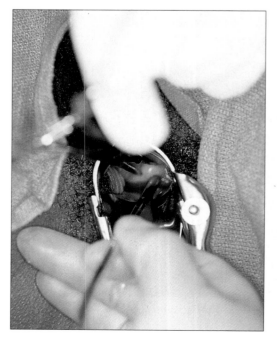

12.12 Insertion of dilator into the cervix.

Step 7

A suction curette commensurate with the gestational age (e.g., a 12 mm suction curette is used for a pregnancy at 12 weeks' gestation) is inserted into the fundus. Some authors suggest that the curette should only be inserted as far as the lower uterine segment to minimize the risk of perforation (*Figs 12.13, 12.14*). The vacuum should not be activated during insertion. After connection to the vacuum machine and the commencement of aspiration, the curette is gently rotated along its longitudinal axis (*Fig. 12.15*) and is then gradually withdrawn. Short, choppy forward and backward movements with the curette should be avoided, as this may predispose to uterine perforation.

Step 8

After completion of aspiration, sharp curettage, using the largest curette that can be introduced into the uterine cavity, should be performed to ascertain whether any products of conception remain within the uterine cavity (*Figs 12.16–12.18*). A "gritty" sensation usually indicates that the uterine cavity is empty. Sharp curettage should not be very vigorous, as this may predispose to uterine scarring and potential problems with dysmenorrhea and infertility in the future. Suction curettage should again be performed if retained products of conception are found. Ultrasonography may be helpful for determining the presence of retained products of conception.

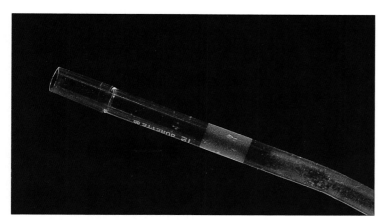

12.13 A curved #10 suction curette.

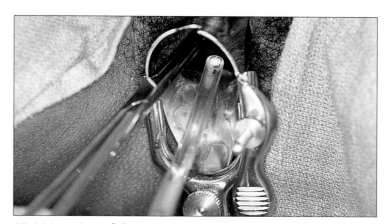

12.14 Insertion of the suction curette through the vagina.

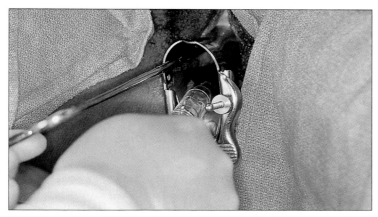

12.15 Insertion of the suction curette through the cervix and into the uterine cavity.

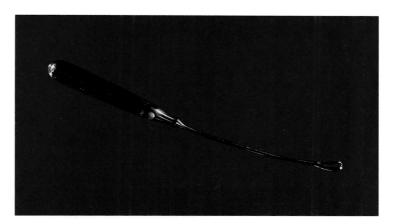

12.16 A sharp metal curette.

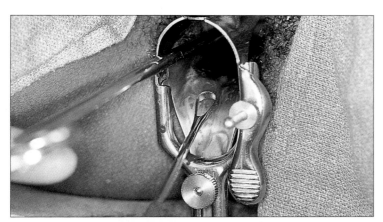

12.17 Insertion of the sharp metal curette through the vagina.

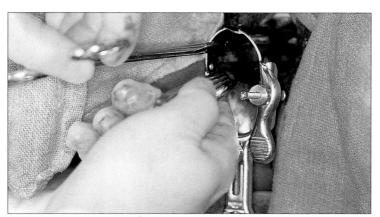

12.18 Insertion of the sharp metal curette through the cervix and into the uterine cavity.

Step 9

Once the uterine cavity is empty, the instruments are removed and a bimanual pelvic examination is performed to assess size and firmness and to evaluate for the presence of adnexal masses, such as a developing broad ligament hematoma. The products of conception are examined to determine if the quantity of tissue obtained is appropriate for the gestational age.

Step 10

A 10-day course of doxycycline (100 mg p.o. b.i.d.) and a four-dose regimen of methylergonovine maleate (0.2 mg p.o. q4h) is started after the procedure. Unsensitized Rh-negative patients should receive 300 μg Rh-immune globulin (Rhogam). Patients should be monitored for 20–30 min for any untoward effects (e.g., bleeding, abdominal pain, hypotension) before discharge and should be encounraged to return in 10–14 days for a post-operative examination.

SECOND-TRIMESTER PREGNANCY TERMINATION BY DILATION AND EVACUATION

The major difference between first- and second-trimester pregnancy termination techniques is that second-trimester pregnancy termination is a two-step procedure, necessitated by the relatively large size of the fetus and placenta. Second-trimester pregnancy termination (i.e., pregnancy termination performed between 14 and 23 gestational weeks) should include placement of osmotic dilators that more slowly and safely dilate the cervix compared with the manual cervical dilation performed in first-trimester procedures. This is done because cervical laceration is more common in procedures that require extensive dilation. Although suction curettage can be used to terminate pregnancies from 14 to 16 weeks of gestation, for pregnancies of these gestational ages curettage should still be preceded by osmotic dilation.

Osmotic dilators can be divided into two types: synthetic (e.g.,

Lamicel and Dilpan) and natural (laminaria tents) (*Fig. 12.19*). Synthetic dilators achieve maximal dilation in a shorter period of time (i.e., 4–8 h), than with natural osmotic dilators (10–14 h). Therefore, synthetic osmotic dilators can be used for 1-day procedures, whereas laminaria tents require the patient to return the next day for uterine evacuation. At our center, synthetic osmotic dilators are used for uterine evacuation procedures performed at 17 weeks' gestation or less and laminaria tents for procedures performed at 18 weeks' gestation or later.

Preoperative information, testing, and informed consent are similar to those for first-trimester procedures. Women undergoing uterine evacuation during the second trimester are candidates for an ultrasound examination before dilator placement to assess gestational age, number of fetuses, placental location, and fetal viability. Introduction of osmotic dilators is as follows.

DILATION

Step 1

A vaginal speculum is inserted (see *Fig. 12.3*).

Step 2

The vagina is washed with iodine-based solution (see *Fig. 12.4*).

Step 3

A singled-toothed tenaculum is placed at the 12 o'clock position of the cervix (see *Fig. 12.8*).

Step 4

The cervix is dilated to No. 7 Hegar or No. 21 French/Pratt size (see *Fig. 12.11*).

Step 5

Either five narrow or three wide laminaria tents or one Lamicel or two Dilapan are inserted through the external cervical os into the internal os, depending on the gestational age and cervical compliance (*Fig. 12.20*). Two folded 4 × 4 sponges are placed within the vagina, with subsequent removal of all instruments.

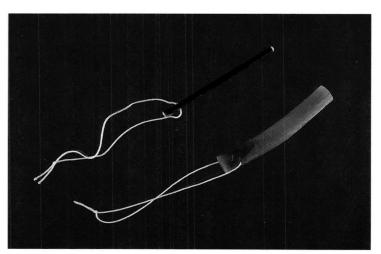

12.19 Laminaria japonicum: undilated (*top*); maximal dilation (*bottom*).

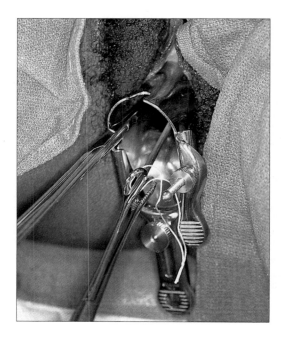

12.20 Insertion of the laminaria into the cervix.

Step 6

The patient is started on a 10-day prophylactic course of doxycycline, with analgesics and anti-emetics provided as necessary.

EVACUATION

Regional analgesia is best for the evacuation procedure, although local (i.e., lidocaine without epinephrine) with system medications (8mg morphine sulfate and 5mg diazepam or intranasal butorphanol tartrate NS [Stadol]) or general anesthesia can be used. Ovum forceps, specifically Sopher (*Figs 12.21, 12.22*) or Bierer forceps (*Figs 12.23, 12.24*), are used to evacuate most products of conception from the uterine cavity.

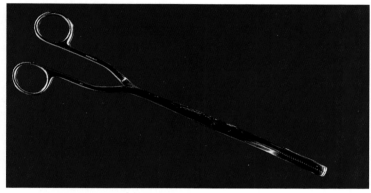

12.21 Sopher forceps (closed).

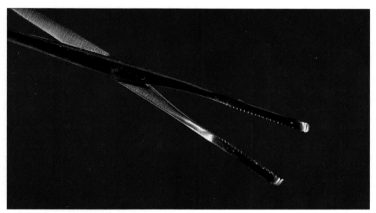

12.22 Sopher forceps (open).

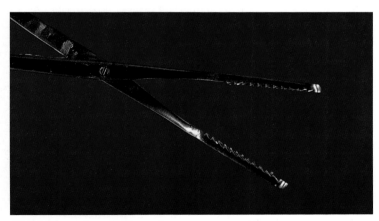

12.24 Bierer forceps (open).

Step 1

A vaginal speculum is inserted and the sponges and osmotic dilators are removed (see *Fig. 12.3*).

Step 2

The vagina is cleansed with an iodine-based solution (see *Fig. 12.4*).

Step 3

A single-toothed tenaculum is placed at the 12 o'clock position on the anterior cervical lip (see *Fig. 12.8*).

Step 4

A paracervical block is used in combination with systemic analgesic (see above) (see *Fig. 12.10*).

Step 5

The cervix is sequentially dilated to accommodate a No. 14 Hegar or No. 43 French/Pratt dilator (see *Fig. 12.11*).

Step 6

Ovum forceps are inserted into the uterine cavity in the closed position (*Fig. 12.25*). The forceps are opened within the endometrial cavity and the products of conception are extracted.

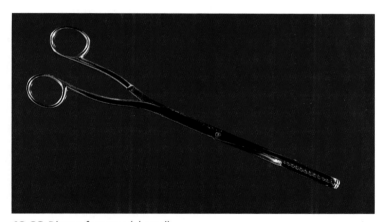

12.23 Bierer forceps (closed).

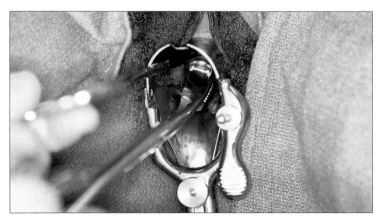

12.25 Insertion of the Beirer forceps, in closed position, through vagina and cervix and into the uterine cavity. Forceps are opened only when within the uterine cavity.

Forceps are maintained in a midline position to decrease the risk of lateral uterine perforation. Concurrent ultrasonography facilitates safe and rapid evacuation of the uterus.

Step 7

When most of the products of conception have been evacuated, suction curettage is performed with either a No. 12 or No. 14 suction curette (see *Fig. 12.15*).

Step 8

Steps 9–12 from first-trimester procedures are repeated.

UTERINE EVACUATION AFTER DEMONSTRATION OF THE NON-VIABLE FETUS

Uterine evacuation after detection of embryonic or fetal demise is performed in essentially the same manner as first- or second-trimester pregnancy termination. The type of termination procedure is determined by the estimated gestational size, as delineated by menstrual history, bimanual pelvic examination, and ultrasonographic fetal biometric and gestational sac measurements. In patients for whom the length of time and fetal demise is unknown, blood tests to detect disseminated intravascular coagulopathy (DIC), such as prothrombin and partial thromboplastin times, fibrinogen or fibrin split products, may be useful in managing uterine evacuation and potential complications arising from the coagulopathic state that may develop as a result of a nonviable fetus remaining within the uterus.

Physicians who elect to use labor induction methods (e.g., intra-amniotic or intravaginal prostaglandin) after detection of fetal demise or for other pregnancy termination indications must be able to provide sharp and suction curettage or manual uterine evacuation with ovum forceps. Retained placenta or other products of conception occurs relatively frequently after labor induction methods; inability to complete the uterine evacuation in a timely fashion could result in serious complications resulting from hemorrhage or infection. Determination of the evacuation method to be used is based on the gestational age of the pregnancy, the amount of tissue remaining within the uterus, and on the operator's own judgement as to the best method for completing the procedure.

Uterine evacuation after ultrasonographic detection of hydatidiform mole should be performed within a hospital; all such patients should have blood product replacement readily available. Suction curettage should be used, and intravenous oxytocin and methylergonovine maleate should be judiciously used to prevent excessive hemorrhage during and immediately after the procedure.

COMPLICATIONS AND THEIR MANAGEMENT

Complications resulting from uterine evacuation procedures can be categorized as immediate and delayed (at least 72 h after the procedure). Immediate complications include hemorrhage and uterine perforation.

The evaluation of hemorrhage immediately following uterine evacuation must include a thorough visual examination of the vagina and cervix, as the source of the bleeding must be determined before treatment is undertaken. Hemorrhage can occur as a result of a cervical laceration, uterine atony or uterine perforation.

A cervical laceration can usually be repaired vaginally, although an extensive cervical laceration may require laparotomy. Uterine atony, or failure of the uterus to contract, may be the result of retained products of conception, use of certain medications, or unknown causes. If retained products of conception are suspected, suction curettage should be immediately undertaken; ultrasonography can be helpful for detecting retained products and guiding suction curettage. Uterine atony caused by medications or unknown factors should be treated by bimanual uterine massage in combination with medications that contract uterine musculature (e.g., methylergonovine maleate).

Intramuscular methylergonovine maleate (0.2 mg) is initially used in tandem with bimanual uterine massage. If bleeding does not abate, an ampule of 15-methyl prostaglandin F2α is administered intramuscularly. If bleeding still does not abate, and especially if bleeding persists with a well-contracted uterus, alternative causes of hemorrhage such as uterine perforation should be entertained.

Hemorrhage may occur immediately after curettage if the uterus has been perforated. Because the uterine vasculature is located primarily in the lateral areas of the uterus, perforations that result in significant hemorrhage usually occur laterally within the uterine cavity. Brisk vaginal bleeding after uterine evacuation that cannot be readily localized and does not respond to the aforementioned treatments should be evaluated by laparotomy.

Uterine perforation is not always accompanied by vaginal bleeding. For example, perforation along the lateral portion of the uterus may result in hemorrhage within the ipsilateral broad ligament. A broad ligament hematoma usually presents as a tense, lateral pelvic mass in a patient with unremitting pelvic pain. In addition, uterine perforation should be suspected if the operator passes an instrument well beyond the length of the uterus. If this happens, the procedure should be stopped and the patient observed for signs of bleeding or intra-abdominal organic injury. Frequently, perforation of the uterine fundus is not followed by vaginal bleeding, as there are relatively few large blood vessels in this portion of the uterus. If perforation occurs during dilation and the patient is found to have suffered no organic injury, she should be asked to return in several days so that the pregnancy termination can be performed; ultrasonographic guidance should be used during this procedure.

If perforation occurs during or at the end of the procedure, signs or symptoms of organic injury will similarly guide the physician as to the need for further surgical evaluation. Specifically, the presence of bleeding or the observation of intra-abdominal contents within the cervical os or vagina (e.g., small bowel, omentum) is an indication for immediate laparotomy. The extent of surgical intervention is determined both by the extent of the perforation and by the location of the uterine rent. A general rule is that the most conservative procedure that quickly halts the bleeding is the surgical management of choice. Conversely, if perforation is suspected and the patient remains stable with no symptoms, close observation for a period of 12 to 24 h usually indicates no further need for surgical intervention. However, irrespective of the management chosen to evaluate and treat the suspected perforation, one must be certain that all products of conception have been evacuated before the patient is discharged.

Delayed complications from uterine evacuation include infection and hemorrhage. Infection or hemorrhage occurring at or after 72 h following the procedure are most frequently the result of retained products of conception. A patient who presents with bleeding, fever, abdominal pain, or leukocytosis should be suspected of having retained products. Ultrasonography can be useful in detecting retained products of conception; however, suction curettage should be performed if there is any indication of retained products of conception, even without conclusive ultrasonographic evidence.

Other causes of delayed post-abortion complications, such as endomyometritis or placental site involution, usually respond to non-surgical management. However, delayed complications may occasionally require laparotomy or hysterectomy. Therefore, physicians should not be cavalier when patients report problems more than 72 h after uterine evacuation procedures.

SUMMARY

All physicians who care for pregnant women must have a thorough working knowledge of uterine evacuation techniques for first- and second-trimester pregnancies, irrespective of the obstetrician/gynecologist's personal decision to perform elective pregnancy termination. Even physicians who use labor induction techniques for second-trimester pregnancy terminations must be well versed in curettage and manual evacuation because of the relatively common occurrence of retained products of conception after expulsion of the fetus.

FURTHER READING

Grimes DA, Schulz KF. Morbidity and mortality from second-trimester abortions. *J Reprod Med* 1985;30:505–14.

Hakim-Elahi E, Tovell HMM, Burnhill MS. Complications of first-trimester abortion: a report of 170,000 cases. *Obstet Gynecol* 1990;76:129.

Hern WM. First and second trimester abortion techniques. In: Leventhal JM, ed. *Current Problems in Obstetrics and Gynecology*. Chicago: Year Book Medical Publishers, 1983:5.

Shulman LP. Pregnancy termination procedures. In: Simpson JL, Elias S, eds. *Essentials of Prenatal Diagnosis*. New York: Churchill Livingstone, in press.

Shulman LP, Ling FW, Meyers CM, Shanklin DR, Simpson JL, Elias S. Dilation and evacuation for second trimester genetic pregnancy termination. *Obstet Gynecol* 1990;75:1037–40.

Stubblefield PG. Pregnancy termination. In: Gabbe SG, Neibyl JR, Simpson JL, eds. *Obstetrics: normal and problem pregnancies*. New York: Churchill Livingstone, 1991:1303.

13

Sterilization Procedures

Gary H. Lipscomb

LAPAROSCOPIC STERILIZATION

Sterilization is a common form of contraception available that uses a variety of methods and approaches (*Fig. 13.1*). This chapter discusses the more popular techniques and methods used for permanent female sterilization.

The only indication for sterilization is the patient's desire to terminate her childbearing potential. These methods of tubal occlusion should be considered permanent by both physician and patient, although failures do occur, and reanastomosis is possible. Factors associated with sterilization regret are presented in *Fig. 13.2*.

The three most commonly used methods of laparoscopic tubal occlusion are electrocoagulation, Falope ring application, and Hulka clip application. When correctly performed these techniques have essentially identical failure rates. The laparoscopic approach to sterilization offers advantages over minilaparotomy or the transvaginal approach, but it, too, has some contraindications (*Fig. 13.3*).

LAPAROSCOPIC ELECTROCOAGULATION

Laparoscopic electrocoagulation is the oldest technique of laparoscopic sterilization. Originally popularized in France by Palmer[1] during the 1960s, unipolar electrocoagulation gained early, widespread popularity[2,3] but fell into disfavor after reports of significant numbers of bowel burns resulting from the procedure. Although most injuries were the result of faulty technique or the use of high-voltage grounded generators delivering thousands of volts of current, unipolar current was eventually replaced with the safer bipolar current. With bipolar current, the operating forceps carries both the active and the return electrode (*Fig. 13.4*). The jaws are isolated from each other so that current passes through one jaw and is retrieved through the other. Thus, the current travels selectively through the grasped tissue, eliminating the possiblity of sparking.

Electrocoagulation requires less precise anatomic placement than other methods and may be useful when the tube cannot be fully mobilized. Electrocoagulation may also be preferable when tubal transection has occurred or when the tubal diameter

---

Permanent Female Sterilization Methods	
Laparoscopic methods	**Hysteroscopic methods**
Electrocoagulation	Occlusion of tubal ostia with silastic plug
Silastic rings	Transcervical
Hulka clip	Indirect tubal injection of cyanoacrylate adhesive
Salpingectomy	
Minilaparotomy Methods	
Pomeroy method	
Uchida method	
Kroener method	
Irving method	

13.1 Methods of permanent female sterilization.

Sterilization Regret	
Factors associated with regret	**Factors not associated with regret**
Marital status change	Religion
Family stress (e.g., death of a child)	Socioeconomic level
Desire for additional children as the "baby" grows up	Educational level
Post tubal ligation syndrome symptoms	Low parity
Postpartum timing	Decision made with husband's approval
Sterilization before age 30	Interval procedure

13.2 Factors associated and not associated with sterilization regret.

Laparoscopic Approach to Sterilization	
Indications	**Relative contraindications**
Desires permanent contraception	May desire future fertility
	Severe cardiac disease
	Severe pulmonary disease
	Severe bleeding diathesis
	Severe adhesive disease
	Massive obesity

13.3 Indications and contraindications for laparoscopic approach to sterilization.

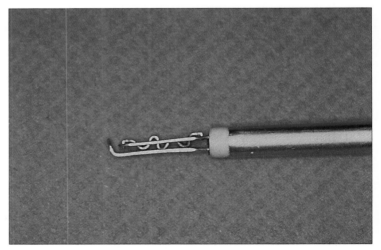

13.4 Bipolar forceps.

prevents correct placement of a ring or clip. Since electrocoagulation destroys the innervation to the coagulated segment of tube, postoperative pain is usually less than with other methods. However, tubal damage is more extensive and sterilization reversal is therefore generally less successful. The ultimate choice of the occlusive method is based on the individual preference of the operating surgeon after consideration of the advantages and disadvantages of each method.

SURGICAL PROCEDURE

Step 1
After insertion of the laparoscope, the uterus is manipulated with the uterine manipulator to expose the fallopian tube (*Fig. 13.5*).

Step 2
The fallopian tube is identified and grasped at the midisthmus with the bipolar forceps, approximately 2 cm from the uterotubal junction (*Fig. 13.6*).

Step 3
The tube is placed on tension to ensure that the forceps are not in contact with any other structure, and the current is then applied until coagulation is complete (*Fig. 13.7*).

Step 4
The tube is regrasped and cauterized at immediately adjacent sites to coagulate 3 cm of tube (*Fig. 13.8*).

Step 5
The same procedure is performed on the contralateral tube.

COMPLICATIONS OF ELECTROCOAGULATION

The most serious complication occurring with electrocoagulation is thermal injury to the bowel. The use of bipolar current minimizes this risk. Taking care to ensure that only the fallopian tube is grasped with the forceps and that the tube is not touching other intra-abdominal structures further reduces the risk of this complication.

Bipolar instruments should be used only with compatible electrosurgical units as recommended by the manufacturer. Incompatible units increase the potential for electrical burns and may provide insufficient current for adequate coagulation, which can be achieved by using an ohmmeter to document cessation of current flow. Alternatively, a timed coagulation period of at least 10 sec will usually ensure complete tubal occlusion.

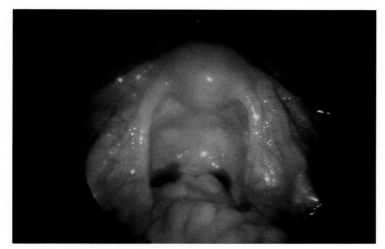

13.5 Panoramic view of uterus and fallopian tubes.

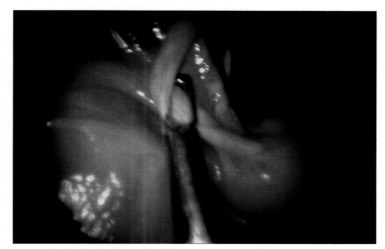

13.6 Electrocoagulation of isthmic segment.

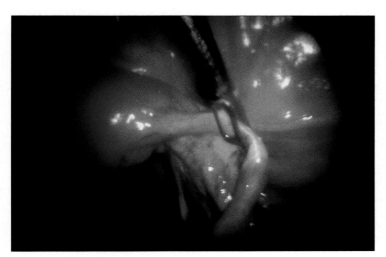

13.7 Electrocoagulation of adjacent segment of tube.

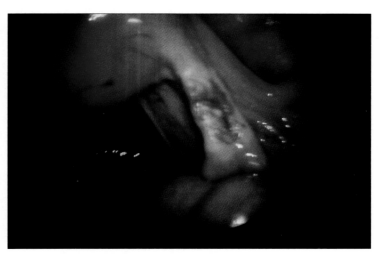

13.8 Appearance of fallopian tube following complete electrocoagulation.

LAPAROSCOPY: FALOPE RING APPLICATION

Laparoscopic sterilization with occlusive devices eliminates the risk of electrical injury to other organs and is potentially easier to reverse. However, these devices require more precise placement and cause more postoperative discomfort unless local anesthetic is also applied to the fallopian tubes. As with electrocautery, the choice of occlusion method is based on the individual preference of the operating surgeon.

The Falope ring is a nonreactive silicone rubber ring with an inner diameter of 1 mm (*Fig. 13.9*). Falope rings are applied with a specialized applicator device consisting of two concentric cylinders; the inner cylinder contains grasping prongs at its distal end (*Fig. 13.10*). The movement of these cylinders is controlled by a single-ring grip (*Fig. 13.11*). A loop of fallopian tube is drawn into the inner cylinder with the retractable prongs, and the Falope ring, which has been stretched over the inner cylinder, is pushed onto the fallopian tube. The loop of tube then undergoes necrosis caused by interruption of its blood supply[4,5].

SURGICAL PROCEDURE

Step 1
After introduction of the laparoscope, the uterus is manipulated with the uterine manipulator to expose the proximal portion of a fallopian tube (*Fig. 13.12*).

Step 2
The preloaded Falope ring applicator may be introduced either through a second suprapubic puncture or through the operating channel of an operating laparoscope. The grasping forceps are extended (*Fig. 13.13*).

Step 3
The fallopian tube is grasped about 2.5 cm distal to the utero-tubal junction (*Fig. 13.14*).

Step 4
A loop of the tube is drawn into the inner sleeve by retracting the prongs until resistance is felt (*Fig. 13.15*).

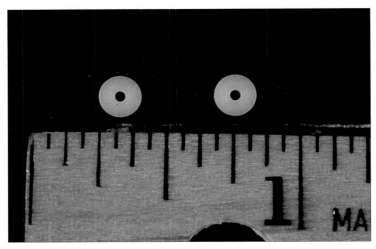

13.9 Falope rings.

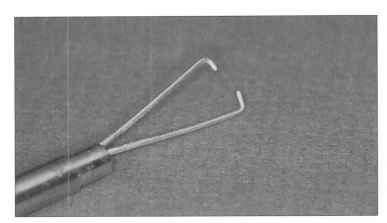

13.10 Grasping prongs of Falope ring applicator.

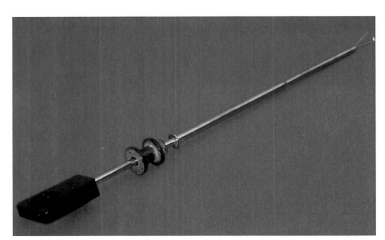

13.11 Falope ring applicator.

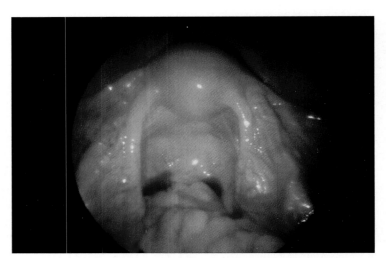

13.12 Panoramic view of uterus and fallopian tubes.

Step 5

The ring is now pushed off the applicator and onto the tube with the sliding mechanism on the applicator. A knuckle of tube 1 cm high should be entrapped by the ring (*Fig. 13.16*).

Step 6

A second Falope ring is applied to the contralateral tube.

COMPLICATIONS

The most common complication occurring with the use of the Falope ring is fallopian tube transection during application. This can be prevented by: slow withdrawal of the tube into the sleeve, thus allowing time for the tube to conform to the sleeve diameter; using a "milking" action with the prongs, which will allow even edematous tubes to be drawn into the sleeve; slightly advancing the entire applicator as the tube is drawn up to avoid counter-traction from the fixed uterine end of the tube; and using another method, such as cautery, on excessively thick, edematous tubes[6].

If the tube is transected, Falope rings can be placed proximal and distal to the transection, thus interrupting blood supply to the rent and occluding both cut ends. Alternatively, cautery can be used to achieve both hemostasis and tubal occlusion.

Another common mistake is improper placement of the ring itself. The ring should be placed 2.5–3 cm from the uterotubal junction. A more distal placement may result in only partial banding of the wider ampullary portion of the tube, and more proximal placement may result in tubal transection due to a lack of tubal mobility at this point. When appropriately placed, a knuckle of tube 1 cm high will be formed. Inability to identify a full double thickness of tube above the ring may indicate inadequate placement.

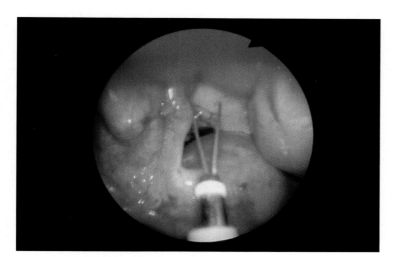

13.13 Loaded Falope ring applicator with prongs extended.

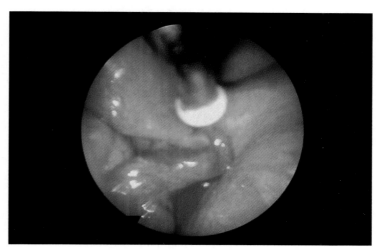

13.14 Isthmic section of fallopian tube grasped.

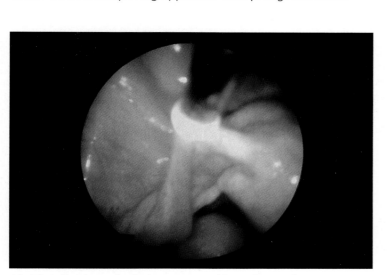

13.15 Fallopian tube being retracted into the applicator.

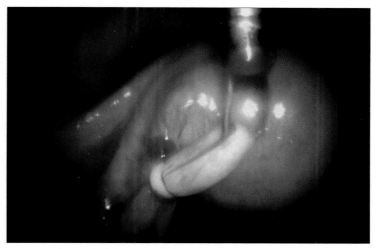

13.16 Adequate knuckle of tube with visible inner loop.

LAPAROSCOPY: HULKA CLIP APPLICATION

Tubal occlusion with the Hulka clip is the most potentially reversible of all the laparoscopic sterilization methods[7,8]. When the clip is correctly placed, only 4 mm of tube and virtually none of the tubal blood supply is destroyed. Therefore, use of this device may be more appropriate in patients who are likely to seek later reversal of sterilization. The disadvantage of this limited destruction is that precise and accurate placement is required to achieve acceptable failure rates. The Hulka clip consists of two toothed jaws of Lexan plastic joined by a stainless steel hinge pin *(Fig. 13.17)*. The pin (gold plated to reduce peritoneal irritation) maintains the clip in an open position. The Hulka applicator is 7 mm in diameter, with a three-ring configuration at the handle *(Fig. 13.18)*. The fixed lower jaw cradles the clip while the mobile upper jaw opens and closes the clip. A center piston, when advanced, closes and then locks the clip closed *(Fig. 13.19)*.

SURGICAL PROCEDURE

Step 1
After introduction of the laparoscope, the uterus is manipulated with the uterine manipulator to expose the proximal portion of a fallopian tube *(Fig. 13.20)*.

Step 2
The loaded Hulka clip applicator is introduced with the clip in the closed position. The clip is opened after the applicator is within the abdomen *(Fig. 13.21)*.

Step 3
The clip is placed perpendicular to the tube at a site 2–2.5 cm from the uterotubal junction *(Fig. 13.22)*.

Step 4
Before locking the clip, recheck for proper placement. The clip can be opened and closed without causing tubal damage until it

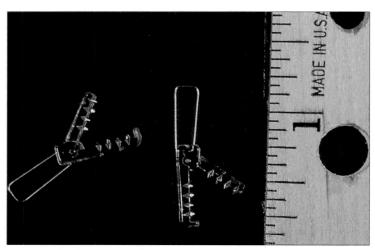

13.17 Hulka clips.

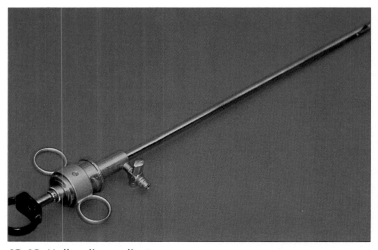

13.18 Hulka clip applicator.

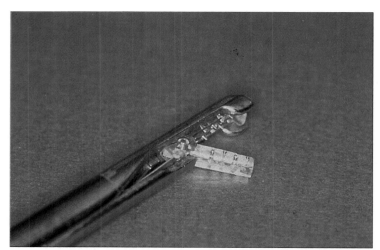

13.19 Loaded Hulka clip applicator with clip in open position.

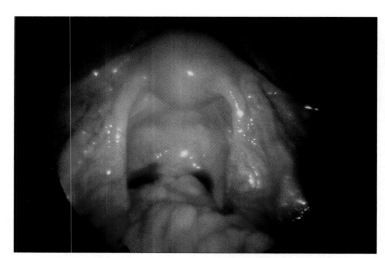

13.20 Panoramic view of uterus and fallopian tubes.

is locked in place. The center piston is advanced to permanently lock the clip and unseat it from the applicator. The applicator is then withdrawn, leaving the clip in place on the tube (*Fig. 13.23*).

Step 6

A second Hulka clip is applied to the opposite tube.

COMPLICATIONS

The most common complication with the Hulka clip is inadequate placement. The clip should be placed on the isthmic portion and perpendicular to the long axis of the tube to ensure complete occlusion by the relatively short clip.

Premature permanent locking of the Hulka clip may occur if the operator is unaccustomed to the device. This complication is the result of overadvancement of the center piston while opening and closing the clip during placement. Careful, slow, deliberate closing of the clip usually prevents premature locking.

LAPAROSCOPIC STERILIZATION UNDER LOCAL ANESTHESIA

Local anesthesia for laparoscopic sterilization is a proven alternative to general anesthesia[9,10]. Although infrequently used in the United States, this technique is successfully employed in many other countries. Local anesthesia offers several significant advantages over general anesthesia: avoidance of risks associated with general anesthesia, decreased anesthesia time, lower cost, rapid recovery, earlier awareness of complications, and less nausea and vomiting. Furthermore, through the use of television technology it is possible for the patient to directly observe the procedure, a factor that enhances her understanding of the operation.

Almost all patients can be considered candidates for laparoscopy under local anesthesia. Local anesthesia may also be appropriate for some patients in whom laparoscopic sterilization under general anesthesia is relatively contraindicated. Indications and relative contraindications for laparoscopic sterilization using local anesthesia are listed in *Fig. 13.24*.

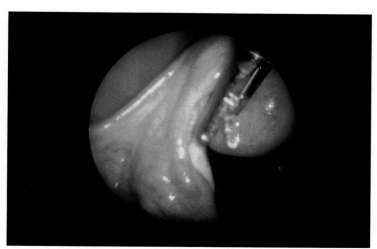

13.21 Intra-abdominal Hulka clip in open position.

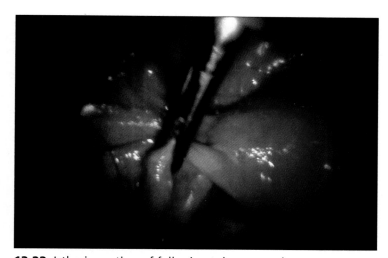

13.22 Isthmic portion of fallopian tube grasped.

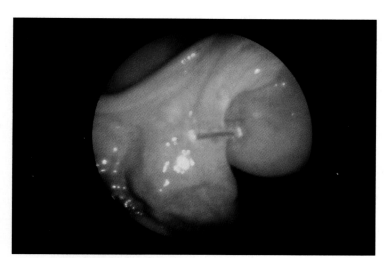

13.23 Perpendicular placement of Hulka clip.

Laparoscopic Sterilization Under Local Anesthesia	
Indications	**Relative contraindications**
Severe cardiac disease	Desires future fertility
Severe pulmonary disease	Severe bleeding diathesis
Patient desires local anesthesia	Possible adhesive disease
	Massive obesity
	Excessively anxious patient

13.24 Indications and relative contraindications for laparoscopic sterilization under local anesthesia.

SURGICAL PROCEDURE

Proper preoperative and intraoperative medication is essential for painless laparoscopic tubal ligation with local anesthesia. The medications required and their timing of administration are listed in *Fig. 13.25*. Although there are few well-controlled studies on the effect of the insufflating gas on operative pain, intra-abdominal nitrous oxide has no systemic effects and its safety is well supported in the literature.

Step 1

With the patient in the lithotomy position, a warmed single-hinged speculum is placed in the vagina and the cervix is cleaned with a prewarmed povidone–iodine solution. A Hulka uterine manipulator is inserted into the uterine cavity and attached to the anterior lip of the cervix. If the uterus is retroverted, the manipulator is placed along the uterine axis and then rotated 180° to antevert the uterus (*Fig. 13.26*).

Step 2

With a 25-gauge, 1-inch needle, the infraumbilical skin is pierced at the planned trocar insertion site and 5 ml of 0.5% bupivacaine HCl is injected radially in all directions just beneath the skin (*Fig. 13.27*).

Step 3

The 25-gauge needle is replaced with a 22-gauge, 3.5-inch spinal needle and a diamond-shaped fascial block is performed. At the same insertion site as the previous skin block, bupivacaine HCl is injected at each corner and at the center of an imaginary diamond. The center point of the diamond should correspond to the point of fascial entry. At each site, 1 ml of 0.5% bupivacaine HCl is injected below the fascia. Another 1 ml of the same solution is injected above the fascia as the needle is withdrawn (*Fig. 13.28*).

Laparoscopic sterilization under local anesthesia		
Drug	**Dose**	**Time and method of administration**
Ibuprofen	800 mg	PO 30 minutes before procedure
Atropine	0.4–0.6 mg	IV on arrival in OR
Midazolam HCl	2.5 mg	IV in divided doses during prep
Fentanyl	0.05–0.1 mg	IV during prep
Fentanyl or alfentanil	0.5–1.0 mg	IV prn pain during procedure

13.25 Drugs used during laparoscopic sterilization under local anesthesia.

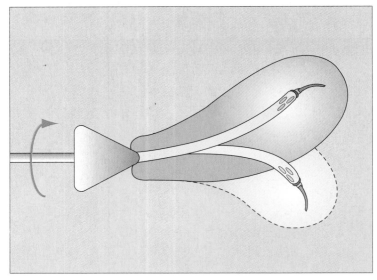

13.26 Uterine manipulator placement in the retroverted uterus.

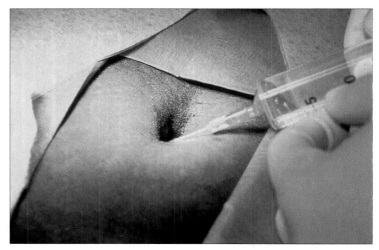

13.27 Initial injection of local anesthetic subcutaneously.

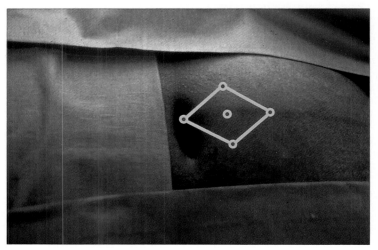

13.28 Diamond-shaped fascial block.

Step 4

A skin incision about 1 cm long is made with a No. 11 scalpel. The tips of a hemostat are placed in the incision and opened to enlarge the incision slightly (*Fig. 13.29*).

Step 5

We prefer to use a direct trocar insertion technique without Verres needle insufflation, but if desired a Verres needle can be used for insufflation before trocar insertion. If direct insertion is used, the well-sharpened trocar is placed in the incision, the abdomen grasped and stabilized, and the trocar then inserted in one quick motion (*Fig. 13.30*).

Step 6

An operating laparoscope is inserted and peritoneal entry confirmed. The abdomen is now insufflated at a rate no faster than 1 l/min. The uterus is slowly positioned with the uterine manipulator to expose one fallopian tube, and 5ml of 0.5% bupivacaine HCl is flowed over and under the tube and round ligament (*Fig. 13.31*).

Step 7

Anesthetic is topically applied on the second fallopian tube. Tubal occlusion can be performed with electrocoagulation, a Falope ring, or a Hulka clip in the same manner described earlier in this chapter[11,12]. If electrocoagulation is used, current should be applied in an intermittent fashion to prevent heat build-up and patient discomfort. Satisfactory coagulation is achieved when current no longer flows, as indicated by an ohmmeter (*Fig. 13.32*).

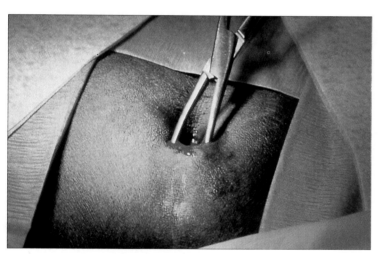

13.29 Incision enlarged with hemostat.

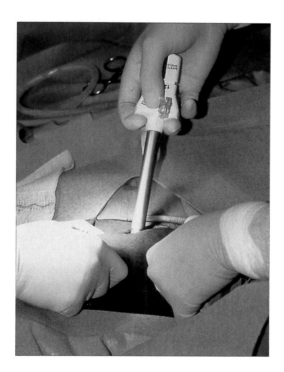

13.30 Trocar junction.

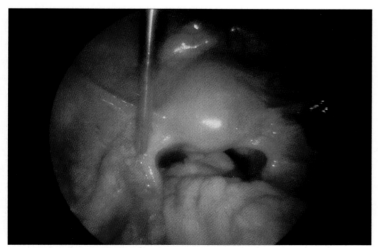

13.31 Topical anesthetic applied to fallopian tube.

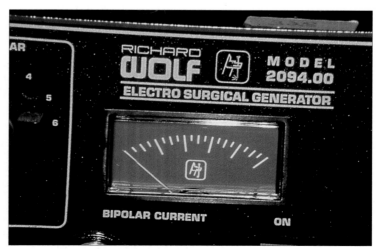

13.32 An ohmmeter.

Step 8

After tubal occlusion the insufflating gas is allowed to escape until gas flow slows. The residual gas is expelled by having the patient cough or by performing a Valsalva maneuver while opening the gas valve only during times of increased intraabdominal pressure. This prevents atmospheric air, which may cause peritoneal irritation, from entering the abdomen after gas expulsion (*Fig. 13.33*).

COMPLICATIONS

A common problem associated with sterilization under local anesthesia is oversedation. In extreme cases this may lead to loss of gag reflex and airway control. These situations usually arise when the anesthesia personnel are concerned for patient discomfort or need to treat severe discomfort, which may be due to inadequate preoperative medications, incomplete fascial field block, or too-vigorous tissue manipulation. Patients who are oversedated as part of local anesthesia may be at even greater risk of anesthetic complications (e.g., aspiration) than when controlled, intubated general anesthesia is used.

Appropriate preoperative and intraoperative medication is essential for painless laparoscopic tubal ligation with local anesthesia. The patient should be given a non-steroidal anti-inflammatory agent, such as ibuprofen 800 mg, 30 minutes before surgery, to reduce the incidence of uterine cramping associated with insertion of instruments and manipulation of pelvic organs. Preoperative medication should include atropine sulphate 0.4–0.6 mg given intravenously for partial vagal blockade; midazolam HCl 2.5 mg given intravenously in divided doses as a tranquillizer/sedative; and fentanyl citrate 0.05–0.01 mg or alfentanil HCl 0.5–1 mg given intravenously for narcosis. An additional 0.5–0.5 mg of alfentanil can be given intraoperatively if needed to relieve patient discomfort (See *Fig. 13.25*).

Many surgeons accustomed to procedures under general anesthesia, commonly forget to talk to the patient during the surgery. A constant stream of information about what is occurring and explanation of when the patient may feel discomfort, and why, are extremely effective in reducing patient anxiety and discomfort. This "vocal" anesthesia should be considered as important to the procedure as the medications previously listed.

Excessive and indelicate manipulation of pelvic structures is common among surgeons unaccustomed to performing procedures under local anesthesia. All manipulations of pelvic and abdominal structures should be kept to a minimum. Necessary manipulation should be slow, gentle, and precise. Rapid laparoscopic movements often cause stretching of the sensitive parietal peritoneum and subsequent pain.

Excessive and rapid insufflation of the abdomen may also cause patient discomfort. The abdomen should be insufflated at a rate of approximately 1 l per minute. Overinsufflation is avoided by stopping the gas flow once the abdomen is sufficiently distended and resuming insufflation only as needed to adequately

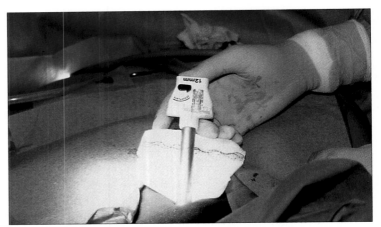

13.33 Insufflating gas released during patient valsalva.

visualize the pelvic organs. Nitrous oxide as the insufflating gas has been suggested to produce less pain than carbon dioxide. The conversion of carbon dioxide to carbonic acid on contact with the moist peritoneum is postulated as the cause of the increased pain. Intra-abdominal nitrous oxide has no systemic effects and its safety is well supported in the literature. Although few well-controlled studies have been done on the effect of the insufflating gas on operative pain, it appears reasonable, on theoretical grounds, to use nitrous oxide if it is readily available.

STERILIZATION BY MINILAPAROTOMY

A minilaparotomy requires basic surgical skills and readily available surgical instruments[13,14]. In addition, a tissue specimen for histologic documentation is commonly taken when a minilaparotomy is performed. It should be noted that it is possible to remove a histologic specimen laparoscopically. Disadvantages include a slightly higher complication rate, greater need for postoperative anesthesia, longer recovery time, and a larger surgical scar.

The most common indication for a minilaparotomy approach to sterilization is in the patient who desires sterilization immediately postpartum. This approach can be used when laparoscopic equipment is unavailable, when the surgeon is not trained in laparoscopy, or when there is morbid obesity or severe tubal or adhesive disease that precludes a successful laparoscopic procedure.

SURGICAL PROCEDURE

Step 1

With the scalpel, a transverse skin incision about 4 cm in length is made two fingerbreadths above the symphysis pubis (*Fig. 13.34*).

Step 2
The fascia is incised transversely with scalpel or scissors (*Fig. 13.35*).

Step 3
The fascia is grasped with two Oschner clamps and dissected from the underlying rectus muscle both superiorly and inferiorly (*Fig. 13.36*).

Step 4
The peritoneum is elevated and entered (*Fig. 13.37*).

Step 5
One tube is identified and ligated. Ligation may be performed with Falope rings, Hulka clips (*Figs 13.38, 13.39*), electro-coagulation, or more traditionally, Pomeroy ligation.

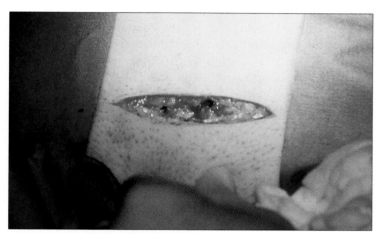

13.34 Incision above symphysis pubis.

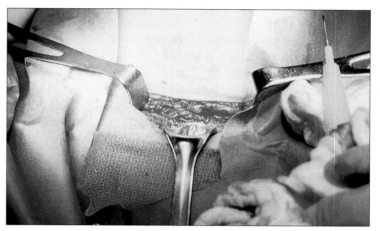

13.35 Transverse fascial incision.

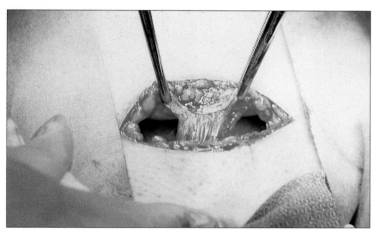

13.36 Dissection of fascia.

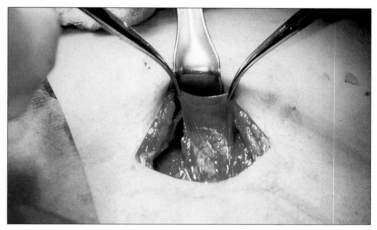

13.37 Elevation of peritoneum.

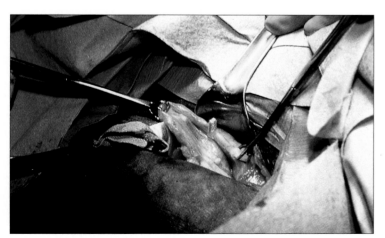

13.38 Grasping of fallopian tube.

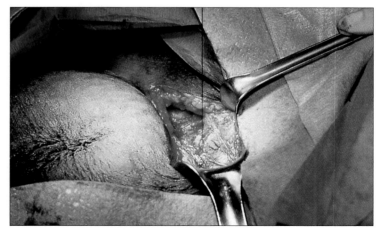

13.39 Ligation of fallopian tube.

Step 6

The peritoneum is left open and the fascia is closed with a running #0 synthetic absorbable suture (*Fig. 13.40*).

Step 7

The skin is closed with a subcuticular stitch of #3-0 or #4-0 synthetic absorbable suture (*Fig. 13.41*).

COMPLICATIONS

The most common problem encountered during sterilization by minilaparotomy is difficulty in obtaining adequate operative exposure. The use of Army–Navy retractors greatly facilitates exposure during the initial incision. Placement of a uterine manipulator before beginning the operation enables the uterus to be manipulated vaginally and allows the tube to be maneuvered into the operative field. The use of Falope rings, electrocoagulation, or Hulka clips further reduces the need for a larger incision.

THE POMEROY TECHNIQUE

In 1930, Bishop and Nelms[15] first reported the sterilization procedure developed by their late associate Dr Pomeroy. Since that initial report, the simplicity and the low failure rate of the Pomery technique for tubal ligation have made this procedure the most common nonlaparoscopic method of surgical female sterilization.

SURGICAL PROCEDURE

Access to the fallopian tubes for the Pomeroy method of tubal sterilization can be obtained through either an abdominal or a vaginal approach. Postpartum sterilization utilizes a periumbilical incision. As this operation is the most common sterilization procedure in which the Pomeroy method is utilized, we have chosen it to illustrate the Pomeroy technique.

Step 1

The inferior skin crease formed by the junction of the umbilical ring and the abdominal wall is identified and elevated with two hemostats (*Fig. 13.42*).

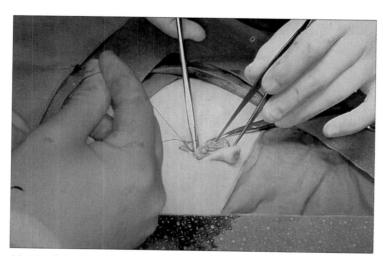

13.40 Closure of fascia.

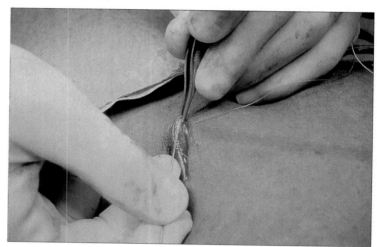

13.41 Closure of skin.

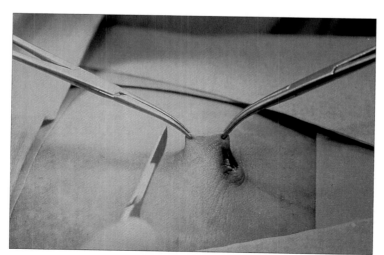

13.42 Identification of inferior skin crease.

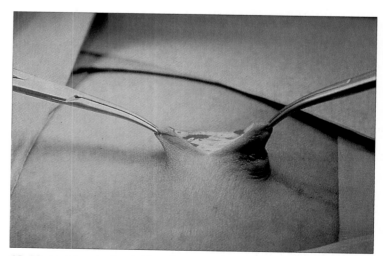

13.43 Incision to fascial level.

Step 2

A scalpel is used to make a 3 cm transverse skin incision between the two hemostats. The incision is continued through the subcutaneous tissue down to the fascia (*Fig.13.43*).

Step 3

The hemostats are repositioned to elevate the fascia. The abdominal cavity is now entered by sharply incising both fascia and peritoneum with a scalpel (*Fig. 13.44*).

Step 4

The fascial and peritoneal incisionis enlarged with Metzenbaum scissors until it is the same length as the skin incision (*Fig. 13.45*).

Step 5

If done as an interval procedure, a uterine manipulator is placed in the cervix as in other sterilization procedures described previously. In the immediate postpartum period, this is not done.

Step 6

With Army–Navy or Richardson retractors, the incision is mobilized towards the fallopian tube to be ligated. The fallopian tube is identified and the midportion of the tube is grasped with a Babcock clamp and elevated into the incision (*Fig. 13.46*).

Step 7

The "knuckle" of the tube held by the Babcock clamp is now double ligated with two #0 plain catgut sutures. The sutures are held in a hemostat to provide traction on the tube (*Fig. 13.47*).

Step 8

The open blade of the scissors is used to pierce the mesosalpinx within the "knuckle" of tube and the ligated segment of fallopian tube is excised and sent for histologic examination (*Fig. 13.47*).

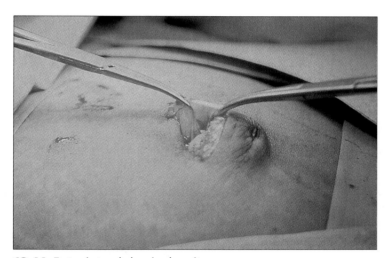

13.44 Entry into abdominal cavity.

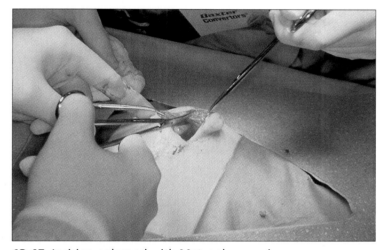

13.45 Incision enlarged with Metzenbaum scissors.

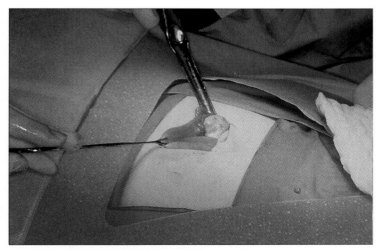

13.46 Elevation of midportion of fallopian tube.

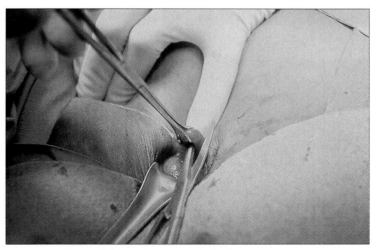

13.47 Excision of ligated segment of tube.

Step 9

The ligated ends of the fallopian tube are now inspected for hemostasis and the presence of visible tubal lumens. After division of the fallopian tube, retraction of the tubal muscularis results in protrusion of the tubal lumen, thus verifying actual tubal excision. The sutures previously used to hold the fallopian tube are cut and the tube is allowed to drop into the abdominal cavity (*Fig. 13.48*).

Step 10

The procedure is performed on the contralateral tube.

COMPLICATIONS

The most common complication is slippage of the ligature securing the severed end of the fallopian tube. The free, bleeding end then retracts into the abdomen. The fallopian tube must be reidentified and religated. This complication can be best prevented by avoiding excessive tension on the suture. Placement of two ligating sutures rather than one, as originally described, further increases knot security. If a second tie is placed, tension should be applied only to the distal suture.

Preventable surgical errors include the ligation and removal of segments of the round ligament or dilated veins and arteries within the broad ligament instead of the fallopian tube. Identification of the fimbriated end of the fallopian tube before ligation should obviate these errors.

The failure rate of the Pomeroy technique is significantly increased if a suture other than plain catgut is selected for ligation of the fallopian tube. Plain catgut is absorbed within 3 to 4 days, allowing the severed ends to retract from each other. The use of a less rapidly absorbed suture allows the two ends of the tube to be held in close approximation for a longer period of time, thus increasing the possibility of fistula formation between the two ends.

THE UCHIDA TECHNIQUE

The Uchida method is a more complex technique of tubal sterilization[16]. The advantage of this method is that failures are extremely rare. For example, Uchida reported no failures in a series of 20,000 sterilization procedures. The disadvantages are that it requires more tubal manipulation and a greater degree of surgical skill to perform than any of the other methods.

SURGICAL PROCEDURE

Step 1

After the fallopian tube has been exposed by the chosen operative approach, the tube is grasped with a Babcock clamp and elevated into the surgical field (*Fig. 13.49*).

Step 2

The fallopian tube is grasped with a second Babcock, and the portion of tube about 2 cm distal to the uterine cornu is placed on tension (*Fig. 13.50*).

Step 3

A 25-gauge needle is used to inject saline into the subserosal area of the tube, ballooning the serosa away from the tubal muscularis (*Fig. 13.51*).

Step 4

The ballooned serosa is incised longitudinally with a scalpel, and a 2 cm segment of tube is dissected free of the serosa with a mosquito hemostat (*Fig. 13.52*).

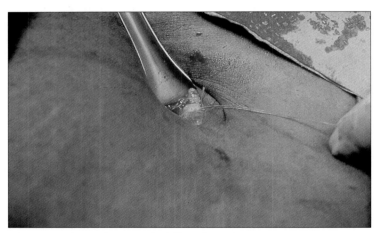

13.48 Cutting of sutures holding the tube.

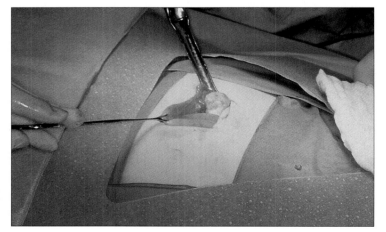

13.49 Elevation of fallopian tube.

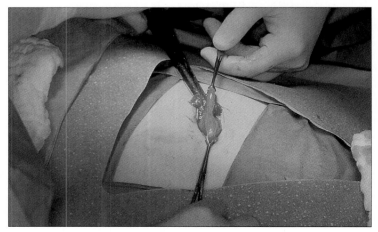

13.50 Tension on portion of tube.

Step 5

Two pieces of plain #0 or #2-0 absorbable suture are passed under the freed segment of tube and tied at both ends of the isolated segment of tube. Both sutures are held with hemostats. The segment of tube between the two ligatures is excised with scissors and sent for pathologic examination (*Fig. 13.53*).

Step 6

The ends of the tube are inspected for the presence of a lumen and for hemostasis (*Fig. 13.54*).

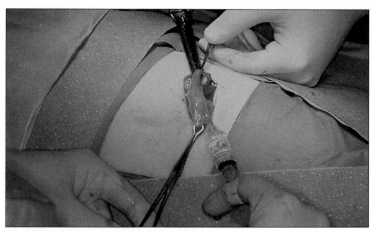

13.51 Injection of saline into subserosal area.

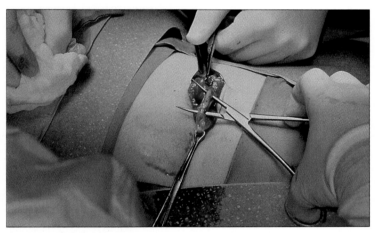

13.52 Incision of serosa.

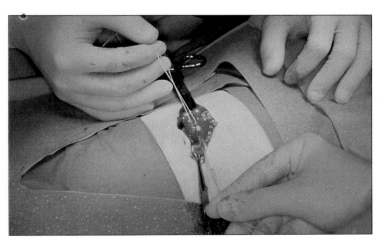

13.54 Inspection of ends of tube.

Step 7

The proximal suture is cut, and this segment is allowed to retract into the mesosalpinx. Traction is applied to the distal tubal segment, elevating it free of the mesosalpinx. A #3-0 synthetic absorbable suture is used to reapproximate the serosa so that the proximal stump is buried within the mesosalpinx and the distal stump is exteriorized (*Fig. 13.55*).

COMPLICATIONS

The most common complication of the Uchida method is bleeding during dissection of the tubal muscularis. Injection of enough saline to cause obvious ballooning of the serosa will decrease the incidence of this complication. A saline–epinephrine or saline–vasopressin solution instead of plain saline can also be used to decrease potential bleeding. If bleeding is encountered that cannot be readily controlled, a hemostat can be passed through an avascular portion of the mesosalpinx beneath the tube and two sutures passed around the bleeding tubal segment. This enables the entire tubal segment to be excised.

Retraction of the distal segment of the tube into the mesosalpinx during reapproximation of the serosa can be prevented by placing a purse-string suture around the distal tubal stump and adjacent serosa before closure of the serosal incision.

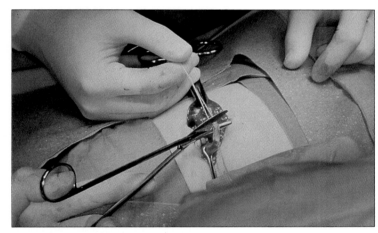

13.53 Excision of segment of tube.

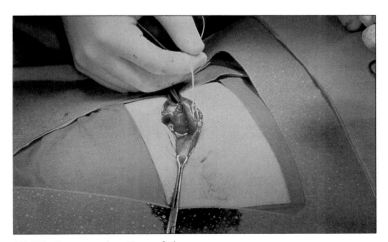

13.55 Reapproximation of the serosa.

MODIFIED IRVING TECHNIQUE

The Irving technique of tubal sterilization was originally developed for use at the time of cesarean section and is not recommended as an interval procedure. It has the advantage of an extremely low failure rate but is associated with an increased incidence of intraoperative bleeding. The original technique, as described by Irving[17], not only buried the proximal tubal stump within the myometrium but also buried the ligated end of the distal tubal segment in the broad ligament. As this step requires additional time and effort without increasing the effectiveness of the sterilization, it is usually omitted today.

Since an abdominal incision large enough to provide necessary exposure is required, this technique is usually performed only when the abdomen has already been been entered for other indications, such as cesarean section. The very low failure rate of this method may be partially due to compression and eventual obliteration of the buried tubal lumen by the involuting postpartum uterus.

SURGICAL PROCEDURE

Step 1

After delivery of the infant and repair of the uterine incision, the uterine fundus is manually delivered into the surgical field. One fallopian tube is identified and grasped with a Babcock clamp (*Fig. 13.56*).

Step 2

A hemostat is passed through an avascular portion of the mesosalpinx in the region of the tubal ampullary–isthmic junction (*Fig. 13.57*).

Step 3

Two #0 synthetic absorbable sutures are passed through this opening, the tube is doubly ligated, and the ends of the suture are left long (*Fig. 13.58*). The tube is now divided between the two ligatures (*Fig. 13.59*). If desired, the segment of tube between the two ligatures can be completely excised for pathologic examination. If inadequate tubal mobility prevents the tubal stump from reaching a suitable avascular area of the uterus, cautery can be used to divide the mesosalpinx, thereby mobilizing the tube.

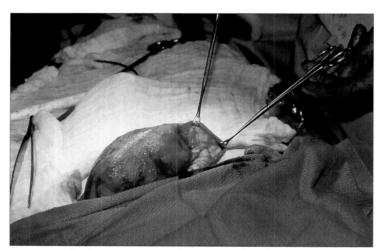

13.56 Identification of one fallopian tube.

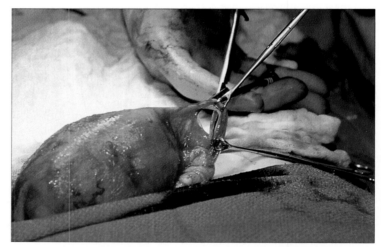

13.57 Hemostat passed through avascular portion of mesosalpinx.

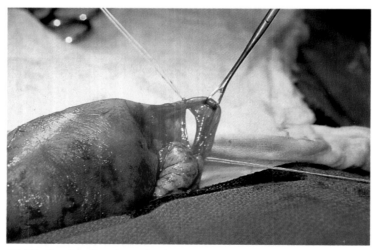

13.58 Double ligation of tube.

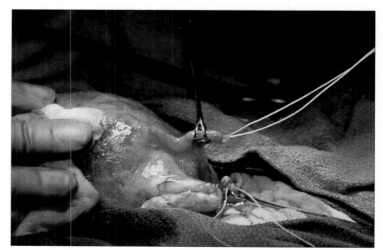

13.59 Division of tube.

Step 4

An avascular area of posterior uterus is now pierced with a mosquito hemostat to create a myometrial pocket about 1 cm deep (*Fig. 13.60*).

Step 5

The sutures attached to the proximal tubal stump are now threaded on eyed, curved needles. The needles are separately passed through the base of the myometrial pocket to exit the uterine surface 1 cm apart *(Fig. 13.61)*.

Step 6

Traction is applied to the sutures, burying the tubal stump in the myometrial pocket, and the sutures are tied (*Fig. 13.62*).

Step 7

The procedure is repeated on the contralateral side (*Fig. 13.63*).

COMPLICATIONS

The most common complication of the Irving method of sterilization is bleeding from the myometrial pocket. Careful selection of an avascular area on the posterior uterus will reduce the incidence of this complication. However, if significant bleeding does occur, it is usually easily controlled with an interrupted figure-of-eight suture over the pocket.

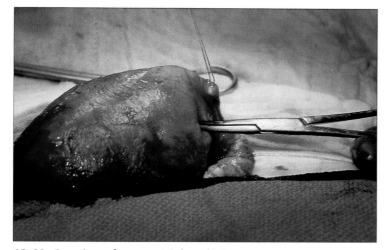

13.60 Creation of myometrial pocket.

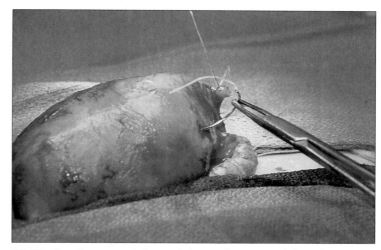

13.61 Needles passed through base of myometrial pocket.

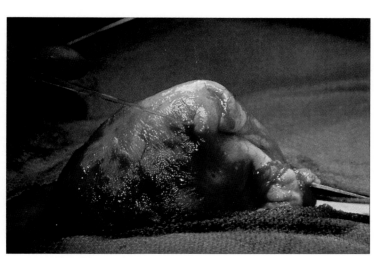

13.62 Completion of procedure on one side.

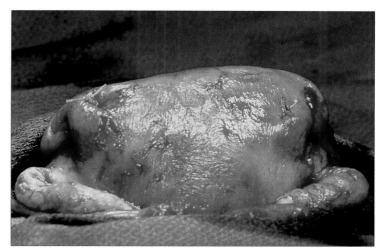

13.63 Procedure repeated on other side.

VAGINAL STERILIZATION

As the safety and popularity of laparoscopic methods of tubal ligation have increased, vaginal sterilization, once a preferred technique[18], has fallen into disuse. The increased incidence of postoperative pelvic infections after vaginal sterilization compared with laparoscopic methods further contributed to this decline in popularity[19]. However, a recent study by Smith *et al.*[20] suggests that the routine use of prophylactic antibiotics can produce a morbidity rate comparable to that of laparoscopic sterilization. The vaginal approach is particularly attractive in very obese patients or those with a retroverted uterus.

SURGICAL PROCEDURE

Possible indications and relative contraindications to sterilization via the vaginal approach are listed in *Fig. 13.64*.

Vaginal sterilization is usually performed with the patient in the dorsal lithotomy position, although the knee–chest position can also be used.

Step 1

Right-angled or Deaver retractors are used to expose the cervix. The posterior cervical lip is grasped with a single-tooth tenaculum. The cervix is then elevated, exposing the posterior fornix of the vagina (*Fig. 13.65*).

Step 2

The vaginal mucosa overlying the cul-de-sac is grasped with forceps and placed on tension (*Fig. 13.66*).

Step 3

A colpotomy incision is performed by transversely incising the tented vaginal wall with Mayo scissors (*Fig. 13.67*).

Vaginal Sterilization	
Potential indications	*Contraindications*
Obesity	Multiple pelvic surgeries
Previous umbilical hernia repair	Endometriosis
	History of pelvic inflammatory disease
	Anteverted uterus
	Uterine immobility

13.64 Indications for vaginal sterilization.

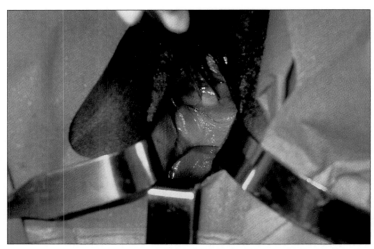

13.65 Exposure of posterior fornix of vagina.

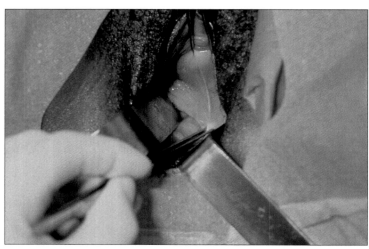

13.66 Vaginal mucosa grasped.

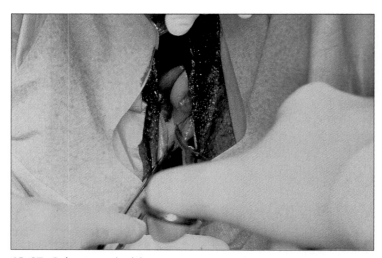

13.67 Colpotomy incision.

Step 4

The points of the Mayo scissors are placed in the opening into the peritoneal cavity and spread to enlarge the incision (*Fig. 13.68*).

Step 5

The anterior retractor is placed posterior to the cervix just within the incision and is elevated, resulting in retroflexion of the uterus. The fallopian tube is delivered into the incision with a Babcock clamp (*Fig. 13.69*).

Step 6

If sterilization is to be performed by the Pomeroy method, the loop of fallopian tube is double-tied with #0 plain catgut sutures, excised, and sent for histologic examination (*Figs 13.70, 13.71*).

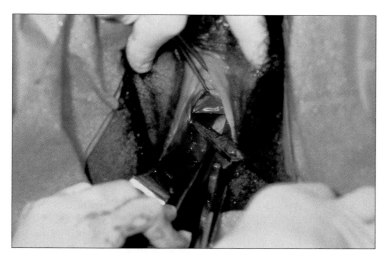

13.68 Enlargement of colpotomy incision.

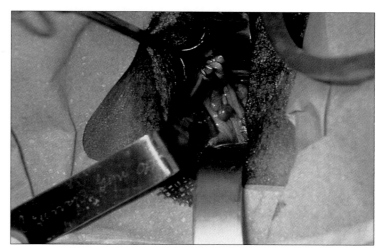

13.69 Grasping of fallopian tube.

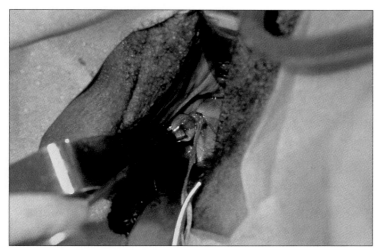

13.70 Suture ligation of tubal segment.

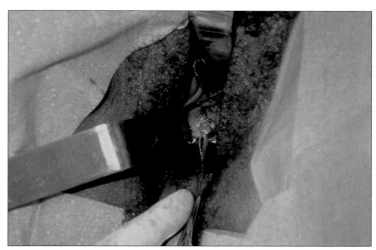

13.71 Tubal segment is excised.

Step 7

At times it may be difficult to mobilize the fallopian tube to easily perform the Pomeroy ligation. In such cases a Kleppinger bipolar forceps can be used to grasp the fallopian tube about 2–2.5 cm from the uterotubal junction and electrocoagulate the tube. The bipolar forceps are reapplied until a 3 cm section of tube is electrocoagulated (*Fig. 13.72*).

Step 8

As an alternative to electrocoagulation, a silastic ring applicator can be used to place a silastic ring 2.5 cm from the uterotubal junction (*Fig. 13.73*).

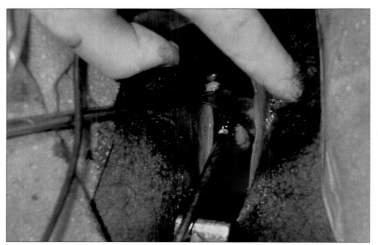

13.72 Use of electrocoagulation forceps.

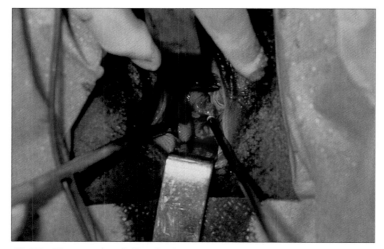

13.73 Placement of silastic ring

Step 9

The colpotomy incision is now closed with interrupted figure-of-eight sutures or a single running suture of an absorbable #0 or #2-0 suture. The underlying peritoneum can either be incorporated with the vaginal mucosa in a single-layer closure or left unclosed (*Fig. 13.74*).

COMPLICATIONS

The most common complication of vaginal sterilization is difficulty in exposing the fallopian tube. Exposure can be facilitated by using ring forceps or curved polyp forceps to bring the tube into the surgical field.

Placing the anterior retractor too deeply into the incision, instead of just under the cervix, will antevert the uterus and hinder exposure. If the uterus remains anteverted after correct retractor placement, retroversion can be accomplished by suprapubic pressure or by sequential placement of Babcock clamps along the posterior uterine wall.

Excessive bleeding may be encountered from the incision edges. Suture ligation may be necessary before proceeding with the surgery.

Postoperative pelvic infection, including tubo-ovarian abscess formation, is one of the most serious complications of vaginal sterilization. One-time intravenous administration of a first-generation cephalosporin for prophylaxis (30 min before the procedure) will minimize the incidence of such infections.

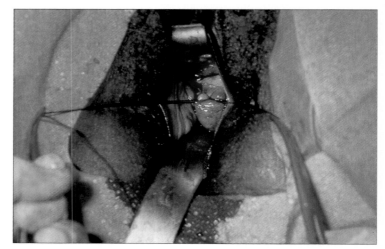

13.74 Vaginal mucosa closure.

REFERENCES

1. Palmer MR. Essais de sterilisation tubaire coelioscopique par electrocoagulation isthmique. *Bull Fed Soc Gynecol Obstet Lang Fr* 1962;14:298.

2. Rioux JE, Quesnel G, Blanchet J, *et al*. Laparoscopie: Sterilisation tubaire: Etude de 1,000 cas et evaluation globale de la methode. *Union Med Can* 1973;102:1865.

3. Yuzpe AA, Rioux JE, Loffer FD, Pent D. Laparoscopic tubal sterilization by the 'burn only' technic. *Obstet Gynecol* 1977;49:106.

4. Yoon IB, King TM. A preliminary and immediate report on a new laparoscopic tubal ring procedure. *J Reprod Med* 1975;15:54.

5. Yoon IB, King T, Parmley T. A two-year experience with the Falope ring sterilization procedure. *Am J Obstet Gynecol* 1977;127:109.

6. Alupert J, Garcia A. Improving Falope ring application in laparoscopic training. *J Reprod Med* 1987;32:340.

7. Hulka JA, Fishburne JI, Mercer JP, *et al*. Laparoscopic sterilization with a spring clip: A report of the first fifty cases. *Am J Obstet Gynecol* 1973;116:715.

8. Lieberman BA, Gordon AG, Bostick JF, *et al*. Laparoscopic sterilization with a spring-clip: Double puncture technique. *J Reprod Med* 1977;18:241.

9. Fishburne JI. Office laparoscopic sterilization with local anesthesia. *J Reprod Med* 1977;18:233.

10. Penfield AJ. Laparoscopic sterilization under local anesthesia. *Obstet Gynecol* 1977;49:735.

11. Lipscomb GH, Stovall TG, Ramanathan JA, Ling FW. Comparison of silastic rings and electrocoagulation for laparoscopic tubal ligation under local anesthesia. *Obstet Gynecol* 1992;80:645.

12. Mehta PV. Laparoscopic sterilization with Falope ring: Experiences with 10,100 women in rural camps. *Obstet Gynecol* 1981;57:345.

13. Penfield AJ. Minilaparotomy for female sterilization. *Obstet Gynecol* 1979;54:184.

14. Lee RB, Boyd JAK. Minilaparotomy under local anesthesia for outpatient sterilization: A preliminary report. *Fertil Steril* 1980;33:129.

15. Bishop E, Nelms WF. A simple method of tubal sterilization. *NY State J Med* 1930;30:214.

16. Uchida H. Uchida tubal sterilization. *Am J Obstet Gynecol* 1975;121:153.

17. Irving FC. A new method of insuring sterility following cesarean section. *Am J Obstet Gynecol* 1924;8:335.

18. Lee JG, Randal JH, Keettel WC. Tubal sterilization: A review of 1,169 cases. *Am J Obstet Gynecol* 1951;62:568–575.

19. Miesfield RR, Giarratano RC, Moyers TG. Vaginal tubal ligation: is infection a significant risk? *Am J Obstet Gynecol* 1980;137:183–188.

20. Smith RP, Maggi CS, Nolan TE. Morbidity and vaginal tubal cautery: A report and review. *Obstet Gynecol* 1991;78:209.

14

Hysteroscopic Surgery

Thierry G. Vancaillie

GENERAL PRINCIPLES

Hysteroscopy is among the very first endoscopic procedures to have been performed in modern medical history. More than a century ago, Pantaleoni wrote a report on a hysteroscopy performed on a woman with postmenopausal bleeding[1]. Hysteroscopy has, however, never reached the level of popularity enjoyed by other procedures such as cystoscopy and gastroscopy. There are two main reasons for this. The first is that another easier procedure had become firmly established, i.e., uterine curettage. The second is that attempts to develop a technique for sterilization have failed.

At present, hysteroscopy faces even stronger competition, resulting from the advent of vaginal ultrasonography[2,3]. The latter method is less invasive and hence more "patient friendly". It can be said, therefore, that diagnostic hysteroscopy will most likely not become a routine gynecologic procedure. On the other hand, interventional hysteroscopy may well reach a level of importance equal to that of transurethral surgery in urology.

INDICATIONS

The indications for diagnostic hysteroscopy are any form of abnormal bleeding in the nonpregnant woman, secondary infertility – hysterosalpingography and hysteroscopy can be considered complementary in these cases – and problems related to foreign bodies, mainly intrauterine contraceptive devices.

As mentioned earlier, the quest for information on intrauterine pathology, which is the primary indication for diagnostic hysteroscopy, can be solved with less burden on the patient by use of methods such as vaginal ultrasonography. The purpose of hysteroscopy has therefore shifted from diagnosis to therapy. The indications for operative hysteroscopy can be summarized as follows: treatment of menorrhagia with endometrial electro-desiccation or resection; treatment of metrorrhaghia by myomectomy; septum division; synechiolysis; tubal cannulation (although fluoroscopy and/or ultrasonography may prove more suitable in this case); and removal of lost or broken intrauterine contraceptive devices (IUCD).

This chapter deals with each of these procedures except for tubal cannulation. The general principles of hysteroscopy are dealt with first, and each procedure is then addressed in detail.

TIMING OF THE PROCEDURE

In general, operative hysteroscopy is best performed during the early proliferative phase of the cycle. The reasons for this are multiple: there is better visualization because the endometrium is less dense and less friable; there is less bleeding because of the vasoconstrictive effects of estrogen; and there is faster healing because the endometrium is in its growth phase. The latter fact is especially important in cases of intrauterine synechiae. The endometrium should cover the raw areas as quickly as possible.

In some cases the surgeon may elect to perform the surgery during menses. The reader's first reaction is probably one of disbelief at the thought of a uterus filled with blood and debris. So it is, but the uterus is easily flushed out with the distension medium. Positive pressure in the uterus will prevent further

menstrual bleeding from occurring during the procedure. Timing during menses is ideal for endometrial ablation or resection.

In cases of amenorrhea it is particularly crucial to avoid the postovulatory period in which the endometrium is not responsive to estrogen stimulation. This can be achieved by natural methods, such as obtaining and charting the basal body temperature curve, or by hormone manipulation. The objective is to be able to stimulate endometrial growth under optimal conditions during the immediate postoperative period. I prefer the basal body temperature method.

No prospective or retrospective studies are available that evaluate the impact of timing of the surgery on complications such as fluid overload. However, in view of the well-known increased incidence of contrast material intravasation during hysterosalpingography when performed in the luteal phase, one can safely predict that fluid absorption is likely to be more pronounced during the luteal phase of the cycle. Fluid overload is a common and worrisome complication of operative hysteroscopy. Possibly reducing its incidence by careful timing of the procedure is worth the effort.

GENERAL SURGICAL PRINCIPLES

The various hysteroscopic surgical procedures share a number of steps in common. The patient is placed in the dorsal lithotomy position. The operative field is prepped and draped in the usual fashion. The surgeon now has the advantage of video technology. The instrument cart is positioned to the left or the right of the patient according to the surgeon's preference. After exposure of the cervix with a speculum, the cervix is stabilized with a tenaculum. It is usually possible to remove the speculum after the endoscope has been inserted into the cervical canal, which enhances maneuverability of the instrument. A cervical block with a local anesthetic is then performed, regardless of whether or not the patient is under general anesthesia. The local block will last several hours beyond the end of the procedure, with significant palliation of postoperative discomfort.

The choice of anesthetic is at the discretion of the surgeon. A combination of short- and long-acting agents may be appropriate. Addition of vasoconstrictors is beneficial in particular procedures such as myomectomy, in which significant blood loss may occur. Whether there is an intrinsic advantage to the use of agents that cause smooth muscle contraction (e.g., Pitressin) is unknown. It has been speculated that such agents in combination with a vasoconstrictor would reduce absorption of distension medium. However, no evidence to support this idea has yet been found.

In general, cervical dilatation is required for hysteroscopic surgery. Exceptions to this include patients with intrauterine synechiae and the presence of a fibroid in statu nascendi. In the latter case, the fibroid causes relaxation of the cervix and widening of the cervical canal. Discussion of the merits of each particular type of cervical dilator is beyond the scope of this chapter. The cervix is dilated to a diameter of 9–10 mm, which is enough to accept the standard-sized resectoscope. Some procedures do not require the use of the resectoscope, and dilatation of the cervix to 10 mm is therefore not necessary.

The resectoscope is completely assembled and the working

element checked for smooth, accurate responsiveness. Light cable, electrical cord, in- and out-flow tubing are connected, as well as the camera.

The instrument is inserted under direct view. Good visualization must be maintained at all times, and surgical maneuver should not be performed until good visibility is obtained. This is especially true when the intrauterine anatomy is severely distorted. An angled optic (15–30°) offers the advantage of an additional dimension in obtaining good visualization. Angulation of the optic allows the operator to scan the area by rotation only of the optic, without moving the endoscope in the cardinal directions. In conditions characterized by reduced intrauterine volume, this feature becomes a real asset.

Intrauterine surgical maneuvers are difficult in themselves because of the reduced space, the relatively long cervical canal, and the difficulty of achieving access to cornual areas. The motions that allow optimal control are those that are executed towards the optic/operator. The preferred approach is therefore to place the active instrument beyond or at the target and to move the instrument towards the operator.

When a video camera is used, care should be taken to maintain good orientation. Operating with the help of a video screen has definite advantages, such as reduced physical strain on the surgeon. However, the level of skill required is increased accordingly.

The details of each hysteroscopic procedure are discussed under their respective subheadings.

COMPLICATIONS

Complications can be divided into two categories: immediate and delayed. The immediate complications include uterine perforation, bleeding, and injury to neighboring organs such as bladder, bowel, and vessels. The most common immediate complication, however, is fluid overload.

Mechanical uterine perforation occurs more commonly during dilatation of the cervix and only rarely during actual hysteroscopy. Electrical perforation occurs when an activated electrode accidentally penetrates the uterine wall. The latter can be avoided by adhering to the general surgical principle of moving an activated electrode only towards the operator.

Bleeding can be caused by a loop electrode cutting too deeply into the myometrium[4]. A more common cause of abnormal bleeding is cervical laceration during dilatation. The latter is innocuous and is bothersome only to the extent that it may somewhat obscure the field during surgery. However, cervical laceration itself can lead to increased fluid absorption, which is more important than the bleeding.

Treatment of bleeding is by electrodesiccation during operative hysteroscopy, if possible, or by placement of an intrauterine balloon immediately after completion of the procedure[5]. In rare cases, bleeding is severe enough to prevent completion of the surgery. The balloon can be commercially purchased or derived from a 30-ml Foley catheter with the tip cut off. The balloon is inserted into the uterine cavity and inflated manually until firm resistance is met. Vital signs should be carefully monitored, because bleeding will not stop if the uterus has been perforated,

which the surgeon may not be immediately aware of. The balloon is left at maximal inflation for at least 2 hours and sometimes for several days (there is no consensus). Deflation of the balloon is done in a stepwise fashion. Several methods are advocated, but all are designed to reduce the intrauterine pressure in two or three successive intervals. Antibiotic coverage has been advocated when a balloon is left in the uterus.

Mechanical or electrical injury to neighboring organs is a serious complication and is not uncommon[4]. Such accidents can be avoided by adhering to the general principles of intrauterine surgery: the electrical wire or other electrode should only be activated when moved towards the operator. In addition, all maneuvers with an activated electrode should be performed under direct visualization. Treatment depends on the site of the injury. Consultation with a general or vascular surgeon may be required.

Fluid overload is the most common and dreaded complication of hysteroscopic surgery, because it is unavoidable and sets in subtly[6,7]. The uterine cavity must be distended during surgery, and a minimum of 35 mmHg is required to achieve that goal. Because the pressure is higher than the capillary and tissue pressures, a positive gradient exists and fluid is therefore absorbed. With increasingly higher intrauterine pressure, even more fluid is absorbed[8]. A threshold in pressure balance is the patient's diastolic pressure (or peripheral vascular resistance): fluid absorption increases significantly once intrauterine pressure exceeds the diastolic pressure. Using the same physical setup in the operating room will lead to significant variability in fluid absorption, owing to differences in peripheral vascular resistance among patients. The surgeon can adapt the settings to the individual patient during the procedure by observing the amount of intrauterine bleeding. Assuming that simple gravity is used to infuse the distension medium, changing the height of the fluid bag influences the amount of bleeding. If the bleeding is completely stopped, the distension medium is freely entering the blood stream. If the observed bleeding completely obscures the field, it is obvious that the vascular pressure is significantly higher than the intrauterine pressure, and absorption is therefore minimal. The bag with distension medium is positioned at a level at which there is some bleeding from cut surfaces but not to the extent that it obscures viewing of the cavity. This is a simple method, under direct control of the surgeon, of regulating the amount of fluid absorption. A little bleeding is better than fluid overload.

Another important aspect is the presence of open vessels, either spontaneously (i.e., during the menstrual phase) or induced by transection with instruments. Clearly, more transected vessels lead to greater fluid absorption. When electrosection techniques with a loop electrode are used, more care must be taken to monitor fluid balance. Although this sounds simple, keeping track of fluid input and output seems to be one of the most difficult things to get organized in the operating room. A simple scheme is to use infusion bags of 3 liters and collection canisters of the same volume. In this way, a quick scan of the number of bags used and full canisters gives a crude idea of the fluid balance. However, this does not replace an accurate determination at regular intervals (e.g., every 10 minutes). There is no absolute level of fluid overload considered acceptable. In a patient with normal kidney function and baseline electrolyte values, an acute infusion of 1000 ml of fluid will bring the sodium level to just around the low end of normal range. More than this should not be tolerated, as an overload of 2000 ml will invariably cause hyponatremia.

Treatment of fluid overload encompasses prevention and correction of acute hyponatremia. Among the factors for prevention of hyponatremia is the choice of distension medium. At present, a combination of sorbitol and mannitol, or mannitol only, is the preferred medium for operative hysteroscopy. Only one medium, Ringer's lactate, is better, but it cannot be used with electrosurgery because it diffuses electrical energy. The advantage of mannitol 5% is that this medium initiates diuresis as soon as it is absorbed. In addition, mannitol 5% maintains serum osmolarity (*Fig. 14.1*) within normal range, notwithstanding the fact that the sodium concentration drops. Therefore there is less transmembranous exchange of electrolytes and free water between the intra- and extracellular compartments. Although there is acute hyponatremia, the lethal consequences of cerebral edema are less likely to occur. Other fluid media commonly used in urology, such as glycine and distilled water, should no longer be used in gynecologic cases, as it has been shown that women of reproductive age are more likely than men to die from the consequences of hyponatremia[9].

It is emphasized that high-viscosity media, such as Hyskon, should be used only in selected cases. These media are hyperosmolar and therefore cause a fluid shift from the intracellular to the extracellular compartment. Moreover, high-viscosity media break down and are eliminated from the circulation only slowly. The volume of Dextran 70 used is capped at 500 ml.

Once dilutional hyponatremia has set in, treatment should be instituted without delay. Data available on dilutional hyponatremia are derived from patients with the syndrome of inappropriate antidiuretic hormone secretion (SIADH) who had received excessive amounts of intravenous fluids[9,10]. The pathophysiologic process consists of water retention caused by lack of renal secretion, paired with intravenous administration of hypotonic fluid such as dextrose 5% in water. This results in excess free water in the extracellular compartment, which diffuses into the intracellular compartment. All organs swell, including the brain. Demise is caused by herniation of the brainstem through the foramen occipitalis. Fluid overload caused by intrauterine infusion of hypotonic solutions follows a similar pathophysiologic process, with the exception that the dilution is far more acute compared to SIADH. It is unclear whether or not this difference is significant with regard to treatment of the condition. Treatment consists of restoring serum osmolarity. This can be achieved by elevation of sodium content and/or elimination of free water. The preferred method is to administer sodium first. It is easier and more predictable, indeed, to elevate serum osmolarity by infusion of sodium than to rely on diuresis. In addition, the mechanism of action of loop diuretics is impeded by low Na^+ concentrations.

The urgency of treatment depends primarily on the type of medium used for distension. Assuming the worst case scenario,

in which glycine was used, Na^+ replacement is initiated immediately. The simplest way to deal with acute hyponatremia secondary to fluid overload with hypo-osmotic media during hysteroscopy is to give the patient 140 mEq Na^+ multiplied by the number of liters unaccounted for. However, because overcorrection of hyponatremia has been equally detrimental[10], it is advisable to give only half the calculated shortage over a short period of time (i.e., 2 hours) and then to measure electrolytes in serum and individualize further treatment. Alternatively, one can calculate the amount of sodium that would bring the patient's serum concentration above the critical value of 125 mEq/l and give only that amount over a short time (e.g., 2 hours).

Swift action is important in these cases. Therefore a rapid short-term treatment should be initiated. One can buy time, for example, by infusing NaCl 3% at a rate of 50–100 ml/h at the time of discovery of the overload. (One ml of NaCl 3% equals 0.5 mEq of Na^+. Therefore 100 ml of NaCl 3% will provide 50 mEq/h. Therefore, infusion of NaCl 3% at a rate of 50–100 ml/h will elevate the sodium concentration at a rate of approximately 1.5–3 mEq/h in a patient of average weight.) After this initial measure, the case is thoroughly reviewed and appropriate action is taken.

Concentrated NaCl in one form or another should be available in the operating room when operative hysteroscopy is performed. It is emphasized again that there is no need for complex calculations: 70 mEq × number of liters of fluid unaccounted for should be replaced within the first two hours or so after discovery of the incident. This will pull the patient out of the danger zone. One should remember that death due to herniation of the pons cerebri can set in within 20 minutes of acute hyponatremia at 120 mEq/l. In many hospitals it will take longer to get the results of an ionogram from the laboratory. Do not waste time! Act as soon as fluid overload is suspected.

Fluid overload that occurs with the use of iso-osmotic media requires less drastic measures. The diuretic action of mannitol 5% will set in immediately to eliminate the excess free water. Some electrolytes are lost in this process as well. There is no consensus among experts and no hard data to indicate the value of Na^+ given intravenously in these cases. The limit of fluid overload can be elevated from 1000 to 2500 ml in a normonatremic patient with normal kidney function. However, when volumes over 2500 ml are unaccounted for, it is the opinion of this author that hypertonic sodium should be administered intravenously at a rate of 50–100 ml NaCl 3% per hour until the calculated value of sodium concentration is over 125 mEq/l. A simplified algorithm for calculation of sodium concentration in serum is shown in *Fig. 14.1*.

Once hyponatremia has been corrected, diuresis will set in spontaneously. Diuresis can be supported with loop diuretics, especially in the presence of pulmonary edema. However, diuretic treatment is associated with additional sodium loss.

Fluid overload causes generalized serum dilution. Other electrolytes are also affected, including potassium and calcium. Hypokalemia and hypocalcemia will cause disturbances of nerve conduction and muscle contraction, first manifested by cardiac dysrhythmias and electrocardiogram alterations. Prompt response to the occurrence of fluid overload will prevent these changes. Administration of dietary potassium supplements in the days before surgery is good practice.

Delayed complications of hysteroscopy are infectious in nature. These complications range from simple endomyometritis to fistula formation between bowel or bladder and the uterus. The main problem is identifying such complications, which may occur several weeks after the surgical event. The patient should be told to report symptoms such as bleeding, fever, diarrhea, and hematuria, which may indicate infection.

Recently, there has been extensive discussion concerning potential for delayed bowel perforation owing to thermal damage without direct contact between the electrode and the bowel. This type of injury is most likely to occur when a large electrode is used in direct contact with the tissue and is activated with a low-wattage, low-voltage current[11]. These electrical parameters produce a low electrodensity that penetrates slowly but deeply into the tissue. Despite the fact that this scenario is indeed possible, it is highly unlikely, because the surgeon would have to hold the electrode in one particular place for as long as a full minute. Under circumstances in which distance between the electrode and the bowel is potentially short because of a thin uterine wall (e.g., at the level of the uterine horn), it is inadvisable to hold the electrode in one particular spot for periods of time exceeding 2 or 3 seconds.

Calculation of Sodium Concentration in Serum

Total body fluid content (TB) = half the body weight in kg
Extracellular fluid (EC) in liters = 45% of total body fluid
Total sodium content in mEq/l = EC × a (preop Na^+ level)
New EC = EC + F (= amount of fluid overload in liters)
New total Na^+ content = unchanged
New Na^+ concentration = total sodium/new EC

Example: weight = 80kg
a = 140 mEq/l
F = 3 l
TB = 40 l
EC = 40 × 0.45 = 18 l
Total Na^+ = 18 × 140 = 2520 mEq
New EC = 18 + 3 = 21 l
New [Na^+] = 2520/21 = 120 mEq/l

To elevate the [Na^+] to 125 mEq/l:
5 mEq × 21 l = 105 mEq
1 ml NaCl 3% = 0.5 mEq Na^+
105 mEq = 210 ml NaCl 3%

14.1 Simple algorithm for calculation of sodium concentration in serum and to calculate sodium replacement.

HYSTEROSCOPIC SEPTAL DIVISION

Hysteroscopic uterine septal resection is a showcase for operative hysteroscopy. Who would hesitate, indeed, in choosing between a Strassman operation and an operative hysteroscopy? Septal resection also demonstrates the range of difficulty that can accompany operative hysteroscopy. One septal resection may require 5 minutes, whereas the next one may be extremely time-consuming. Nevertheless, septal resection is commonly ranked as one of the less complicated hysteroscopic interventions.

INDICATIONS
Repeated pregnancy loss, typically in the second trimester, is the cardinal indication for correction of the septate uterus[12,13]. Because of the minimally invasive nature of the procedure, it is best to schedule immediate intervention without waiting for a second or third loss of pregnancy.

It has been questioned whether or not a septum in a nulliparous woman, discovered during investigation of infertility or abnormal bleeding, should be treated despite the absence of pregnancy loss. It is open to debate that a septate uterus is the cause of the infertility. However, one may want to consider sparing the patient the risk of pregnancy loss after exhaustive treatment for infertility.

CHOICE OF EQUIPMENT
The standard-sized resectoscope (24–26 Charriere) is routinely used for these procedures. It is sometimes necessary to use the smaller so-called pediatric resectoscope, which is especially useful in nulliparous patients or in patients with a large septum and small uterine horns. The electrode of choice is the knife electrode. The knife electrode is typically in the shape of a right angle, which is seen as a transverse bar through the optic. Although a needle electrode is sometimes available, it requires far more control than the knife electrode and therefore should be chosen only when the knife electrode cannot be used because of space constraints.

SURGICAL PROCEDURE
Some steps of the procedure have been described previously and are briefly summarized here. The procedure using the resectoscope is described. Alternative methods, such as the use of a fiber laser, are discussed later.

It is assumed that the diagnosis of a septate uterus has been made either by preoperative investigations, such as ultrasonography, or by laparoscopy before or at the time of operative hysteroscopy.

Step 1
Local anesthesia: A paracervical block is performed. The use of vasocontrictors such as Pitressin is not a requirement.

Step 2
The cervix is dilated up to 10 mm.

Step 3

The equipment is assembled and the resectoscope is inserted under direct view.

Step 4

Assessment of the anatomy: The operator locates both tubal ostia and both hemicavities, noting how far the septum reaches. In the case of a uterus didelphus (two cervices, single fundus) the operator will be unable to visualize both cavities. To facilitate localization of the hemiuterus that cannot be viewed, a probe is inserted into that hemiuterus and pressed against the middle. The operator should be able to see the indentation caused by the probe.

Step 5

Delineation of the septum: Lack of depth perception prevents the operator from identifying the corner made by the fundus and the septum. However, gentle probing with the electrode enables the surgeon to feel the transition. In some instances there is little space between the ostium and the septum, preventing passage of the knife electrode. The electrode, which is usually bent at a 90° angle, can be more or less straightened to reduce the transverse diameter and enable the surgeon to reach the base of the septum without touching the lateral wall of the uterus or the ostium.

Step 6

Section of the septum (*Fig. 14.2*): The ideal method is to start cutting the septum at the fundus and to move the activated electrode towards the optic, which obeys the general rules for operative hysteroscopy. The best approach for a right-handed

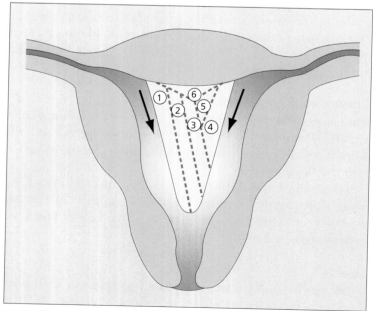

14.2 Schematic representation of the successive incisions made into a uterine septum with the resectoscope. Arrows indicate direction.

physician is from the patient's right. Each progressive cut is started slightly more proximal from the start of the previous cut. This will result in a convex fundus. The left lateral edge of the septum is transected last. The convexity of the fundus can be remodeled.

Estimating when to stop cutting is the challenge in septal resection. Three structural signs can guide the hysteroscopist. First, there is the difference in consistency and structure of tissues: the septum is fibrous, hard, and noncompliant, whereas the myometrium is trabecular, soft, and compliant. The two types of tissue also differ in electrical resistance: myometrium conducts well and is easily cut, whereas the septum presents more resistance to the advancing electrode. Finally, there is a difference in vascularization: sectioning of the septum causes only very minor bleeding, whereas myometrium bleeds profusely. The use of vasoconstrictors should be avoided so that this difference is not attenuated.

In some cases the septum is so wide that the endoscope and electrode can not be advanced to the fundus. In such cases the surgeon has no choice but to start cutting the septum from the cervical edge onward. This requires the cut to be made while moving the electrode away from the optic, which goes against the general surgical principles for operative hysteroscopy. However, as the section progresses, the uterine cavity distends and the surgeon can convert to the technique described previously.

ALTERNATIVE PROCEDURES

Correction of a septate uterus can be performed alternatively by laparotomy (Strassman procedure) or by hysteroscopy with the use of a fiber laser. For all practical purposes, the Strassman procedure has now been abandoned. Using laser to transect a septum is technically feasible, and the general surgical principles remain the same. The advantage of the laser fiber is that it can be introduced through a flexible endoscope, adding maneuverability. The disadvantage is that the fiber laser procedure is slower than electrosurgery and, in most countries, is substantially more expensive.

COMPLICATIONS

All complications previously described can occur during septal resection. The most common complication is fundal perforation with the knife electrode. It has been suggested that concomitant laparoscopy would prevent this from happening. Laparoscopy confirms the diagnosis of a "single fundus". However, it does not prevent perforation, but merely confirms the fact. Intermittent viewing of the fundus in diaphanoscopy (i.e., without a light cable attached to the laparoscope, looking at the uterus glowing in the dark) may help the surgeon to decide when to stop sectioning the septum. It can be assumed that when transluminescence of the uterus is uniform, the septum is completely transected. With experience however, the hysteroscopist will be able to rely on hysteroscopic features only to decide when the section has been completed.

HYSTEROSCOPIC SYNECHIOLYSIS

Synechiolysis is a procedure that taxes the surgeon's skill to the greatest extent, because the anatomy of the uterine cavity is severely distorted. However, it is also the most rewarding procedure. There is a wide range of difficulty levels. Some cases can be handled in the office with minimal sedation. Others may require several frustrating hours in the operating room. In some cases, reconstruction of the uterine cavity will take several successive sessions.

INDICATIONS

The main indications for synechiolysis are secondary infertility and pregnancy loss caused by intrauterine adhesions[14]. It is debatable whether reduced menstrual flow resulting from intrauterine adhesions is an indication in itself for intervention. However, a young woman unsure about future childbearing should be given the benefit of the doubt and should undergo the procedure even if pregnancy is not planned in the foreseeable future. Ethnic background must be considered in making the decision for intervention. In some North African populations, cessation of menses is a reason for the woman to be repudiated by her husband. In general, however, hypo- or amenorrhea does not in itself justify the real risk of a surgical intervention.

SURGICAL PROCEDURE

Some steps of the procedure have been described previously and are briefly summarized here.

Timing

It is important to schedule the procedure during the proliferative phase of the cycle, either natural or induced. An unopposed estrogen environment is the desired milieu. Enhanced healing, firm myometrium, and a rapidly growing endometrium are a few of the reasons why an unopposed estrogen environment is preferred. In the presence of amenorrhea it is recommended that the patient record her basal body temperature and that the day of surgery is selected according to the temperature curve.

Equipment

Synechiolysis is a procedure that is best not performed with a resectoscope. Use of simple mechanical devices, such as scissors or graspers, is the preferred modality because these cause the least tissue destruction. These instruments can be introduced through the operating channel of a rigid endoscope, the operating port of a flexible endoscope, or can be passed along the outer sheath of a rigid endoscope. None of these methods is superior, and all of them require extensive practice before they can be mastered.

Synechiolysis sometimes requires the use of fluoroscopy. A "C-arm" or mobile fluoroscopy unit should be available[15]. This implies that the operating table is radiolucent. The patient is placed in the dorsal lithotomy position with the legs suspended in "candy cane"-type stirrups. The head of the C-arm is passed over the patient's abdomen and inclined cephalad, so that the

direction of the X-ray beam is perpendicular to the hollow of the sacrum, allowing optimal viewing of the uterus. An appropriate distension medium is required to allow visualization with fluoroscopy and hysteroscopy simultaneously. One possibility is to mix Dextran 70 (Hyskon) with Renographin at a ratio of 1:1 (v/v). This medium is still viscous enough to be minimally miscible with blood and is sufficiently radiopaque to allow delineation of the contour of the uterine cavity and synechiae sufficiently to guide the surgeon. The purpose of real-time hysterography during hysteroscopic visualization is that sometimes the endoscopic view is confusing. When several tracts are visible, the surgeon does not have any anatomic indication as to which of these tracts is connected to a sequestered part of the cavity or leads to a plane between layers of myometrium. Real-time hysterography gives the operator the desired information, to facilitate the choice of which tract to explore surgically. In cases where the outer contour of the uterine cavity is visualized, fluoroscopy is not required.

Step 1

Local anesthesia: A paracervical block is performed. The use of vasoconstrictors, such as Pitressin, is not recommended, because the surgeon must rely to some extent on the occurrence of bleeding to judge whether or not the surgical plane is suitable.

Step 2

Passage of the cervical canal: The use of cervical dilators in patients with intrauterine adhesions is contraindicated, because the uterine walls are significantly weakened by the disease process that caused the synechiae. Blind transcervical manipulation is associated with a risk of perforation and reduces the chances that the uterus will ever again be functional. The cervical canal is passed under direct view only. Once explored and its dimensions known, the canal can be enlarged mechanically to accommodate larger instrumentation.

Step 3

Assembly of equipment: The simplest setup is the rigid 5-mm diagnostic hysteroscope with a 1.6-mm rigid instrument held alongside the outer sheath of the endoscope. An assistant holds the tenaculum, which is applied to the anterior lip of the cervix, allowing the surgeon to use both hands. The surgeon manipulates the endoscope in one hand and the syringe with distension medium in the other, or else operates the mechanical instrument used to break up the adhesions. When ancillary instruments are used free alongside the endoscope, the operator holds the endoscope in front of the eyepiece with the palm facing up. The fingers of the hand close on the upper side of the endoscope and hold the mechanical instrument by its shaft. The hand holding the endoscope guides not only the endoscope but also the mechanical instrument used to operate on the synechiae. This is a true challenge to fine motor control! The other hand controls the two other dimensions of the ancillary instrument: the back-and-forth motion and the opening and closing of the jaws.

Step 4

Assessment of anatomy: No other surgical situation in operative hysteroscopy is characterized by such distorted anatomy. This is the main reason why it is advisable to combine two imaging methodologies in real time. There are two critical areas: the internal cervical os and the cornual area. The posterior wall of the internal cervical os is the most common site for perforation in patients with Ashermann syndrome because it is located on a straight line from the external cervical os. The surgeon has a tendency to miss the curvature of the ante- or retroversion. In the presence of a closed cervical canal and internal cervical os, the use of fluoroscopy is mandatory. The surgeon should remember that the intrauterine pressure will drive the blood out of the capillaries, causing the mucosa to appear pale and indistinguishable from fibrous scar tissue. Intermittent reduction of pressure will facilitate recognition of mucosal surfaces and of vessels that have been severed but prevented from bleeding by the elevated intrauterine pressure.

The other challenging anatomic areas are the cornua and the tubal ostium. Lack of depth perception makes it difficult to determine whether the curvature of the lateral uterine wall is normal or whether there are residual marginal adhesions. Fluoroscopy is once more the solution. In some instances, the scar tissue comes close to the tubal ostium or actually includes it. There is little that can be done in such a situation except for careful dissection. A fully occluded cornua and ostium cannot be cured hysteroscopically. In such a case, the cavity is made functional first. In the event that both ostia are found to be closed, a choice must be made between reconstructive tubal surgery with tubocornual anastomosis or *in vitro* fertilization.

Step 5

Lysis of adhesions can be effected in different fashions. On the assumption that scar tissue is more friable than healthy tissue, blunt mechanical energy is most widely used to separate the anterior uterine wall from the posterior wall. Blunt mechanical energy can be provided by the tip of the endoscope. Graspers can be used to disrupt fibrous bands by spreading the jaws or by grasping and gently avulsing adhesions, or by a combination of both. Adhesions can be divided sharply with scissors, and scissors can also be used for blunt dissection.

The difficult areas are along the fundus and the side walls. The difficulty resides in reaching these areas and/or lack of adequate depth perception. The preferred method for lysis of adhesions in these areas is to attempt to find the plane between the adhesion and the uterine wall first by sharp dissection, so as to isolate the synechia and then to transect it. The most challenging location is the central fundal synechia. This is one situation in which the cardinal rule of safety in hysteroscopy must be violated, because the only feasible way to transect the adhesion is with a cutting instrument moving away from the endoscope, which has the potential to cause a perforation.

Step 6

In some cases there is complete obstruction of the uterine cavity, either at the level of the isthmus or at the internal cervical os.

Fluoroscopy reveals only a blind pouch. In such a situation an additional procedure can be used to obtain visualization. Fine needles are available that can be introduced either through the operating channel of an operative hysteroscope or even through the resectoscope. These needles were originally designed to deliver local anesthesia; however, they can also be used in this situation to probe the blind pouch in search of a hidden cavity. The fluid used can be radiopaque to facilitate identification with fluoroscopy. Some vital dye is added to color the mucosa, enhancing visual identification during further hysteroscopic dissection. Intravascular injection will be identified on fluoroscopy. Once a cavity has been located, injection of fluid increases its volume and thereby the chance that further dissection will unroof the enclosed area. This procedure is excruciatingly slow and unnerving. Probing with a needle is not immediately successful and is sometimes extremely frustrating. In some advanced cases, one should retain the option of postponing further exploration and dissection of the cavity until a later date. It may require up to four sessions of operative hysteroscopy before the cavity is completely restored.

Step 7

Recurrence of synechiae is common, as with every condition involving scar tissue. Early second-look hysteroscopy is therefore advisable. Intrauterine adhesions are usually present at the time of second look but can easily be broken down, even by mere distension of the cavity. In patients with ambivalence about future pregnancy, one can postpone second-look hysteroscopy until after menstrual problems recur.

ALTERNATIVE PROCEDURES

There is no true alternative procedure. The best treatment for intrauterine adhesions is the hysteroscopic approach. Blind insertion and avulsion of adhesions no longer have a place in modern medicine. Discussion persists as to whether one hysteroscopic modality is superior to the other but too few cases of intrauterine adhesions have been reported to allow comparative prospective studies. The combination of direct visualization with fluoroscopic imaging is the most accurate method at present to achieve optimal characterization of the anatomic distortion with ensuing optimal capability to correct it.

COMPLICATIONS

All complications previously described can occur during surgery on a patient with Asherman syndrome. The most common complication is perforation of the uterine wall during attempts to lyse synechiae or while engaging in a fausse route. This happens most often at the level of the internal cervical os and the tubal ostium. Lack of depth perception is the main cause, in addition to lack of surgical common sense and experience. Few patients present with intrauterine synechiae, and consequently few physicians are experienced in treating the condition. Many complications can be avoided by recognizing and referring cases that require the attention of an experienced hysteroscopist.

The potential for perforation will persist regardless of the physician's level of experience. Judicious use of combined imaging techniques is the surgeon's sole safeguard.

HYSTEROSCOPIC IUCD REMOVAL

The removal of a lost IUCD used to be the principal indication for operative hysteroscopy in many European countries before the advent of endometrial ablation[16]. It certainly provided impetus for the development of hysteroscopic equipment. In the United States, litigation involving the Dalkon shield has impeded widespread use of intrauterine devices. Operative hysteroscopy for a problem such as retrieval of a lost IUCD or part of a broken device is therefore not widely performed.

INDICATIONS

Loss of an IUCD is defined as the inability of the physician to ascertain that the device is well positioned inside the uterus. During speculum examination of the cervix, the physician checks whether the strings attached to the device are visible and whether any part of the IUCD is protruding from the cervix. In China, IUCDs are made of flexible metal rings, which are inserted into the uterus during the postpartum (12 weeks) or postabortem period. No string is attached to these devices, and they are allowed to remain *in utero* throughout the entire period of childbearing age into menopause. Chinese doctors advise against regular changes of the IUCD because they have noted that side effects of IUCD use, such as an increased incidence of tubal pregnancy, decrease with duration of use. They have not observed the occurrence of unusual infectious complications that has been reported in the Western literature and which appears to be related to increasing duration of use, hence the recommendation to replace an IUCD every 2 years.

Inability to find the string of the IUD is not in itself an indication for hysteroscopy. Noninvasive imaging techniques are available to ascertain the appropriate location of the IUCD. Ultrasonography, transvaginal or abdominal, is the best method because it allows visualization of the contour of both the uterine cavity and the device. Two features are looked for: the distance between the fundus and the transverse arm of the IUCD and the distance between the internal os and the tail of the IUCD in the cervical canal. Both features can provide an indication of incorrect placement owing to disproportion between the size of the IUCD and the uterine cavity, a congenital abnormality of the cavity (subseptum), or acquired organic pathology (fibroid).

It is a common misconception that an IUCD can wander easily through the uterine wall. It is far more likely that the uterine wall is damaged during insertion and that the IUCD becomes partly embedded in a resulting breach at the time of its insertion. The device can then penetrate and sometimes pass entirely through the uterine wall. It is therefore important to check the positioning of the IUCD immediately after insertion.

An alternative method for locating an IUCD is fluoroscopy. The patient is positioned on the table, a speculum is inserted to place a tenaculum on the cervix, and the speculum is subsequently removed. The operator holds the tenaculum while the fluoroscopy monitor is switched on. Once the IUCD has been located, the operator manipulates the tenaculum while observing the screen. The position of the image of the IUCD in relation to the cervix gives a crude idea of its location. Note that a plain KUB film has only limited value.

SURGICAL PROCEDURE

The initial steps of operative hysteroscopy are only briefly repeated.

Timing

The general rule of scheduling surgery during the proliferative period of the cycle applies. However, there is no contraindication to performing the surgery during the luteal phase, although the latter is technically more difficult.

Equipment

The resectoscope is not the ideal instrument for removal of an IUCD. The simplest setup is a diagnostic endoscope along which a grasper is introduced. The grasper is used to draw forward the threads attached to the IUCD and sometimes for blunt dissection of embedded parts of the IUCD. The distension medium of choice is Dextran 70, but any fluid medium is acceptable.

Step 1

Local anesthesia: Paracervical block is an adequate form of anesthesia.

Step 2

Cervical dilatation is required only when the cervix does not allow the passage of a diagnostic hysteroscope. The majority of IUCD wearers are multiparous and such insertion is usually not a problem. If dilatation is required, it can be limited to 7 mm.

Step 3

The equipment is assembled and the hysteroscope is inserted under direct visualization.

Step 4

Assessment of the anatomy: Both tubal ostia are located first. The IUCD is then identified. Before any attempt is made to remove the device, the operator verifies that the entire IUCD is located within the cavity. Minimal embedding in the uterine wall is acceptable. If it appears that a significant portion of the IUCD is buried in the uterine wall, attempts to forcefully remove the device from the uterus should be halted, and dissection to free the device should be carried out first.

Step 5

Removal of the non-embedded IUCD: If it appears that the IUCD is well positioned in the uterine cavity and that the only problem is that the strings attached to it are folded up into the cavity, one should consider leaving the device *in situ*, depending on the clinical situation. The strings can be brought out without removing the IUCD. This is also the easiest method of actually removing the device. Once the strings are visible in the cervical canal, one can use them to remove the IUCD itself in the old-fashioned way. If the strings are missing, the operator should first identify the smallest diameter of the IUCD and attempt to grasp it at that point. It is sometimes sufficient to align the IUCD correctly by positioning its tail along the longitudinal axis. A long thin polyp forceps can then be introduced and the IUCD removed.

Step 6

Removal of the embedded IUCD: On panoramic overview; the operator may be unable to identify the entire device or in rare instances, a small piece of the device may protrude from the uterine wall while the majority of it remains embedded in the myometrium. These two situations may be difficult to distinguish. However, a judgment must be made because subsequent action is dependent on it. The issue is whether the device can be extracted from below or whether laparoscopy must be done to extract the IUCD from the uterus. Gentle manipulation of the device hysteroscopically will enable the operator to evaluate whether this is indeed feasible. Knowledge of the exact shape of the IUCD is helpful. Some devices have thickenings at their extremities, which make removal difficult once they have traversed through the myometrium. In this situation, a blunt grasping forceps is used to dissect the myometrium around the embedded parts of the IUCD. It may be necessary to introduce an electrical probe to desiccate the myometrium around the object before dissection. Desiccation alone will often dislodge the device. Once it is free, it can be retrieved as described above. The operator can stop the dissection at any time if it is estimated that the IUCD has migrated through the entire thickness of the uterine wall. It will then be necessary to stop the hysteroscopic surgery and to proceed to laparoscopy for removal of the device.

ALTERNATIVE PROCEDURES

Again fluoroscopy is the alternative to direct visualization. Provided the device is radio-opaque, it can be visualized on the fluoroscope. In most cases, the operator will be able to grasp the IUCD and to remove it. However, when resistance is felt, one should refrain from pulling with excessive force. Operative hysteroscopy is far more difficult for removal of a broken piece rather than an entire device.

COMPLICATIONS

Every complication mentioned above can occur with removal of the embedded intrauterine device. Because of the fact that dissection of the myometrium is sometimes required, perforation is the most common mishap.

HYSTEROSCOPIC FIBROID RESECTION

Doctor Neuwirth in New York is certainly to be commended for initiating the development of hysteroscopic myomectomy[5,17]. For more than a decade he struggled against the disbelief of his colleagues until the advent of endometrial ablation widened the indications for hysteroscopic myomectomy. Initially, myomectomy was reserved for treatment of submucous fibroids in patients who desired continued fertility. At present, conservative surgery of the uterus has gained more ground. Myomectomy in combination with endometrial ablation may represent an acceptable treatment for abnormal bleeding in a patient who does not desire further fertility. Acceptance of this procedure will depend largely on the availability of training for physicians in this type of intervention. Because a hysteroscopic myomectomy involves sectioning of large surfaces, the procedure puts the patient at greatest risk of fluid overload. Note that differences in size measured by ultrasound are one-dimensional, whereas the corresponding differences are three-dimensional in hysteroscopic resection. The difference between resection of a 2-cm fibroid and a 3-cm fibroid is a lot of sweat and experience[18].

INDICATIONS

The indication for hysteroscopic myomectomy is removal of submucous fibroids with conservation of the uterus. Hysteroscopic myomectomy is the classic example of "uterus sparing" surgery. The foremost indication for myomectomy is a history of infertility or pregnancy loss. Abnormal uterine bleeding due to a submucous fibroid is now becoming a second indication for myomectomy. In most of the latter cases, endometrial ablation and resection should be performed concomitantly, because the abnormal bleeding is the main reason for the patient to seek medical help.

SURGICAL PROCEDURE

Timing

Myomectomy is best performed during the early proliferative phase when the endometrium is thin and bleeding is less profuse than at other phases of the menstrual cycle.

Equipment

The standard resectoscope (26–28 French) is the instrument of choice. The preferred fluid distension media are sorbitol, mannitol, or a combination of both. A pump to instil the fluid is not necessary. Gauged gravity is equivalent and is less subject to technical failure. There are many different electrodes to choose from. The most commonly used electrode is the loop electrode bent at 90°. This electrode allows resection of most fibroids of the anterior and posterior uterine walls, the most common locations. Technical problems arise with tumors growing at the level of the fundus and within the cervical canal. The angled loop electrodes cannot then be used efficiently because the electrode cannot be brought behind the tumor. In such cases the straight loop electrode should be used. This electrode forces the operator to work against the general principles of operative hysteroscopy, however, because the electrode is not moved towards the optic when activated. If no information regarding location is available, one should load the resectoscope with the standard 90° loop electrode.

Step 1

Local anesthesia: A paracervical block is performed regardless of whether the patient is under general anesthesia or not. Addition of a vasoconstrictive agent such as Pitressin is helpful, because blood loss can be substantial. Prospective studies to validate that vasoconstrictors do indeed reduce blood loss during hysteroscopic myomectomy are lacking. However, it seems logical that they would and their use has become widely accepted.

Step 2

The cervix is dilated to 10 mm.

Step 3

The equipment is assembled and the resectoscope is inserted under direct visualization. A large amount of fluid is used during hysteroscopic myomectomy. It is therefore important that collection of fluids be done with a minimum of leakage. A drape that fits underneath the patient's buttocks, far enough so that there is minimal loss of fluid, is recommended.

Step 4

Assessment of the anatomy: The size and the exact location of the fibroid are noted. In addition, it is important to determine whether or not the largest diameter of the fibroid lies within the uterine cavity. When this proves to be the case, the surgical procedure is relatively simple for a fibroid less than 3 cm in diameter. Larger fibroids are a challenge no matter where they are located. When the largest diameter is not directly visible to the hysteroscopist, determination of size is difficult and can lead to serious underestimation. In addition, the surgery is significantly more complicated because of the difficult access to the intramural part of the tumor and the rich vascular supply of the fibroid and the surrounding myometrium.

Step 5a

Resection of a submucous fibroid of the anterior or posterior wall (*Fig. 14.3*): The right-angled loop electrode is used. The surgeon executes a "dry run" first, moving the electrode over the tumor without activating it, to "feel" the microanatomy of the uterine cavity. It is also important to assess whether the active element of the resectoscope will move without resistance over the desired distance.

A high wattage pure cutting current is used (e.g., 140 W at 1000 V continuous output). The current is activated before the electrode touches the tissue. The time necessary for the electrode to penetrate into the fibroid is significantly longer than that necessary to maintain a smooth cut through the fibroid. The current is maintained until the electrode is guided outside the tissue. Interrupting the current before the electrode is retrieved outside the tissue will cause the electrode to become stuck in the tissue, with ensuing difficulty in releasing the instrument, accompanied by frustration and delay.

An initial incision is made longitudinally in the middle of the fibroid. This initial incision can be made deep. The lateral edges of the incision will tend to bend inward, as if the fibroid was folding. This enables the operator to take large strips along these edges. After three passes, the top of the fibroid becomes a flat surface. Depending on the dimensions of the fibroid, there will be one or two incisions in the middle before the edges can be shaved off again. The general principle remains, however, to core out the middle of the fibroid first and then to proceed to the lateral edges to obtain a flat surface. One should refrain from the temptation to attack the fibroid at the base, for two reasons. First, there are large veins around the base of the fibroid, which, once transected, become the gate to fluid overload. Second, the fibroid loses part of its attachment to the uterine wall and therefore becomes mechanically unstable. Electrical pathways also become less efficient.

The uterus represents only a small reservoir, and tissue strips must be removed periodically. This can be accomplished with a polyp forceps in a blind fashion.

Once the outer shell of the fibroid has been reached, the remaining peel of fibroid can be removed with the loop electrode used as a mechanical device. The shell of tissue is loosened by blunt dissection from all sides. Occasionally, some fibrous attachments must be transected electrically.

When the fibroid has been resected and the tissue strips have been removed, the surgeon should check for hemostasis. This is done by reducing the pressure of the fluid inflow by lowering the i.v. fluid bags. It will be noted that the size of the tumor bed will be significantly reduced by myometrial contraction. Bleeding is minimal. The bleeding is substantially less after the fibroid has been removed in its entirety compared with the blood loss during resection of the fibroid itself.

Step 5b

Resection of a fibroid implanted at the fundus of the uterus (*Fig. 14.4*): The surgical principles described above can obviously not

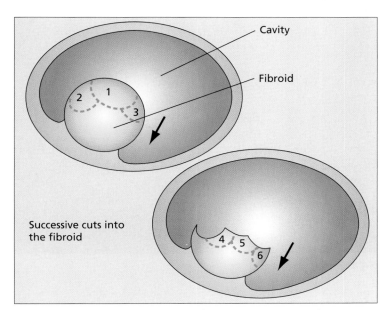

14.3 Schematic representation of successive incisions for resection of a submucous fibroid of lateral walls. Arrow indicates direction.

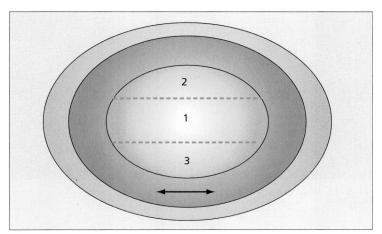

14.4 Schematic representation of successive incisions of a fundal fibroid. Arrow indicates direction.

be observed when the fibroid is located in line with the endoscope as opposed to a 90° angle. The preferred approach is to use a straight-loop electrode and to resect the fibroid by making horizontal passes. The sequence of the cuts is the same as described above, although it is much more difficult to maintain a systematic approach to resection of the fundal fibroid. An additional difficulty is the fact that with the endoscope held in a horizontal plane there is more difficulty in maintaining distension, because the ports for distension at the distal end of the instrument are located anteriorly and posteriorly. A vertical approach to resection of the fundal fibroid is possible. However, the distance between the anterior and posterior walls is significantly shorter than the distance between the left and right lateral walls. Longer strips of tissue can therefore be resected in the horizontal approach.

Step 5c

Resection of a partly intramural fibroid: There is a significant step upwards in degree of difficulty between resection of the submucous firboid and the partly intramural fibroid. One of the reasons is that partly intramural fibroids have a tendency to be discovered later and therefore to be larger. The main difficulty, however, is that part of the fibroid is embedded within the uterine wall.

The uterus will try to expel fibroids. Therefore, when the myometrium is cut around the insertion of the fibroid, the latter will start to migrate toward the uterine cavity. This does not justify cutting around the base of the fibroid first, however. The initial steps as described above should be followed. When the fibroid has been resected to a level flush with the uterine cavity,

some myometrium surrounding the cut surface of the fibroid is resected to allow access to the base of the fibroid. Cutting of myometrium must be kept to a minimum, involves only the edges around the base of the fibroid, and affects only the very surface of the myometrium. Lowering the intrauterine pressure at this time is helpful in permitting the remainder of the fibroid to be expelled from its bed. The base of the fibroid is teased out of its attachments. One should be aware of the fact that the myometrium at the level of the base of the fibroid can be extremely thin. Caution is therefore advised. Because large chunks of tissue are difficult to remove, it is preferable to avoid teasing out the base of the fibroid too soon which results in an oversized piece of tissue that will be difficult to remove and difficult to cut further into smaller pieces. *Figs 14.5–14.12* illustrate the systematic approach to submucous fibroid resection.

ALTERNATIVE PROCEDURES

Alternative procedures to hysteroscopic myomectomy are hysterectomy and myomectomy by uterotomy. In a patient with further desire for pregnancy, the hysteroscopic route is indisputably preferred. Another alternative is to perform a myomectomy vaginally by blind manipulation. When the fibroid is small or when the cervix has significantly softened, the latter method is certainly attractive and is an acceptable alternative in experienced hands. Vaginal myomectomy, which requires incision of the cervix and even the isthmus of the uterus, is less advisable, although no clinical studies exist that compare these two methods. I avoid incisions of the myometrium in patients who intend to become pregnant.

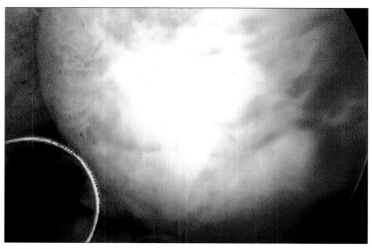

14.5 Submucous myoma.

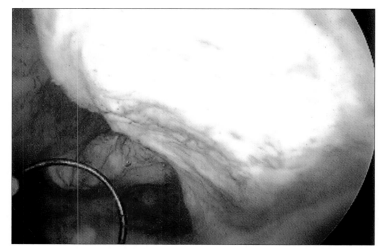

14.6 Initial pass with loop.

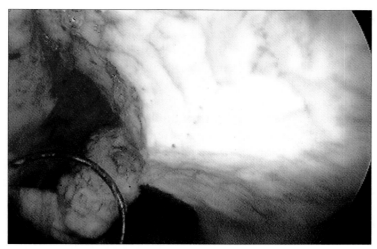

14.7 Successive portions of the myoma are removed.

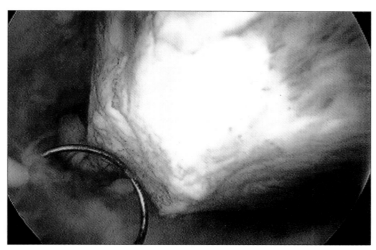

14.8 Systematic shaving of the submucous myoma.

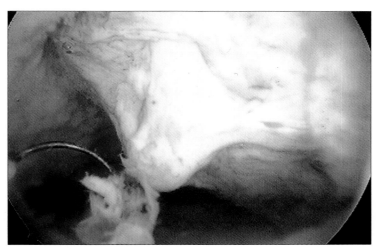

14.9 The myoma is removed near its base.

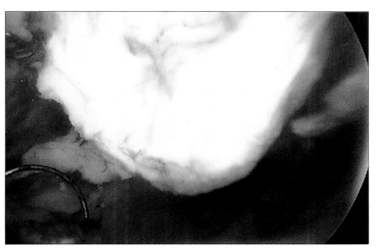

14.10 The shaving process should be done in full view.

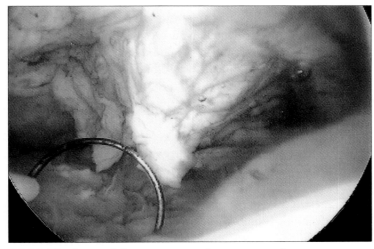

14.11 The base of the myoma can be very vascular.

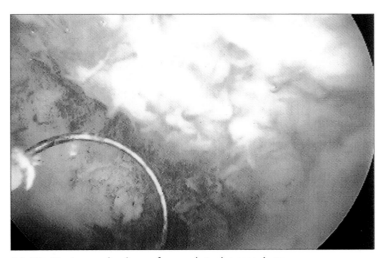

14.12 Hystoscopic view of completed procedure.

COMPLICATIONS

The main complication of hysteroscopic myomectomy is probably the inability of the surgeon to complete the procedure owing to its complexity. Next comes fluid overload. A fibroid is surrounded by a fibrous capsule. Within this capsule are found many large veins. Incision with the loop electrode at the implantation site of a fibroid opens a number of such veins, which in turn leads to fluid overload. The fluid overload will continue until the myometrium is able to contract around the vessels, which occurs only after the fibroid has been completely resected. Therefore, it is important to avoid cutting the base of the fibroid early in the procedure and to debulk the fibroid in a timely fashion. However, fluid absorption will always occur and the amount of such absorption must always be closely monitored.

All other complications mentioned earlier can occur during myomectomy. The third most common complication is perforation of the uterine wall with the activated electrode. This can be avoided by following the general rules of intrauterine surgery.

HYSTEROSCOPIC ENDOMETRIAL RESECTION/ABLATION

Endometrial ablation has saved hysteroscopy from oblivion. It is the large-scale procedure needed by a technique to become widely accepted. Although methods of endometrial ablation have been performed for many decades[19], the overall procedure has met significant resistance within the scientific community. The aura of laser surgery has captured the attention of the public, however, thereby forcing the medical establishment to increase its interest in the methodology.

Many different methods are available for endometrial ablation, and more are under development[20]. No one method has a clear advantage over another. Yag-laser has the advantage of the longest follow-up. Roller-ball ablation is technically the easiest to perform[21]. Finally, resection of the endomyometrium allows histologic examination of a specimen. It is probable that all three methods will continue to be performed, although the current financial crisis argues in favor of the electrosurgical methods. Within a few years, additional instrumentation will be available that will enable endometrial ablation to be performed as an office procedure. Let us hope, however, that operative hysteroscopy will remain. The following description of the technique will be limited to the electrosurgical methods.

INDICATIONS

Endometrial ablation is a conservative treatment for excessive but regular bleeding (i.e., menorrhagia). Other bleeding abnormalities can be treated with endometrial ablation, with the understanding that the procedure addresses the volume of bleeding and not necessarily the cyclicity. In end effect, any abnormal bleeding of benign etiology can be treated conservatively by reduction of the endometrial tissue, which is the source of the bleeding. Endometrial ablation is a symptomatic treatment, not a causative one.

What are the limits? Is a 12-week-sized uterus myomatosus a contraindication for endometrial ablation or not? This discussion is not intended to answer these questions. The limitations of the technique are dictated mainly by the skills of the surgeon. The true contraindications are pregnancy and cases of uterine, cervical, or endometrial malignancy. Under benign conditions it is possible to reduce the amount of uterine bleeding in almost all cases. This was the original purpose of endometrial ablation, which started as an emergency procedure: reduction of flow, either in an acute or a chronic situation. The subsequent need for hysterectomy in a small subset of patients is predictable and should not be used as an argument against the legitimacy of the procedure. Hysterectomy is a topic of heated debate at the time of writing. It is true that in earlier generations only a few hundred hysterectomies were performed in the USA, whereas that number has risen to the present level of half a million per year. As with many other aspects of medicine, hysterectomy has shifted from a life-saving operation to a commodity of modern life. Endometrial ablation may provide that desired quality of life with less invasive surgery.

SURGICAL PROCEDURE

Timing

The procedure is best performed in the proliferative phase of the cycle. In many instances it is advisable to administer suppressive therapy. Good, consistent suppression of the endometrium is obtained with medication such as depot Lupron. GnRH agonists and antagonists are the most reliable agents for obtaining a thin endometrium, provided that the endometrium is allowed to slough away after administration of the drug.

Equipment

Endometrial ablation can be obtained by electrodesiccation, electrosection, or a combination of both. For electrodesiccation, a large surface electrode is used, such as the roller ball or bar. Any electrode with a large contact surface will produce desiccation. Electrosection is performed with a wire loop electrode for controlled resection of the endomyometrium. For electrosection of the uterine walls, the right-angled loop electrode is most appropriate. The distension medium is nonconductive, preferably sorbitol, mannitol, or a combination of both. The fluid balance is carefully monitored. The settings on the electrosurgical generator depend on the desired bioeffect. Desiccation is best performed with a low-wattage, medium- to high-voltage current, such as 60 W of "maximum blend" or "coagulation" current. Section is done with a high-wattage, low-voltage continuous current (e.g., 140 W of cutting current).

Step 1

Local anesthesia: A combination of short-acting, long-acting anesthetic and vasoconstrictor is ideal for endometrial ablation. The anesthetic is administered for every case, even if the patient is operated on under general anesthesia, because it will help to control postoperative pain, which is most severe during the first 2 hours after the procedure.

Step 2

Passage of the cervical canal: The cervix is first dilated to a diameter of 10 mm. The resectoscope can then be introduced under direct vision. Some surgeons may prefer to use laminaria, which are inserted on the evening preceding the procedure or, if the surgery takes place in the evening, on the morning of the surgery.

Step 3

Assembly of equipment: The appropriate electrode is connected to the working element of the resectoscope. Maintaining accurate determinations of the fluid balance is important, especially during electrosection.

Step 4

Assessment of the anatomy: It is important for the operator to survey the anatomy carefully. Unless the patient is known to have a particular abnormality, the operator expects to see the fundus and two ostia. Any congenital or acquired anomalies are noted. Obviously, the latter are the most common. At least 20% of patients undergoing endometrial ablation have had cesarean sections, the scars of which present two potential problems. First, they are sites of lesser resistance, and there is therefore the potential for perforation. Second, the anatomy around the isthmus can be distorted to such a degree that it becomes difficult to ablate the entire endometrium. Any suspect lesion is biopsied at this time.

Step 5

Setting the electrosurgical generator: There is a wide variation among different electrosurgical generators and also among generators from the same manufacturer. The standard setting of, for example, 60 W of damped current for electrodesiccation is not always optimal. An effort should be made to have the same electrosurgical generator in the operating room for every case of operative hysteroscopy. However, this goal may not always be realistic. Therefore, the operator must test the equipment in every single case as if the energy source were new. Electrodesiccation is obtained by an electrode in contact with the tissue. Contact is established before the instrument is activated. The operator should observe no sparking while the electrode is active. Sparking is detrimental to the process of electrodesiccation because it induces changes to the surface of the tissue that prevent further penetration of the electrical current. The typical changes observed in tissue during the process of desiccation are blanching, which occurs slowly and expands progressively, and the formation of small gas vacuoles that arise from the tissue undergoing desiccation.

Step 6a

Electrodesiccation of the uterine walls: The surgery is performed in a standardized fashion. No particular sequence is better than another. I prefer to desiccate the fundus and the ostia first and then the anterior wall, the posterior wall, and finally the cornual areas. In a small uterus the strokes can be guided from fundus to cervix, whereas in a larger uterus the surgeon may elect to divide the process into two halves, with the fundal half done first. The electrode is moved slowly while the operator observes the changes occurring in the tissue. The blanching caused by heating of the tissue should be seen preceding the electrode. The electrodesiccation process occurs simultaneously all around the electrode, and therefore also in front of it. When the electrode is moved too quickly, the tissue in contact with the electrode does not become desiccated.

Step 6b

Electrosection of the uterine walls (*Fig. 14.13*): The procedure is performed in an equally standardized fashion. I prefer to delineate the fundus and tubal ostia with the roller-ball electrode before resecting the walls. The desiccation forms a "white line" at the fundus, which helps in orientation. There are two additional advantages. First, the desiccation adds to the destruction of the endometrium at a site that is difficult to resect well with a right-angled electrode, which is the one to choose for resection of the uterine walls. Second, during desiccation of the fundus, the electrode causes some dehiscence between the anterior and posterior walls at the level of the fundus, which facilitates access to the upper edge of the endometrial lining of the anterior and posterior walls with the loop electrode. Resection of the endomyometrium is started at the posterior wall of the uterine cavity, because the strips of tissue produced tend to settle down at the fundus along the posterior wall, thus preventing access to the posterior wall. Further resection is then done in a clockwise fashion. The strips of tissue are removed with polyp forceps on a regular basis, because the uterine cavity is small and has a low capacity for storage of tissue strips.

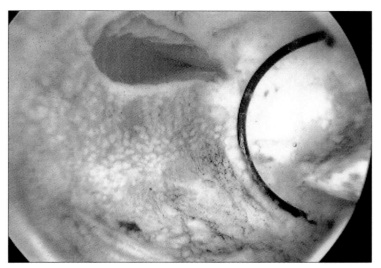

14.13 Electrosection of the endomyometrium. The glandular structure of the endometrium around the right ostium is obvious.

Step 7

During resection of the endomyometrium, the surgeon may unroof small cystic areas of glandular tissue (*Fig. 14.14*). This is ectopic endometrium and therefore represents adenomyosis. Taking a separate biopsy of the area will provide histologic confirmation of the diagnosis. I perform a complete resection of the endomyometrium first and remove all strips of tissue. Then I inspect the cavity and resect all areas that could possibly correspond to glandular tissue. This specimen is submitted separately for histologic diagnosis of adenomyosis.

Step 8

After resection has been completed, the surgeon may choose to desiccate the cut surface (*Figs 14.15, 14.16*). The objective is to reduce the amount of postoperative bleeding. Whether there is any additional benefit in terms of procedural outcome is unclear.

ALTERNATIVE PROCEDURES

Endometrial ablation is a procedure that has only recently enjoyed popularity. Alternative procedures do not truly exist. Curettage and hysterectomy are interventions with different objectives. Alternative procedures to the one described here are those using laser energy sources or a combination of laser and electrosurgery. These are probably only variations rather than true alternatives.

COMPLICATIONS

Complications of endometrial ablation and resection are similar to those that occur during myomectomy. Resection of the endometrium is quite similar to myomectomy. Electrodesiccation of the endometrium with a large-surface electrode is less likely to disrupt the vasculature, and therefore fluid absorption is less pronounced.

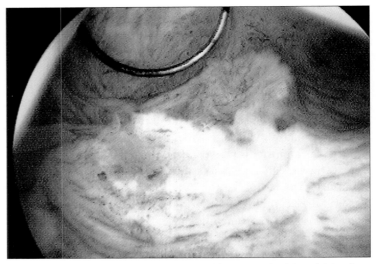

14.14 An area of adenomyosis is easily recognizable within the myometrium after resection of the endomyometrium.

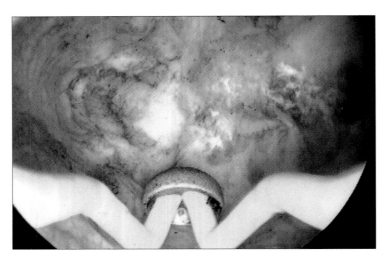

14.15 The cut surface is desiccated with a large-surface electrode.

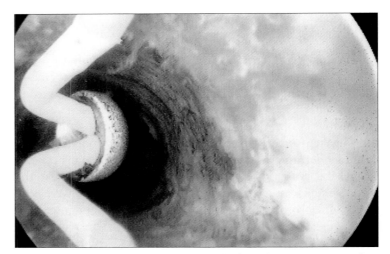

14.16 View of the endocervical canal after electrosection and desiccation have been completed.

REFERENCES

1. LaMorte AI, DeCherney AH. History of operative hysteroscopy. In: *Endometrial Ablation*. Lewis BV, Magos AL, eds. Edinburgh: Churchill Livingstone, 1993:1–6.

2. Reuter LK, Daly DC, Cohen SM. Septate versus bicornuate uteri: errors in imaging diagnosis. *Radiology* 1989;172:749–52.

3. Querleu D, Brasme TL, Parmentier D. Ultrasound-guided transcervical metroplasty. *Fertil Steril* 1990;54:995–8.

4. McDonald R, Phipps J, Singer A. Endometrial ablation: a safe procedure. *Gynecol Endosc* 1992;1:7–9.

5. Neuwirth RS. A new technique for and additional experience with hysteroscopic resection of submucous fibroids. *Am J Obstet Gynecol* 1978;131:91–4.

6. Arieff AI, Ayus CA. Endometrial ablation complicated by fatal hyponatremic encephalopathy. *JAMA* 1993;270:1230–2.

7. Baggish MS, Brill AI, Rosensweig B, Barbot JE, Indman PD. Fatal acute glycine and sorbitol toxicity during operative hysteroscopy. *J Gynecol Surg* 1993;9:137–43.

8. Garry R, Hashman F, Kokri MS, Mooney P. The effect of pressure on fluid absorption during endometrial ablation. *J Gynecol Surg* 1992;8:1–10.

9. Ayus CA, Carlos C, Wheeler JM, Arieff AI. Postoperative hyponatremic encephalopathy in menstruating women. *Am J Intern Med* 1992;117:891–7.

10. Arieff AI. Treatment of symptomatic hyponatremia: neither haste nor waste. *Crit Care Med* 1991;19:748–51.

11. Odell RC. Electrosurgery. In: *Endoscopic Surgery for Gynaecologists*. Sutton C, Diamond M, eds. London: WB Saunders, 1993:51–9.

12. DeCherney AH, Russell JB, Graebe RA, Polan ML. Resectoscopic management of Mullerian fusion defects. *Fertil Steril* 1986;45:726–8.

13. Valle RF, Sciarra JJ. Hysteroscopic treatment of the septate uterus. *Obstet Gynecol* 1986;67:253–7.

14. Valle RF, Sciarra JJ. Intrauterine adhesions: hysteroscopic diagnosis, classification, treatment and reproductive outcome. *Am J Obstet Gynecol* 1988;158:1459–70.

15. Wamsteker K. Hysteroscopy in Ashermann's syndrome. In: *Hysteroscopy, Principles and Practice*. Siegler IM, Lindeman HJ, eds. Philadelphia: JB Lippincott, 1984:198–203.

16. Van Der Pas H. Conception and Contraception. In: *Manual of Hysteroscopy*. Van Der Pas H, Vancaillie TG, eds. Amsterdam: Elsevier Science Publishers, 1990:174–87.

17. Neuwirth RS, Amin HK. Excision of submucous fibroids with hysteroscopic control. *Am J Obstet Gynecol* 1976;126:95–9.

18. Loffer FD. Removal of large symptomatic intra-uterine growths by the hysteroscopic resectoscope. *Obstet Gynecol* 1990;76:836–40.

19. Bardenheuer FH. Elektrokoagulation der Uterusschleimhaut zur behandlung klimakterischer Blutungen. *Zentralblatt Gynaekol* 1937;59:209–16.

20. Loffer FD. A comparison of hysteroscopic techniques. In: *Endometrial Ablation*. Lewis BV, Magos AL, eds. Edinburgh: Churchill Livingstone, 1993:143–50.

21. Vancaillie TG. Electrocoagulation of the endometrium with ball-end resectoscope. *Obstet Gynecol* 1989;74:425–7.

15

Laparoscopy

Brian M. Cohen

LAPAROSCOPIC TECHNIQUE

Laparoscopy facilitates detailed examination of most abdominal structures with a telescope inserted through the umbilicus. This easy visualization of the pelvis permits a thorough inspection of the female reproductive organs.

The advent of miniaturized, lightweight microchip cameras and high-wattage lighting systems has resulted in excellent optical resolution of the pelvis and has facilitated an increased number of laparoscopic diagnostic and operative procedures, thus avoiding the need for laparotomy. In recent years, the development of functionally efficient laparoscopic instruments, together with laser systems and endoscopic sutures, has totally revolutionized the practice of surgical gynecology. These innovations, fueled by the need for non-invasive surgical methods and coupled with a trend towards ambulatory surgical procedures, have led to the development of many endoscopic operations for the surgical correction of gynecologic disorders. This section reviews the available instrumentation, basic techniques of laparoscopic entry of the abdomen, and the pre-, intra-, and postoperative care of patients undergoing gynecologic endoscopy.

INDICATIONS FOR LAPAROSCOPY

The indications for laparoscopy, diagnostic and therapeutic, are summarized in *Fig. 15.1*.

SURGICAL PROCEDURE

Laparoscopic procedures are usually carried out under general anesthesia, with the patient intubated to facilitate adequate control of her cardiorespiratory status.

All instruments are prepared and checked before the patient is anesthetized. Specific requirements anticipated for a particular procedure dictate the need to ensure that instruments not usually used are present and available in the operating room.

Step 1

The patient is placed in the lithotomy position with the buttocks well over the end of the operating table. This position ensures adequacy of uterine anteversion and elevation without restriction caused by the end of the operating table. The patient's legs are moderately abducted, well padded, and supported from the buttocks to the ankles. The staff checks to see that no pressure points that might cause neurologic, muscular, or skin damage are present. The arms and hands are placed at the patient's side and appropriately padded to ensure that there is no strain on the joints or pressure damage to any area.

Step 2

A pelvic examination is completed, the bladder is drained, and the abdomen is mapped. Vital landmarks are checked before the beginning of any laparoscopic procedure (*Figs 15.2, 15.3*). Such checks include assessment of the patient's aorta and vena cava, her sacral promontory, the site of the umbilicus, and the ability to move it below the aortic bifurcation. Percussion of the lower abdomen excludes possible major adhesions or omentoabdominal wall fixation, in which there is unexpected dullness in the

---

Indications for Laparoscopy

Diagnostic

Pelvic pain, dysmenorrhea, dyspareunia, pelvic masses, possible endometriosis

Congenital anomalies of the pelvis commonly associated with primary amenorrhea

Complications of pregnancy (suspected ectopic pregnancy)

Pelvic inflammatory disease (acute and chronic, possible pelvic abscesses)

Infertility (tubal anomalies or occlusion)

Possible appendicitis

Acute abdomen and its multiplicity of causes

Therapeutic Indications

Correction of congenital pelvic anomalies (e.g., cystic paroophoron or epoophoron, elongated fimbria ovarica)

Excision of dysgenetic gonads (e.g., XY, and/or blind tubal or müllerian remnants)

Lysis of adhesions, including lysis of organs (tube, ovary, and uterus)

Management of pelvic inflammatory disease (acute and chronic drainage of pelvic abscesses)

Correction of endometriosis, including removal of endometriomas; laser ablation, coagulation, or excision

Removal of ovarian cysts and benign ovarian tumors

Harvesting of oocytes for assisted reproductive technology

Completion of gamete intrafallopian tube procedures (GIFT)

Myomectomy

Correctional removal of a portion of ovary or oviduct

Uterosacral nerve ablation

Presacral neurectomy

Management of ectopic pregnancy, including salpingotomy, partial or total salpingectomy

Variations of tuboplasty, including fimbriolysis, fimbrioplasty, and salpingoneostomy

Sterilization procedures, including Hulka clip, Yoon rings, and variations of unipolar and bipolar electrosurgical coagulation

Appendectomy

Salpingectomy

Oophorectomy

Salpingo-oophorectomy

Ventrisuspension

Assisted hysterectomy

15.1 Diagnostic and therapeutic indications for laparoscopy.

lower abdomen. This is particularly important in patients who have undergone previous pelvic or abdominal surgery.

Some surgeons prefer to empty the stomach with a nasogastric tube, using gentle suction. The surgeon can facilitate this by placing gentle pressure on the epigastrium and left upper abdominal quadrant. A preoperative enema helps to ensure that the rectosigmoid is empty and not prominent.

In patients undergoing laparoscopy for infertility, the procedure is usually begun after the completion of hysteroscopy (see Chapter 14). An appropriate uterine cannula is placed in the cervix and attached to a single-toothed tenaculum.

Step 3

The lower abdomen is prepared and draped and the patient is placed in a Trendelenburg position. The umbilicus is examined: a wide umbilicus facilitates a transverse infraumbilical incision, whereas a small, pencil-like opening indicates the need for a longitudinal, lower umbilical incision. This permits placement of the trocar and cannula in the abdomen.

Step 4

In extremely thin and in obese patients, the umbilicus is elevated together with the upper abdominal skin. The skin is incised with a No. 11 scalpel blade and the Verres needle passed with elevation of the lower abdomen. The needle is held between the thumb and first finger; the anatomy should be felt, i.e., transection of the fascia and "popping" of the peritoneum as the needle passes through these layers. Utilization of the Verres needle is unnecessary when direct trocar placement is utilized.

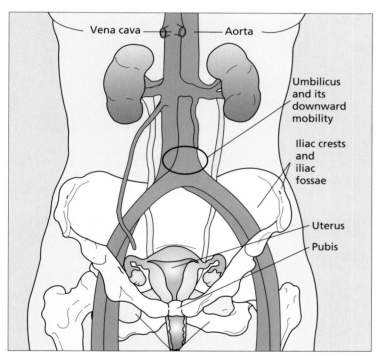

15.2 Vital landmarks checked prior to commencement of laparoscopy procedure. Note level of umbilicus and its downward displacement relative to major blood vessels and the sacral promontor.

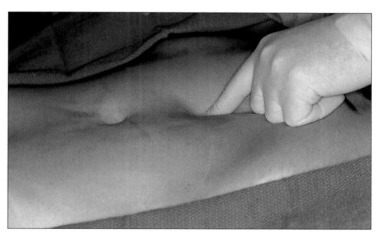

15.3a End of aortic bifurcation.

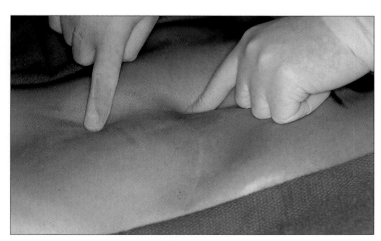

15.3b Umbilicus and aortic bifurcation.

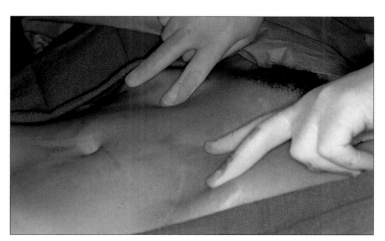

15.3c Iliac fossae.

Step 5

The fluid check test is then completed. A syringe filled with saline is attached to the Verres needle and the fluid is gently pushed into the abdomen. There should be no resistance to this maneuver. The tap is shut and the plunger removed; a column of free fluid should now demonstrate free flow into the abdomen as the lower abdominal wall is elevated with the left hand (*Figs 15.4–15.6*).

Step 6

The tubing connecting the Verres needle with the insufflator is attached and pressures are checked in the non-flow mode. These pressures should register 0–4 mmHg and below zero if the lower

abdomen is elevated to create a vacuum within the abdominal cavity (*Fig. 15.7a*).

Step 7

With the insufflator set at 1 l/min, CO_2 is insufflated into the abdomen and intermittent checks are made on the manometer. At approximately 3 liters of CO_2, abdominal pressures should be 8–11 mmHg (*Fig. 15.7b*). During insufflation, the abdomen is observed and percussed to ensure total generalized distension of the abdominal cavity. Any localized distension indicates the possibility of extraperitoneal location of the needle, usually identified by elevated pressure (*Fig. 15.7c*), and dictates the need to check and/or recommence the insufflation procedure.

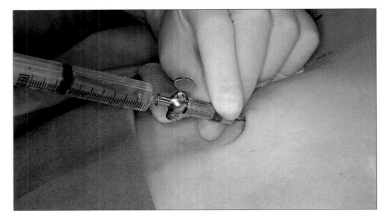

15.4 Verres needle inserted into abdomen, open position.

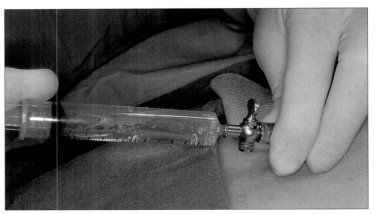

15.5 Verres needle, closed position.

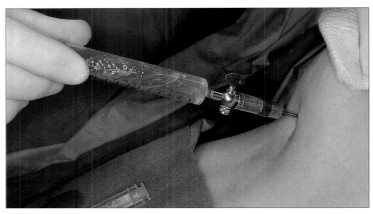

15.6 Fluid test.

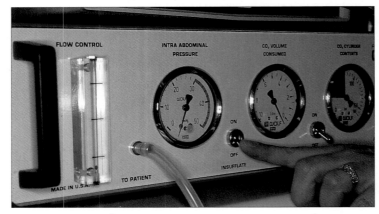

15.7a Manometric pressure.

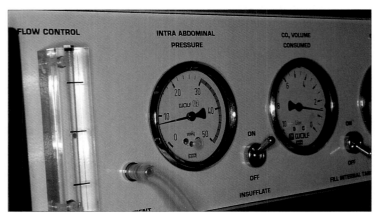

15.7b Normal insufflation.

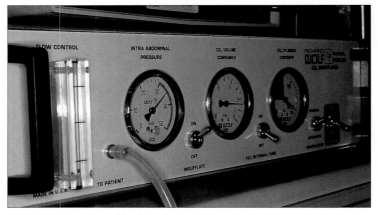

15.7c Manual insufflation: intra-abdominal pressure is high.

Step 8

Once an adequate, generalized pneumoperitoneum has been established, the Verres needle is removed, the umbilical incision is symmetrically enlarged with the No. 11 scalpel, and the laparoscopic trocar and cannula are gently inserted, with elevation of the lower abdomen and with the entry portals in the open position. These maneuvers produce an auditory sound of the gas exiting the abdomen as soon as the CO_2 pocket is entered by the trocar and cannula. At this stage, further entry is stopped, the trocar is removed, and the laparoscope with its light attached, is inserted through the cannula into the abdomen under direct vision (*Fig. 15.8*).

Step 9

A panoramic examination of the upper abdomen and subsequent detailed assessment of the pelvis is completed as a routine in every case. The pelvic exam commences anteriorly and goes in a full circle from the bladder to the pelvic sidewall to the posterior cul-de-sac, the opposite pelvic sidewall, and back to the anterior pelvis. Each oviduct is thoroughly explored from the uterine attachment to its fimbrial end, and the ovary is mobilized to examine each aspect above and below it (*Fig. 15.9*).

Once the abnormalities present have been reviewed and the decision has been made to proceed to operative endoscopy, second, third, and sometimes fourth lower pelvic cannulas are inserted. Conical trocars are preferred. These should also have open portals that provide an audible emission of gas when they communicate with the pneumoperitoneum. Usually at least one additional puncture site must be used during a diagnostic procedure so that a probe can be inserted and the under surface of each ovary examined.

Step 10

With the knife ready, the lights are switched off. Guided by the laparoscopic light, the anterior abdominal blood vessels are defined with transillumination (*Fig. 15.10*). Lower abdominal

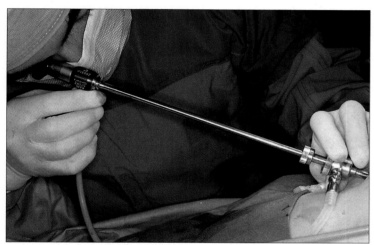

15.8 Cannula advanced under direct vision.

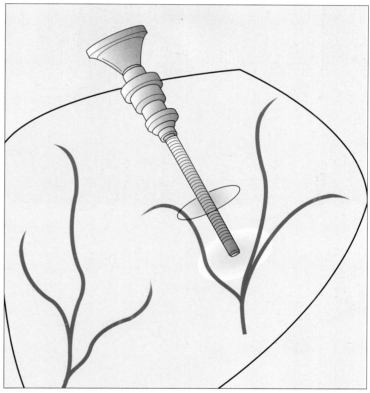

15.10 Transillumination of lower abdomen allows definition of anterior abdominal blood vessels.

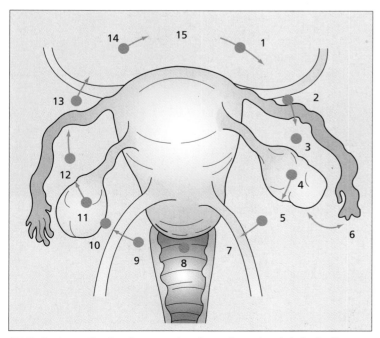

15.9 Systematic circular examination of total pelvis including each fold and tubogonadal relationships.

incisions are made in the defined avascular areas. The entry of each accessory trocar and cannula is observed directly through the laparoscope (*Figs 15.11, 15.12*) and as the peritoneum is entered the corresponding trocar is removed and its cannula secured.

The decision as to the width of cannula used is dependent on the pathology present. Most secondary cannulas are 5 mm in diameter. However, when removal of pelvic pathology is anticipated, an 11- or 12-mm cannula is placed to permit removal of tissues such as excised ectopic pregnancy, uterine fibroids, and/or ovarian lesions.

Where necessary, cannula dilators can be used, e.g., to convert a 5-mm cannula placement to an 11-mm cannula. Such conversion is facilitated by increasing the size of the lower abdominal incision and applying the appropriate dilator over the smooth, guiding rod (*Fig. 15.13*).

In all cases, the main cannula for the laparoscope is metallic, to facilitate electroconduction and to minimize the accumulation and transmission of capacitance energy in the lower pelvis. Once the main cannula is inserted and the secondary trocars and cannulas have been safely placed under direct vision, each is held by painting the abdominal wall with benzoin and securing the cannula with sterile adhesive tape (*Fig. 15.14*). The peritoneum is barely penetrated by the cannula, to avoid complications that may be caused by the cannula, e.g., avulsion of a cyst wall or laceration of the mesosalpinx.

Step 11

In the extremely thin patient, particular caution must be exercised because the umbilicus is adjacent to major posterior abdominal blood vessels. The upper abdomen is elevated by an assistant, who grasps the upper abdominal wall at two sides. The surgeon also elevates the abdomen before beginning the umbilical skin incision. Once this incision is completed, the Verres needle tip is

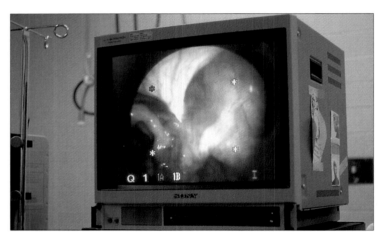

15.11 Entry of trocar.

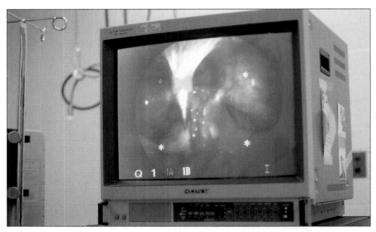

15.12 Entry monitored under direct visualization.

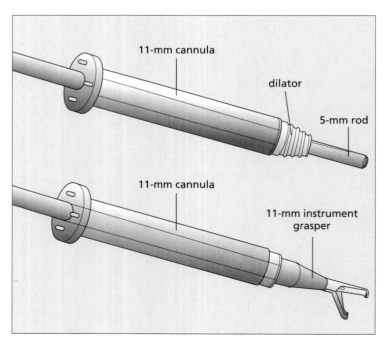

15.13 Use of dilator set to convert 5-mm to 11-mm cannula for operative laparoscopy.

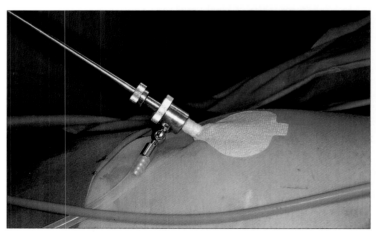

15.14 Cannula taped to abdominal wall.

placed within this cut. The lower abdominal wall is elevated anteriorly and the needle is directed just beneath the skin level into the pelvic cavity.

In extremely obese women, it is essential that the lower umbilical edge, where all layers come together and unite, is precisely identified. Once this has been accomplished, the umbilicus is elevated at the same time that its lower edge is pulled down. An incision is made directly through the umbilicus. This incision guides the Verres needle directly into the abdomen. The incision within the umbilicus is enlarged after the pneumoperitoneum is established so that the abdomen is entered directly by the trocar and cannula. These are gently inserted, aiming towards the anterior pelvis and away from the posterior vertebrae and sacral promontory. These two maneuvers are critical caveats with respect to safe insertion of trocar and cannula in obese patients.

OPEN LAPAROSCOPY: THE HASSON TECHNIQUE
In this method, there is no placement of a Verres needle or a sharp trocar. A vertical incision is made in the umbilical area to facilitate placement of a blunt-ended trocar and cannula directly into the abdomen. Pneumoperitoneum is completed only after the cannula has been secured. The Hasson technique is accepted as an alternative method of laparoscopic umbilical entry and has gained in popularity among surgeons since its introduction by H.M. Hasson in 1971.

SURGICAL PROCEDURE
Step 1
The umbilicus is grasped with two Allis forceps and a vertical incision is made from within the umbilicus to just above its lower edge (*Fig. 15.15a*). This incision maintains direct contact with the rectus fascia and the linea alba at the lower edge of the umbilicus. It is particularly useful for the obese patient, as it avoids the hazards associated with entering the infraumbilical subcutaneous tissues.

Step 2
Once the vertical incision has been completed, the wound edges are kept apart with specialized, S-shaped, small retractors (*Fig. 15.15b*).

Step 3
The linea alba–central fascia is defined within these retractors and grasped both superiorly and inferiorly with curved Kocher's forceps (*Fig. 15.15c*).

Step 4
The fascia is then transected in the horizontal plane and a hemostat is used to enlarge the incision. The S-shaped retractors are placed on each edge of the umbilicus in a horizontal manner, the fascial edges are held with traction sutures (*Fig. 15.15d*), and as the incision is probed with the hemostat it is common to enter the peritoneal space (*Fig. 15.15e*).

Step 5
One of the retractor blades is placed in the peritoneal space to facilitate subsequent placement of the cannula together with its cone, which is secured at a distance compatible with the thickness of the patient's abdominal wall (*Fig. 15.15f*).

Step 6
The cannula and its blunt-edged probe are placed into the peritoneal cavity as the retractors are withdrawn, and the fascial placement sutures are secured around the V-shaped suture holders of the Hasson cannula. The smooth trocar is withdrawn and gas is insufflated through the side portal of the cannula.

DIRECT TROCAR INSERTION
Placement of the sharp, laparoscopic trocar and cannula directly into the abdomen has also been advocated. This procedure has been carried out in many patients with good results. To date, this author has preferred the open Hasson method if problems and/or difficulties are anticipated with closed insertion of the Verres needle.

USE OF DISPOSABLE TROCARS AND CANNULAS
In recent years, disposable trocars and cannulas have been designed in an effort to improve safe entry into the abdominal cavity. As these instruments are developed, it is of particular importance that they be lightweight, electrically conductive, and of a suitable length to be securely fixed in the abdominal wall with minimal penetration into the peritoneal cavity. Although they offer no specific advantages over carefully maintained re-usable trocars and cannulas, they have gained popularity among surgeons.

Some of the new disposable instruments, e.g., mobile, multi-angled grasping forceps, Allis forceps, and angled staplers, are positive innovations that permit improved laparoscopic surgical techniques. If their use is anticipated, they should fit the cannulas available.

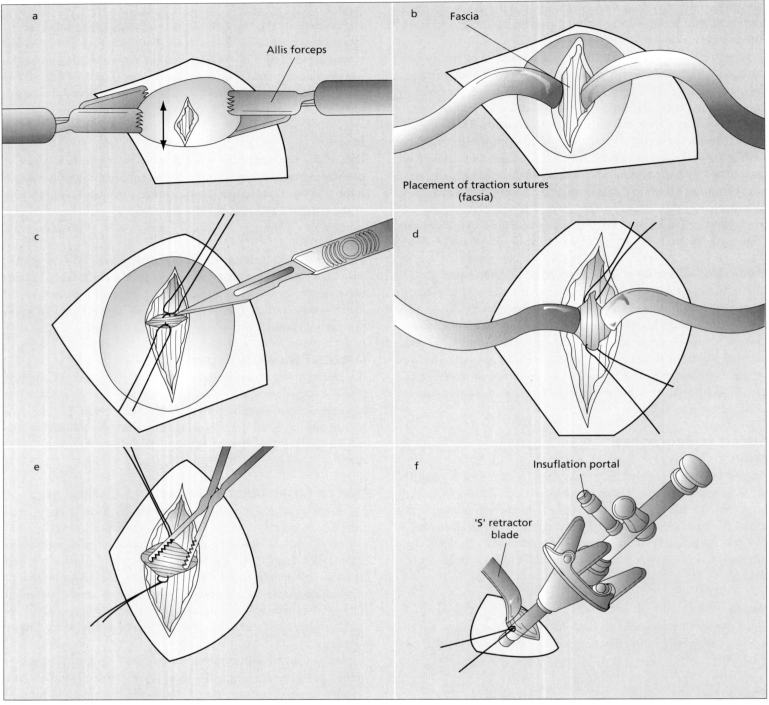

Allis forceps

Fascia

Placement of traction sutures
(facsia)

Insuflation portal

'S' retractor
blade

15.15 Principles of dissection and direct entry insertion of
Hasson cannula (open laparoscopy)
a. Longitudinal incision of skin.
b. Use of S-shaped retractors.

c. Transverse incision of fascia with scalpel.
d. Re-insertion of retractors into fascia.
e. Mosquito forceps enter peritoneum.
f. Direct insertion of round-ended trocar.

ABDOMINAL CLOSURE AND POSTOPERATIVE CARE

After completion of any laparoscopic procedure, hemostasis must be checked and unquestionably secured. Thereafter, all secondary cannulas are removed under direct vision to ensure that there is no vascular perforation or bleeding from the anterior abdominal wall. Immediately before removal of the main laparoscopic cannula, all CO_2 is exsufflated, with persistent pressure on the upper and lower abdomen by both the surgeon and the assistant to ensure maximal removal of gas from the abdomen. Once this has been completed, the minimal number of subcutaneous sutures are inserted and steristrips are applied to the skin, secured with tincture of benzoin. If a cannula larger than 10 mm has been used, a specific attempt is made to suture the fascia in addition to the subcutaneous tissues.

The vagina is checked, instruments are withdrawn, hemostasis is ensured, and the bladder catheter removed. Once recovered, the patient is discharged, with adequate oral analgesics and antibiotics when indicated. She is advised to report any rise in temperature >99°F and any problems with urination or defecation. She is kept at strict bedrest for 24–48 h, depending on the extent of the operative procedure. The operative wounds are kept dry with plastic tapes, thus enabling the patient to shower as desired. She is seen a week after surgery, at which time the steristrips are removed and the abdomen is checked in the routine manner.

Details of the operative procedure, together with review of video tape or video photographs, are completed at this visit, and the patient's future reproductive health care is planned at this time.

Laparoscopy is presently an active therapeutic, gynecologic operative modality which has passed beyond being solely a diagnostic procedure. Many operations can be performed through the laparoscope and these are presently being evaluated in a prospective manner.

In the years to come, only those procedures that are truly an advance over previous surgical methods will stand the test of time and will become commonplace, routine gynecologic operations.

LAPAROSCOPY: DIAGNOSTIC USES

The advent of laparoscopy and the further development of instrumentation for this procedure represent a major advance in avoiding the need for laparotomy. Laparoscopy affords detailed, generalized intraperitoneal examination and specifically facilitates excellent visualization of the pelvic organs to enable accurate diagnosis of any pathology present. Once the laparoscope has been inserted, a systematic examination is carried out. This includes brief exploration of the upper abdominal contents, the liver, stomach, omentum, gallbladder, and subphrenic areas, together with the cecum and appendix.

The pelvis is examined in a routine clockwise fashion, e.g., from anterior vesical fold to right adnexa, anterior and posterior folds of the mesosalpinx, the upper and under surfaces of the ovaries, and the lateral right cul-de-sac over the bowel and cul-de-sac to the left lateral cul-de-sac/uterosacral area, the under surface of the left ovary, upper surface of the left ovary, both sides of the mesosalpinx, and the left pelvic sidewall, returning to the left anterior vesical space.

Photo documentation is facilitated by a beam splitter. Video examination of the pelvis can be followed by the surgeon and assistants. Timely and selected photographs are taken to highlight and define the pre-, intra-, and postsurgical status of the reconstructed pelvis.

Common diagnostic findings are listed in *Fig. 15.16* and illustrate the multiple pathologies that are easily discernable at laparoscopy. In the case of laparoscopy for infertility, details of the tubo-ovarian relationship must be documented. A patulous,

Diagnostic Findings

- Pelvic inflammatory disease, acute salpingitis, subacute inflammatory disease with pyosalpinx and/or pelvic abscess, chronic pelvic inflammatory disease (including tuberculosis and actinomycosis)

- Endometriosis, mild, moderate, and severe (see Fig. 15.15). This includes periovarian endometriosis, peritoneal deposits and distortion, ovarian endometriomas, and cul-de-sac obliteration (partial or complete)

- Adhesions (mild, moderate, and severe), peritubal, periovarian, periuterine, and/or involving the bowel to any pelvic organ

- Congenital anomalies of the Mullerian system, including those found on the oviducts at the level of the fimbria, paroophoron, epoophoron, and intramesosalpingeal cysts, cystic hydatids of Morgagni

- Congenital atresia of the oviduct, DES anomalies of the oviduct, accessory oviducts, accessory ovaries, and duplication of the tubal ostium

- Variations of adhesive disease related to prior surgical procedures

- Pelvic neoplasms, benign or malignant, primary and secondary (e.g., deposits in the cul-de-sac) following breast, bronchial, thyroid, or renal carcinoma

- Fibromyomata: fibroids (subserous, intramural, ligamentary, submucous, diagnosed at hysteroscopy)

- Ovarian anomalies, including cysts, follicular or luteal, and neoplasms (benign or malignant)

- Complications of pregnancy (e.g., all varieties of ectopic pregnancy and ruptured corpus luteum cysts)

- Torsion of each or any of the pelvic organs, primarily the ovary, tube, and common portions of the tube and ovary together

15.16 Common diagnostic findings of laparoscopy.

wide opening of the fimbrial ostium should be present. The relationship between this ostium and the ovarian surface should be uninterrupted by any adhesive process, e.g., periovarian adhesions or endometriosis. The ostium should also be close to the ovarian surface, e.g., within a distance of 2 cm.

MANAGEMENT OF ADNEXAL MASSES

In the case of an adnexal mass and the possibility of ovarian carcinoma, routine management as for ovarian carcinoma should be instituted. If there is any doubt about the status of the lesion, frozen sectioning should be performed. If there is any doubt concerning the histopathology of the tumor, laparotomy and routine staging and management under the guidance of a gynecologic oncologist should be instituted, as would occur under normal circumstances in the investigation of such a pelvic mass.

When an ovarian cyst has been observed prospectively and is considered functional on the basis of detailed, ultrasound examination combined with normal blood count, sedimentation rate, and CA-125, laparoscopic intervention and cystectomy may be considered.

When there is difficulty in stripping a cyst, particularly in the absence of endometriosis, carcinoma should be suspected. Gynecologic oncologic management should be instituted.

A major technical difficulty is that encountered during the management of a fresh corpus luteum cyst mistakenly suspected of being an endometrioma. A true corpus luteum cyst is an extremely friable, hemorrhagic lesion. Ideally, this is diagnosed preoperatively by a detailed history and physical examination, together with an adequate sonographic evaluation. When a cystic corpus luteum is suspected and the patient is absolutely stable with no free fluid in the abdomen but the dominant clinical feature is pain, this should be managed conservatively with suppression of the lesion. This is accomplished by administration of a combination estrogen/progesterone pill and/or a GnRH agonist. Ideally, these lesions and active endometriomas are first suppressed in this fashion so that any subsequent laparoscopic intervention is facilitated by the now quiescent and relatively ischemic pathology.

Operating on an acute hemorrhagic corpus luteum carries a risk of major hemorrhage and may necessitate the untimely removal of an otherwise healthy ovary. This should not be undertaken in the young or infertile patient unless absolutely necessary. If major hemorrhage occurs, laparotomy with wedge excision of the hemorrhagic tissue, assisted by a suitable ovarian vascular clamp, is the procedure of choice (*Fig. 15.17*).

LAPAROSCOPIC INTERVENTION FOR ENDOMETRIOSIS

The therapeutic modalities of laparoscopic intervention for endometriosis are listed in *Fig. 15.18*. Both electrosurgery and various laser systems have a major role in the surgical correction of this disease.

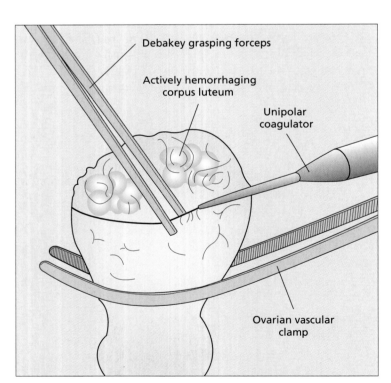

15.17 Laparotomy for procuring hemostasis and preservation of ovary in active hemorrhage of vascular ruptured corpus luteum.

Therapeutic Modalities of Laparoscopic Intervention for Endometriosis
• Bipolar electrosurgery: the button electrode, Kleppinger-type grasper, or bipolar needle transection
• Laser systems
Carbon dioxide (CO_2)
Argon
KTP-532
Sapphire-tipped Yag varieties
• Unipolar electrosurgery

15.18 Therapeutic modalities of laparoscopic intervention in endometriosis.

Advantages and Disadvantages of Varying Modalities Used in Laparoscopic Treatment of Endometriosis

1. Bipolar button electrode

Advantages:

- Most superficial
- Electrosurgical safety
- Ease of use at all angles

Disadvantages:

- Cannot specifically get to deeper areas of endometriosis
- Potential lateral spread at higher wattages

2. Bipolar graspers/needle

Advantages:

- Grasper holds and coagulates most blood vessels up to 2 mm in diameter
- Needle valuable in transection of adhesions

Disadvantages:

- Potential deep and increased lateral spread
- Uncontrolled thermal spread

3. CO_2 laser

Advantages:

- Precision with minimal deep or lateral spread
- Well visualized — "What you see, is what you get"
- Defined tissue effects. Can penetrate deeper with direct control as required

Disadvantages:

- Angulation for tissue effect sometimes difficult (the laser travels in a direct mode)
- Water backstop required for safety
- Careful control necessary to avoid laser damage beyond the target zone
- Particular care needed when transecting adhesions with respect to organs or tissues behind the adhesions being divided
- No color-specific sensitivity
- Cumbersome delivery system
- Smoke plume requires repeated suction from the peritoneum

4. KTP-532 (Yag modified fiberoptic laser)

Advantages:

- Simplified delivery system
- Ease of application
- Wavelength preference, color-sensitive for dark colors, e.g., in endometriosis.

Note: Argon fiber may be classified with the KTP

Disadvantages:

- Significant deeper and lateral spread (not visible)
- Repetitive cost of disposable fibers
- Need to prepare the fiber repeatedly in moderate to major cases
- Smoke plume suction from the pneumoperitoneum

5. Sapphire-tipped Yag laser

Advantages:

- Fiberoptic delivery system
- Multiple variety of tips provide specific advantages, e.g.:

  > Sharp, non-frosted – for precise dissection and minimal lateral spread
  >
  > Frosted – lateral spread with excellent hemostasis
  >
  > Blunt or rounded – excellent hemostasis

Disadvantages:

- Sharp tip: no lateral spread, and non-hemostatic. Frosted tip: lateral spread could damage lateral structures not visualized
- Rounded area, poor vaporization, easy destruction of tips renders this instrument highly expensive to replace during surgery

(The instrument must be in direct contact with tissue at all times to avoid destruction of tip)

6. Unipolar coagulation

Advantages:

- Ability to work at multiple angles
- Ease of use via direct or secondary cannulas

Disadvantages:

- Imprecise regarding depth of penetration and possible excess lateral and deep tissue destruction
- Greater thermal hazard and theoretical increased electrical risk of capacitance or spark jumping

15.19 Advantages and disadvantages of varying modalities used in laparoscopic treatment of endometriosis.

BASIC LAPAROSCOPY FOR ENDOMETRIOSIS

The pelvis is explored in a methodical and detailed fashion. Documentation of the extent of endometriosis is completed using the American Fertility Society (AFS) scoring system (*Fig. 15.20*). In general, multiple superficial deposits are coagulated using the bipolar button or one of the laser systems. Specific precautions with any method are taken when the endometriosis lies over major lateral pelvic blood vessels, particularly at the ovarian fossa, because of

THE AMERICAN FERTILITY SOCIETY
REVISED CLASSIFICATION OF ENDOMETRIOSIS

Patient's Name _____ Date _____

Stage 1   (Minimal)   - 1–5
Stage 11   (Mild)   - 6–15   Laparoscopy _____ Laparotomy _____ Photography _____
Stage 111 (Moderate) - 16–40   Recommended treatment _____
Stage 1V   (Severe)   - >40   _____

Total _____ Prognosis _____

PERITONEUM	ENDOMETRIOSIS	< 1cm	1.3cm	> 3cm
	Superficial	1	2	4
	Deep	2	4	6

OVARY		< 1cm	1.3cm	> 3cm
	R Superficial	1	2	4
	Deep	4	16	20
	L Superficial	1	2	4
	Deep	4	16	20

	POSTERIOR CUL-DE-SAC OBLITERATION	Partial		Complete	
		4		40	

OVARY	ADHESIONS	< 1/3 Enclosure	1/3-2/3 Enclosure	>2/3 Enclosure
	R Filmy	1	2	4
	Dense	4	8	16
	L Filmy	1	2	4
	Dense	4	8	16

TUBE	R Filmy	1	2	4
	Dense	4*	8*	16
	L Filmy	1	2	4
	Dense	4*	8*	16

* If the fimbriated end of the fallopian tube is completely enclosed, change the point assignment to 16.

Additional endometriosis: _____ Associated pathology: _____
_____ _____
_____ _____
_____ _____

To be used with normal
tubes and ovaries

To be used with abnormal
tubes and/or ovaries

15.20 American Fertility Society scoring system to classify endometriosis.

the relationship to the ureter. At the uterosacral ligaments, the areas lateral to or below these structures have a specific anatomic relationship to the ureter and major blood vessels. These must be carefully checked and negotiated. Particular caution is also exercised with endometriosis over the bowel or bladder.

THE USE OF TISSUE IRRIGATION AND SUCTION

Heparinized solutions, e.g. 2,000 IU heparin in 1 l Ringer's lactate, together with 100 mg ampicillin and 100 mg hydrocortisone succinate, are preferable to saline, as they do not cause peritoneal edema. Scattered peritoneal endometriosis is coagulated or vaporized lesion by lesion in a systematic, organized fashion.

In the infertility patient, concentration is focused on repairing tubo-ovarian surfaces and relationships. Superficial endometriosis is vaporized or coagulated. Deeper lesions are vaporized or coagulated and excised wherever possible (*Fig. 15.21*). If the fimbria

ovarica is elongated to greater than 4 cm, the tubal ostium should be reapproximated close to the ovary by using the Bruhat technique. This method has the objective of partial vaporization and cicatrization of the overlying peritoneum adjacent to the fold of the fimbria ovarica. This causes shortening of this structure. Bruhat shortening may be effected by the defocused laser beam, particularly the CO_2 laser, but it is also accomplished using the KTP-532 laser, the bipolar button electrode at a low-wattage setting, or the endotherm at about 75°C (*Figs 15.22, 15.23*). Care is exercised to avoid excess damage at this site, thereby avoiding compromise to the fimbrial blood supply.

LAPAROSCOPIC SURGERY FOR ENDOMETRIOMAS

Preoperative suppression of confirmed endometriomas facilitates hemostasis, and thus ensues an improved surgical result. It should be noted that many patients with endometriosis are in the habit of taking an abundance of analgesics, including non-steroidal analgesics and aspirin products. These may affect platelet function and blood clotting and can contribute to excessive blood loss at laparoscopy. All patients should be cautioned to avoid these products for a minimum of 2 weeks before surgery.

The endometrioma should be removed. Total removal is undertaken if the lining of the cyst strips easily (*Fig. 15.24*).

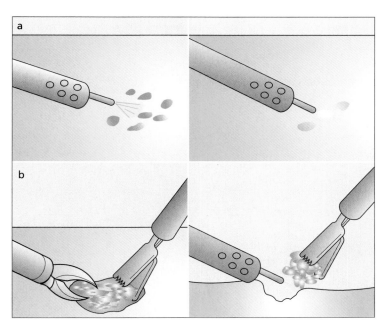

15.21 Laparoscopic treatment of endometriosis: **a.** superficial lesions vaporized; **b.** deep lesions vaporized, dissected free and excised.

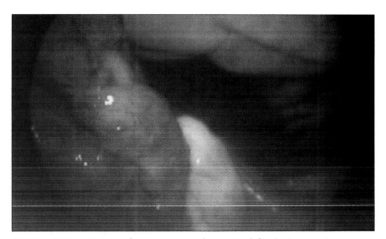

15.22 Ostium away from ovary: elongated fimbria ovarica.

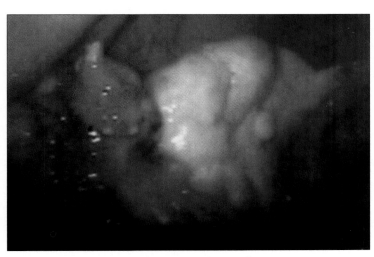

15.23 Tubal approximation to ovarian surface.

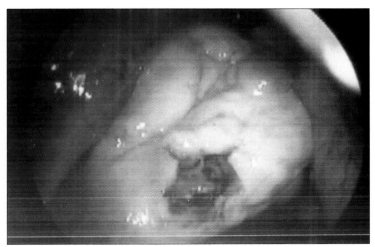

15.24 Excision biopsy benign ovarian cyst.

Step 1

The surface of the endometrioma is coagulated using a bipolar button, defocused CO_2 or a KTP-532 laser beam (*Fig. 15.25a*).

Step 2

Once an ischemic incision line has been created, the endometrioma is entered and a plane of cleavage is found between the outer ovary held by toothed, grasping forceps and the inner endometrioma (*Fig. 15.25b*).

Step 3

If the endometrioma strips easily, it is removed *en toto* (*Fig. 15.25c*), hemostasis is checked, and the ovary if left to heal without any sutures, as these may precipitate greater adhesion formation (*Fig. 15.25d*).

Step 4

The pelvis is irrigated continuously with the heparinized Ringer's lactate solution.

Step 5

When there is difficulty in stripping the endometrioma, intermittent lines of hemostasis are made on its outer surface with the bipolar button, the sapphire-tipped Yag laser, or the endotherm. An overlying cap of tissue is then removed with a laser or scissors after penetration and suction aspiration of its fluid contents. Extensive irrigation and suction of the endometrioma cavity is completed. The cavity is then entered with the laparoscope and thoroughly explored (*Fig. 15.26a*).

Step 6

Its inner layers are vaporized or coagulated under direct vision (*Fig. 15.26b*). A significant opening (at least 1 cm in diameter) is created over the lesion to facilitate postoperative drainage and healing.

Step 7

Simple drainage of an endometrioma with a needle is not helpful, as this usually permits recurrence of the endometrioma. It is preferable to create a wide opening to enter the endometrioma with the laparoscope and to complete vaporization and coagulation of its inner wall under direct vision.

In selected patients with extensive endometriosis, postoperative suppression with GnRH agonists or Danazol therapy is advisable for 2–3 months. Such suppression is usually indicated if there has been significant bowel involvement and resection of bowel has not been undertaken. Bowel resection is usually not indicated in patients intent on pursuing further fertility, but is commonly reserved for the later hysterectomy procedure. This is often necessary in patients with extensive endometriomas and associated bowel involvement.

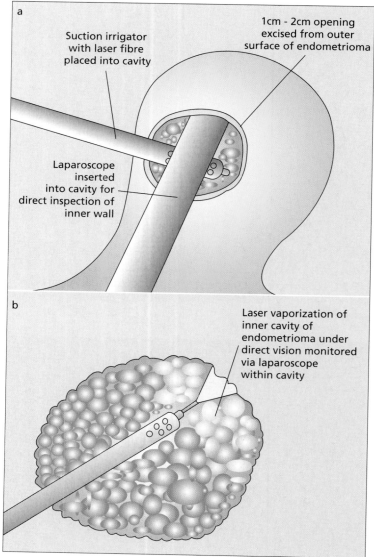

15.26 Laser vaporization of inner wall of endometrioma.

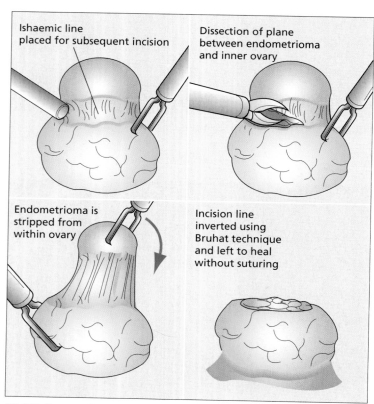

15.25 Removal of an endometrioma.

LAPAROSCOPIC MYOMECTOMY

INDICATIONS

Laparoscopic myomectomy is indicated in patients who present with symptomatic fibroids and who are opposed to hysterectomy. These symptoms include menorrhagia, dysmenorrhea, and dyspareunia. In women who do not desire future pregnancy, hysterectomy is the procedure of choice.

Fibroids can be classified as subserous, intramural, or submucous, together with other varieties, e.g., intraligamentous (*Fig. 15.27*). Where future pregnancies are intended and significant intramural fibroids are present, i.e., greater than 4 cm, these should be removed at formal laparotomy. This open procedure facilitates adequate uterine suturing and reconstruction, minimizing the risks of uterine rupture in a future pregnancy. Submucous fibroids are removed at operative hysteroscopy using the rectoscope.

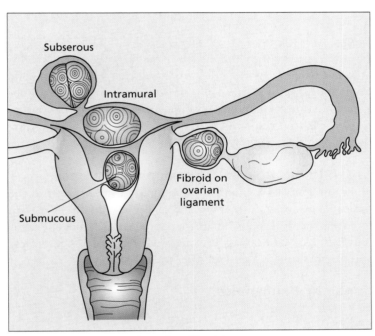

15.27 Basic location of uterine fibroids.

SUBSEROUS OR WIDELY PEDUNCULATED MYOMAS

These lesions represent the "classic" tumors that can be safely removed at operative laparoscopy.

SURGICAL PROCEDURE

Step 1

Once the pelvis has been explored and the tumors have been reviewed, the blood supply of each fibroid must be carefully assessed and defined.

Step 2

Vasopressin 5 IU in 50 ml of saline is carefully injected around the base of the fibroid, using a fine 20-gauge needle passed through a protective shield via a secondary cannula (*Fig. 15.28*). Particular care to avoid blood vessels and close cardiovascular monitoring is accomplished by alerting the anesthesiologist before injection of this potentially cardiostimulatory drug.

Step 3

The bipolar button electrode or endotherm coagulator is used to coagulate and effect a peripheral layer of ischemia around the base of the fibroid (*Fig. 15.28*).

Step 4

The lesion is then transected from within this ischemic area layer by layer, using the bipolar button electrode or the endotherm knife, assisted by hook scissors. A KTP, sapphire-tipped YAG, or CO_2 laser can also be used at this stage.

Step 5

Intermittent hemostasis is accomplished at each stage, layer by layer. The tumor is grasped with solid, locked grasping forceps (*Fig. 15.29*) through a second or tertiary portal and the dissection and coagulation with the bipolar button and scissors or endotherm knife are completed.

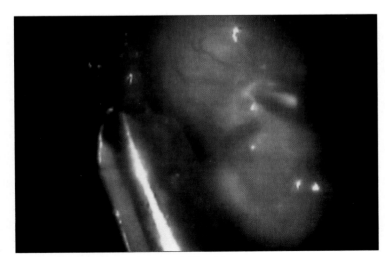

15.28 Coagulation of base of fibroid.

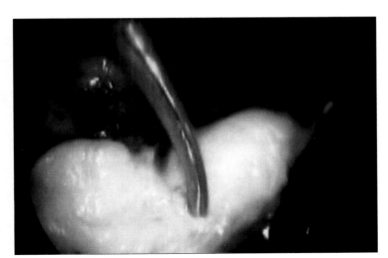

15.29 Scissors morcellation of fibroid.

Step 6

Once the fibroid has been removed from its base, liberal irrigation is directed at the bed of the lesion to ensure that there is total and absolute hemostasis (*Fig. 15.30*). Each individual fibroid is subsequently removed in the same manner, i.e., by ensuring an ischemic layer at its base and subsequent layer-by-layer dissection and coagulation.

Step 7

Large fibroids can be left in the cul-de-sac until the end of the procedure. Fibroids less than 2 cm in diameter can be easily divided in halves and removed through an 11-mm channel. Larger fibroids can be removed via the cul-de-sac or morcellated with a mechanical morcellator. The morcellated segments are then withdrawn through the anterior abdominal wall via the 11-mm cannula (*Fig. 15.31a*). After completion of the procedure, the base of each fibroid is checked for hemostasis. When wide-based lesions are observed, particularly on the posterior uterine surface, an anti-adhesive barrier material can be placed via a secondary cannula (*Fig. 15.31b*).

INTRAMURAL FIBROIDS

Intramural fibroids can be removed in women who do not contemplate further childbearing or for lesions that do not

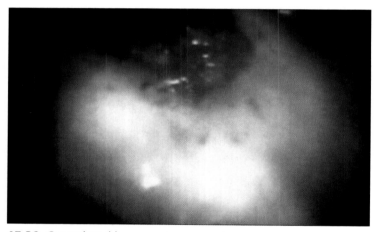

15.30 Coagulated base: post-myomectomy.

traverse more than one-third to one-half of the myometrial layer, with fibroids less than 4 cm in diameter. The operative technique is modified as follows.

SURGICAL PROCEDURE

Step 1

The periphery of the lesion is injected with vasopressin 5 IU in 50 ml saline (*Fig. 15.32a*). The fibroid becomes ischemic.

Step 2

The lesion is transected by a longitudinal incision on the uterus (*Fig. 15.32b*). The fibroid is dissected from within this lesion held by a locked, grasping forceps (*Fig. 15.32c*).

Step 3

Once again, removal is accomplished in a layer-by-layer, repetitive hemostatic fashion. Once the fibroid has been removed, sutures are inserted. A single layer of #3-0 absorbable suture is placed (*Fig. 15.32d*).

Step 4

Hemostasis is checked and the lesion may be covered by an anti-adhesive barrier (see *Fig. 15.31b*). In patients who contemplate pregnancy, removal of an intramural fibroid in this manner would indicate a 4–6 month postponement of attempting conception to ensure adequate healing and in the hope of avoiding possible uterine rupture.

LASER REDUCTION OF INTRAMURAL FIBROIDS

Some surgeons have provided preliminary evidence that in the patient considering further childbearing and who does not wish to have a major or open laparotomy procedure, a 4–6 cm intramural fibroid can be significantly reduced and rendered less vascular by using a Yag laser fiber at laparoscopy.

SURGICAL PROCEDURE

Step 1

The patient is prepared for this operation by 2 months of pre-operative GnRH agonist administration to reduce leiomyomata size.

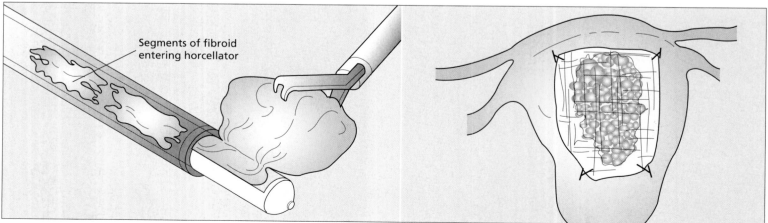

15.31a Fibroid morcellation.

b Adhesion barrier placed and held in place with absorbable clips.

Step 2

The fibroid is injected with a 1:10 solution of vasopressin and is partially coagulated around its base to facilitate ischemia and hemostasis (*Fig. 15.33*).

Step 3

The fiber is advanced to half the diameter of the fibroid, at which time the laser is activated (*Fig. 15.34a*) and slowly withdrawn.

Step 4

Hemostasis is completed at the puncture sites (*Fig. 15.34b*). The GnRH agonist is continued for 1 month postoperatively. In most patients there is approximately a 50% reduction in fibroid volume. It is possible that prior diversion of vascular perfusion of the endometrium to the fibroid can now be corrected so that there may be redirection of blood flow to the endometrium, with positive effects on the patient's reproductive status. In particular, this may reduce the incidence of miscarriage.

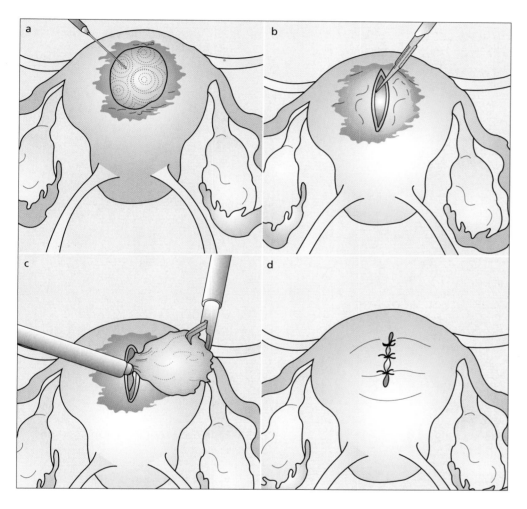

15.32 a. Injection of vasopressin 5 i.u. in 50ml saline into periphery of lesion.
b. Longitudinal incision to transect lesion on the uterus.
c. Dissection of fibroid from within lesion using locked grasping forceps.
d. A single layer of synthetic absorbable sutures.

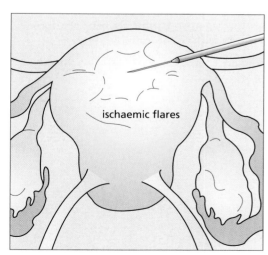

15.33 Injection of vasopressin.

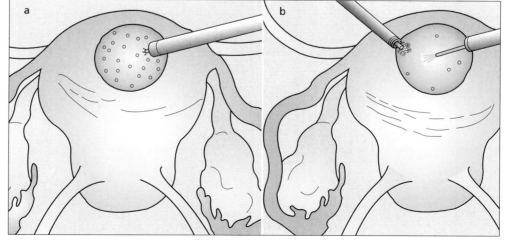

15.34 a. Hemostasis of puncture site with bipolar button electrode.
b. Fibreoptic laser advanced, fiber activated at depth of fibroid and withdrawn.

In women with fibroids greater than 4 cm in diameter who intend future childbearing, the author's opinion remains to proceed to laparotomy (*Fig. 15.35*) and reconstruction of the uterine wall in multiple layers (*Fig. 15.36*).

In patients over the age of 35 who intend to attempt conception after only 3–4 months, a permanent suture material such as polypropylene is inserted in the uterine musculature. The outer serosal layer is repaired in a subcuticular fashion (*Fig. 15.37a*). An adhesive barrier material is spread over the uterine incision and sutured in placed with #6-0 absorbable sutures (*Fig. 15.37b*).

Perioperative prophylactic antibiotics are administered and careful observation of postoperative hematocrit is essential. If the fibroid is subserosal and the myometrium has not been significantly entered or divided, the patient may proceed to conception from the next menstrual cycle.

LAPAROSCOPIC UTEROSACRAL NERVE ABLATION

This procedure has different results reported for the relief of pelvic pain and dysmenorrhea, particularly in patients with endometriosis. The operation is completed as an adjunct to meticulous reduction and division of peritoneal adhesions, laser and/or bipolar coagulation of endometriosis, and removal of periovarian adhesions, laser and/or intraovarian endometriomas or ovarian cysts. The classic indication is to relieve severe dysmenorrhea, although some surgeons prefer to carry out nerve ablation by dissection of the presacral nerves at the sacral promontory.

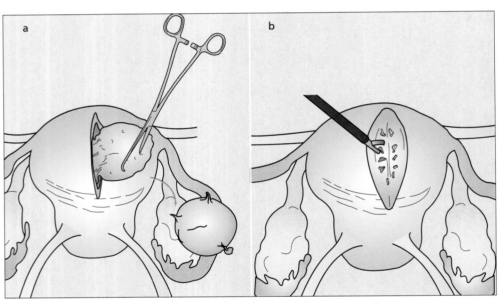

15.35 a. Removal of fibroid. **b.** Bipolar hemostasis in cavity wall.

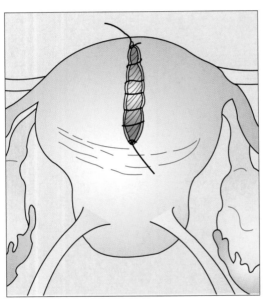

15.36 Repair of uterine walls in multiple layers.

15.37 a. The outer serosal layer is subcuticularly repaired and an adhesive barrier material spread over the uterine incision.
b. The adhesive barrier material is sutured in place with 6-0 absorbable sutures.

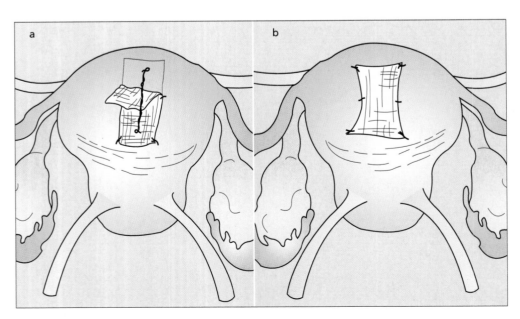

SURGICAL PROCEDURE

Step 1

The cul-de-sac is defined and the uterus is elevated to define the uterosacral ligaments. If necessary, the lateral peritoneal wall is divided above the uterosacral ligaments to ensure that the ureters are not displaced close to the lateral and/or inferior aspect of the uterosacral ligaments. There is commonly a major cervical artery lateral to the uterosacral ligament, and this must be watched for and avoided (*Fig. 15.38*).

Step 2

The uterosacral ligament is coagulated with a bipolar coagulator immediately adjacent to its attachment to the uterine cervix (*Fig. 15.39*). This minimizes the risks of ureteral damage and of traumatizing the cervical artery. Once the uterosacral ligament has been coagulated, it is divided with the laser (CO_2, KTP, or sapphire-tipped Yag).

Step 3

The ligament is divided slowly and carefully in multiple shallow layers so that hemostasis is effected throughout the procedure (*Figs 15.40a, 15.40b*). No more than 0.5 cm of the ligament is totally transected (*Fig. 15.40c*), and when this is completed, coagulation of the proximal uterosacral ligament is effected with a bipolar electrode (*Fig. 15.40d*).

Step 4

Hemostasis is checked, the ureters are confirmed to be well displaced from the operative site, which is irrigated once more, and the procedure is completed. It should be noted that uterosacral

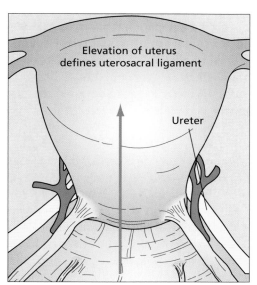

15.38 Anatomy of uterosacral ligament. Note underlying branches of uterine artery and contiguous ureter.

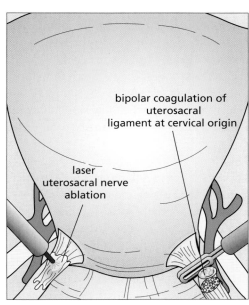

15.39 Laser or electrodessication of the uterosacral ligament,

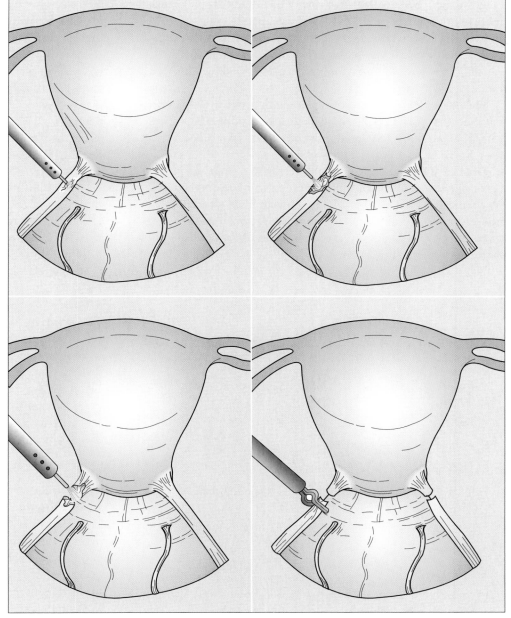

15.40 Use of laser and electrosurgical dessication for division and hemostasis of uterosacral ligament.

nerve ablation is not performed in patients who have previously undergone this procedure. A repeat operation has been the classic setting for vascular or ureteral damage.

In general, the procedure is reserved for those with severe dysmenorrhea or central pelvic pain. The operation is executed in a conservative fashion because of the presently unknown status of long-term possible contributions to or causations of utero-vaginal prolapse.

LAPAROSCOPIC TUBOPLASTY

At the turn of the century, tuboplasty was permitted only when laparotomy was necessary for another reason. The very low success rate for this procedure did not indicate that such an operation was ethically justifiable.

Between 1911 and 1940, the success rates for tuboplasty ranged from about 5–25%. The advent of magnification in the 1950s brought about better success rates, with the result that pregnancies followed tuboplasty in 20–35% of those operated on.

In the 1980s, microsurgery facilitated success rates averaging close to 50% for all tuboplasty procedures. In reversal of sterilization, isthmo-isthmic anastomosis was followed by a live birth rate of 80% of patients.

The advent of *in vitro* fertilization, with progressively improving success rates, now 20–25% per cycle in some centers, indicates that we should reconsider the indications for tuboplasty at present.

Operative laparoscopy permits successful tuboplasty in most patients who require surgical intervention for correction of mechanical infertility (*Fig. 15.41*). Indeed, if the procedure can no longer be competed via the laparoscope, one must seriously question whether or not one should be considering *in vitro* fertilization in preference to laparotomy.

Common Laparoscopic Tuboplasty Procedures

- Excision of congenital tubal anomalies, large cystic hydatids of Morgagni or accessory tubal stalks
- Removal of paratubal cysts
- Salpingectomy, partial or total
- Salpingotomy for tubal pregnancy
- Tubal mobilization by lysis of peritubal and periovarian adhesions
- Fimbriolysis and division of fimbrial bridges and adhesions
- Salpingoscopy
- Salpingoneostomy
- Laparoscopic assisted transvaginal tubal cannulation for proximal tubal occlusion

15.41 Common laparoscopic tuboplasty procedures.

At the present time, therefore, excluding reversal of sterilization and microsurgical tubal anastomosis, most patients awaiting surgery for mechanical tubal disorders have their procedure completed at operative laparoscopy.

LYSIS OF ADHESIONS: SALPINGOLYSIS

If there are significant peritubal and periovarian adhesions, adhesions covering the adnexa, and/or adhesions to the anterior abdominal wall, consideration is given to the safe placement of second, third, and fourth operative cannulas as needed.

SURGICAL PROCEDURE
Step 1
Through the use of a beam-split telescope or the video monitor, adhesions are directly observed and put on traction by grasping around the oviduct and/or ovarian ligaments assisted by counter uterine displacement. These procedures facilitate definition of the adhesions and adhesive layers. Where necessary, Ringer's lactate is injected into adhesive layers to aquadissect and separate them and thus to define the underlying organ structure.

Step 2
All of the blood vessels within the adhesions are coagulated along the lines of intended incision and then divided using the operating scissors (*Fig.15.42*) and a fiberoptic or a CO_2 laser (*Fig. 15.43*). It is essential that the adhesions are divided layer by layer. One must always be aware of both sides of the adhesion, particularly at sites related to the lateral pelvic sidewall, the ureter, or blood vessels, or adjacent to the uterosacral ligaments, the cul-de-sac, or bowel. In this manner, adhesions are divided until the oviduct is adequately mobilized.

Step 3
The primary focus is on the distal oviduct and tubo-ovarian relationships. Reproduction and subsequent pregnancy are primarily dependent on restoring normal fimbrial–gonadal activity. Significant adhesions that are not related to the fimbrial ovum pickup mechanism are ignored if they are not thought to be causing any clinican symptoms. Extensive dissection at sites unrelated to ovum pickup may cause further adhesion formation and this may be counterproductive to the operative procedure.

Step 4
The ovarian surface is dissected free of adhesions, taking particular care to avoid traumatizing the hilar ovarian veins (*Fig. 15.44*). Transection of these veins may result in major hemorrhage necessitating oophorectomy to accomplish hemostasis, unless the abdomen is opened and the veins are specifically repaired using classic microvascular technique (*Fig. 15.45*). This specific problem is emphasized because the primary goal is reproduction. Loss of an ovary is a major negative event in any reconstructive reproductive surgical procedure.

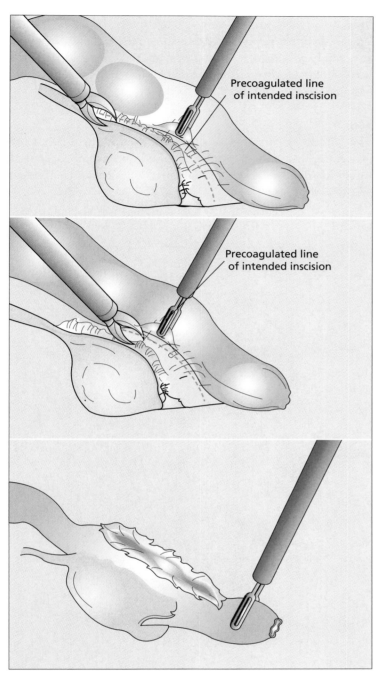

15.42 Lysis of peritubal and ovarian adhesions.

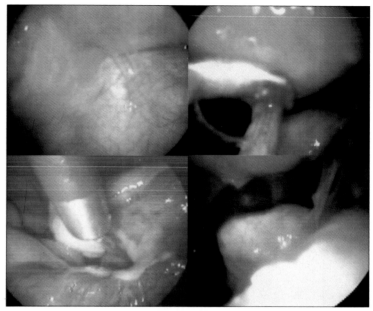

15.43 Lysis of peritubular adhesion with CO_2 laser.

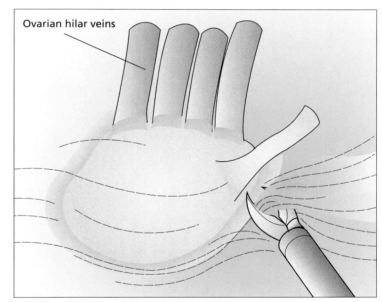

15.44 Anatomy of ovarian hilar veins.

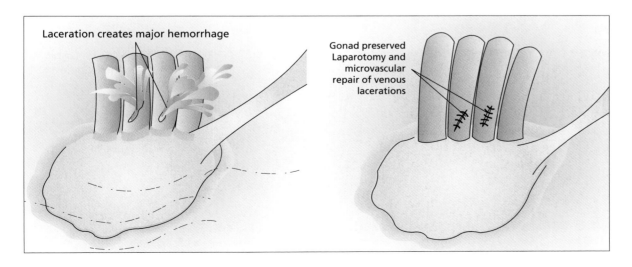

15.45 Laceration and repair of ovarian hilar veins.

Step 5
Periovarian adhesions are best removed by laser vaporization. The vaporized adhesive films are gently rubbed off the ovarian surface with small, moistened Kitner sponges (*Fig. 15.46*).

Step 6
The end of the oviduct is defined and its fimbrial edges are grasped at the serosa (*Fig. 15.47*). A smooth-ended dilating forceps is placed in the distal ostium and gently dilated on withdrawal. This technique effectively separates adhesive fimbria, resulting in a more patulous tubal ostium (*Fig. 15.48*).

Step 7
When specific bridges are noted or major adhesions between fimbria have solid and sometimes vascular bands, these are precoagulated with bipolar coagulation and divided, using the operating scissors or a fiberoptic or CO_2 laser.

Step 8
The oviduct is chromotubated intermittently throughout the procedure. Mass irrigation of 200–300 ml of the heparinized solution is passed through the Fallopian tubes before completion of any tuboplasty.

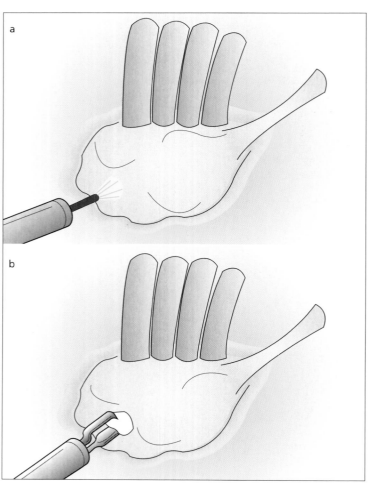

15.46a. Laser vaporization of ovarian adhesion.
b. Blunt dissection of ovarian adhesions.

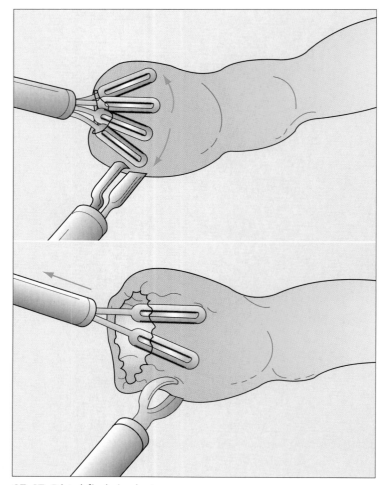

15.47 Distal fimbrioplasty.

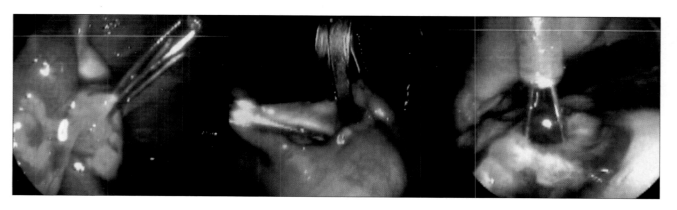

15.48 Distal fimbrioplasty.

Step 9

The specific bands of scarring that cause narrowing of the tubal ostium are defined and transected (*Fig. 15.49*), after which the tube is gently dilated with grasping forceps.

Step 10

In many instances, the fimbria are everted by partially coagulating and/or vaporizing the overlying serosa just behind the fimbrial opening (*Fig. 15.50*). This technique, originally described by Bruhat, effectively allows the distal ostium to peel back like the petals of a flower and is more likely to maintain the oviduct with an everted fimbrial opening.

SALPINGONEOSTOMY

The objective of laparoscopic salpingoneostomy is to provide an adequate opening of the totally occluded distal oviduct, usually a hydrosalpinx. Hydrosalpinges present in various forms, ranging from maximal tubal preservation in a normal-sized but totally occluded oviduct to large, dilated, water-filled, retort-shaped organs. The objective of the procedure is to open the oviduct, ensure eversion of the distal endosalpinx, which may heal as neofimbria and, whenever possible, to explore the endosalpinx. This assessment is helpful for advising the patient regarding her prognosis for subsequent conception.

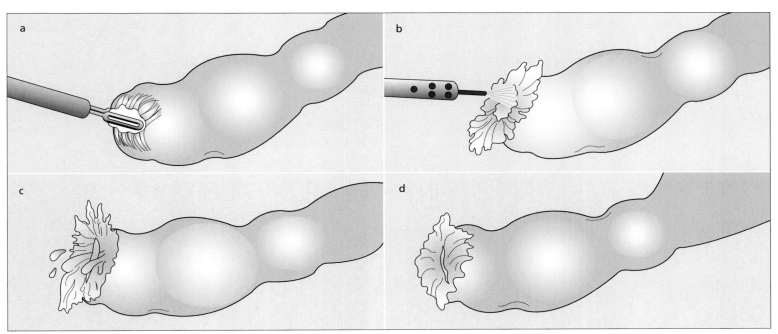

15.49 Bruhat technique of fimbrioplasty: **a** precoagulation of vascular adhesive bands; **b** transection with fiberoptic laser; **c** completion of technique, ostium widely patent; **d** everted ostium after serosal eversion.

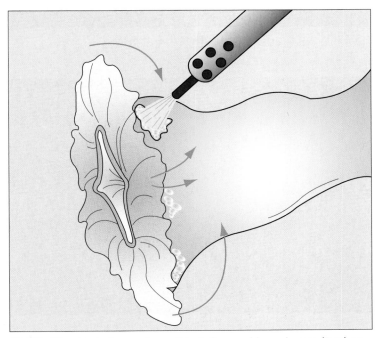

15.50 Distal tubal eversion with defocused laser beam (Bruhat technique).

Success rates for salpingoneostomy range from 10 to 30%, with most women conceiving within 1–3 years after the procedure. Early conceptions occurring within 6 months of the operation during the healing phase are more likely to be ectopic.

SURGICAL PROCEDURE

Step 1

Neosalpingostomy is best carried out using three lower abdominal cannulas (*Fig. 15.51*). Once the oviduct has been defined, it is chromotubated to more effectively enlarge it and to facilitate definition of the avascular lines between the occluded fimbria. The oviduct is elevated into the anterior and medial pelvis above the uterus to avoid the lateral pelvic sidewall, the posterior cul-de-sac, and the bowel.

Step 2

The distal tube is grasped with fine, Addison-like forceps and the intended lines of dissection are precoagulated with a bipolar button electrode (*Figs 15.52–15.57*). This prehemostasis may be completed with the endocoagulator.

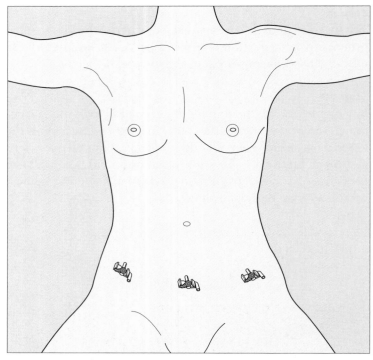

15.51 Cannula placement for neosalpingostomy.

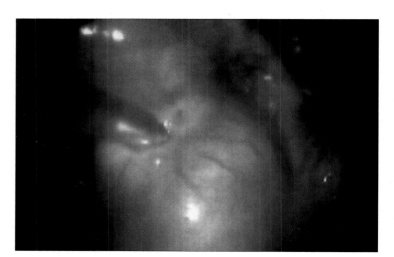

15.52 Hydrosalpinx.

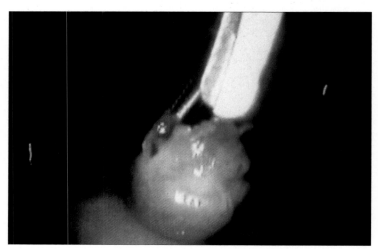

15.53 Distal tube grasped with Addison forceps.

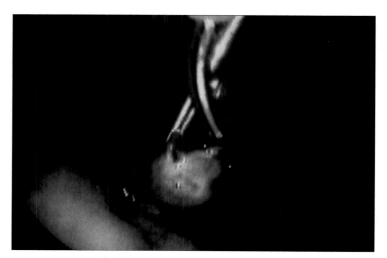

15.54 Precoagulation of intended lines of dissection.

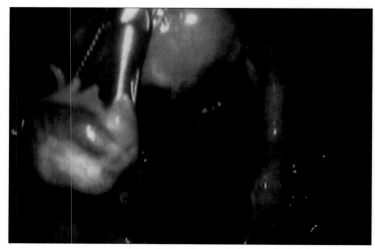

15.55 Opening of the distal tube.

Step 3

A CO_2, a KTP fiberoptic, or a sapphire-tipped Yag laser is used to open the distal oviduct through the avascular lines of the incision along the prior precoagulated areas (*Fig. 15.58*). As the oviduct is opened, some of its fluid contents are collected and submitted for culture and sensitivity, including chlamydial culture.

Step 4

The open ends of the oviduct are now everted using the Bruhat technique. Selected sites of serosa are cicatrized using the bipolar button electrode, the endotherm, or a defocused laser beam (*Fig. 15.59*). This effects significant eversion with total opening of the oviduct. Some surgeons have chosen to evert the distal oviduct on itself in a bent-back, rolled-up fashion.

Step 5

The endosalpinx can be viewed with a salpingoscope or a 3–4 mm hysteroscope. This is placed in the distal oviduct via one of the lower abdominal portals. Ringer's lactate is used as a suitable distension irrigation medium and the distal oviduct is explored in its ampullary segment as far as the endoscope can be advanced. Such exploration provides insight regarding the risk of ectopic pregnancy, which is higher in patients who have endosalpingeal damage and increasing areas of transtubal fibrotic folds. Both oviducts are opened in a similar fashion and mass hydrotubation using a solution of Ringer's lactate containing an antibiotic and a corticosteroid is continued until the end of the procedure. All fluid is then suctioned from the pelvis and hemostasis is checked once more before completing the procedure.

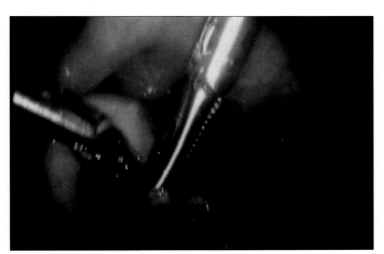

15.56 Opening of the distal tube.

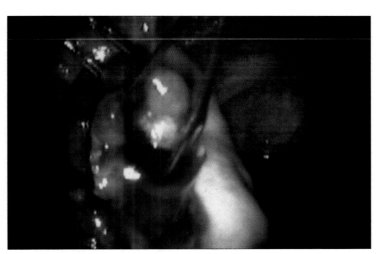

15.57 Completion of fimbrioplasty.

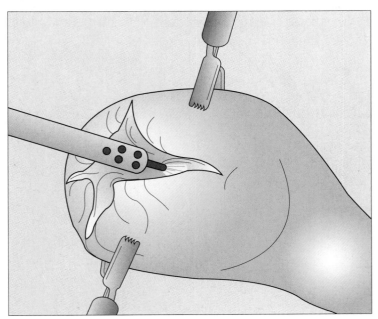

15.58 Use of laser to open fimbriae.

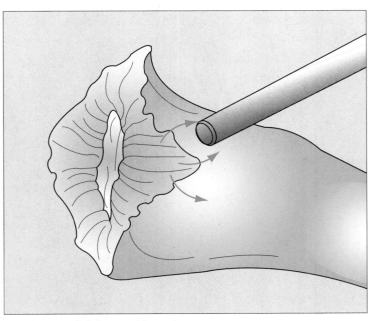

15.59 Use of defocused laser beam.

LAPAROSCOPIC USE OF THE ENDOLOOP

The endoloop is a suture innovation based on the principles applied in the tonsil snare. A hangman's knot is present on the suture material and, using a synthetic plastic rod through which the suture runs, the knot can be firmly secured around tissue or a pedicle (*Fig. 15.60*). A modification of this principle facilitates extracorporeal knot-tying into a hangman's knot which is then pushed back into the abdomen to effectively achieve the same end (*Fig. 15.61*).

The endoloop is indicated for ligation of vascular pedicles, e.g., significant omental adhesions but, more specifically, the vascular pedicles of organs such as the oviduct in partial and total salpingectomy, the ovary in oophorectomy, and both tube and ovary in salpingo-oophorectomy.

SURGICAL PROCEDURE

Step 1

Use of the endoloop is facilitated by use of at least two lower abdominal 5-mm cannulas. One part is used for the knot-passing cannula to protect the suture material and to prevent significant loss of pneumoperitoneum during suture insertion. The second cannula facilitates placement of a grasping instrument to hold the organ tissue or pedicle to be ligated.

Step 2

The tissue is mobilized by dissection and the pedicle defined. The pedicle must be fully mobile and free of contiguous tissues so that a secure knot can be obtained. The endoloop is passed into the pelvis and the loop is opened. The grasping forceps enters the abdomen from the opposite side and is passed through the open end of the loop to grasp the organ or pedicle to be ligated (see *Fig. 15.60*).

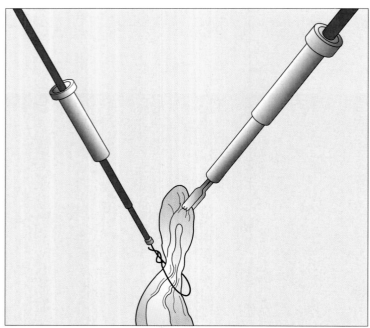

15.60 Pre-tied surgical loop.

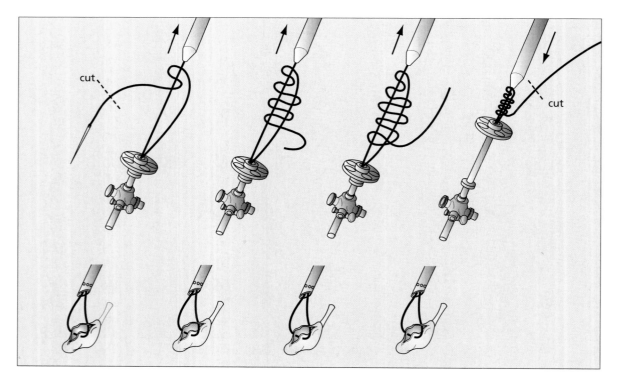

15.61 Endoscopic knot tying.

Step 3

Once the suture has been placed in a good position, the upper plastic union is snapped and the long plastic rod is steadily and firmly pushed down into the abdomen (*Fig. 15.62a*). The knot is firmly secured by this placement, which is facilitated in multiple short, firm thrusts.

Step 4

When the knot is absolutely secure, it is transected with the hook scissors (*Fig. 15.62b*). Suture material available includes plain catgut, chromic catgut, and polydioxanone.

Step 5

After transecting the first suture, second and third endoloops are passed and placed in a similar fashion. After completion of three sutures and transecting their ends, the organ or pedicle is divided with a suitable scissors, needle coagulator, or laser device. The residual pedicle is coagulated electrosurgically or with the endotherm when indicated (*Fig. 15.62c*).

LAPAROSCOPIC OOPHORECTOMY

Instrumentation for this procedure includes three lower abdominal portals, one 11 mm in diameter, as well as claw forceps, grasping forceps, hook scissors, bipolar coagulating button, bipolar forceps, endoloops, and morcellator.

Atrophic, non-vascularized ovaries and those related to congenital dysgenesis can be removed with a totally electrosurgical technique after defining the major pelvic blood vessels and ureter on the ipsilateral pelvic sidewall.

SURGICAL PROCEDURE

Step 1

Aquadissection of the sidewall with injection of 50–100 ml of Ringer's lactate in the extraperitoneal space may facilitate this dissection in certain cases.

15.62 Use of pre-tied surgical loop: **a.** snapped plastic sheath pushes knot firmly at pedicle as inner suture is pulled outwards; **b.** suture transected with scissors; **c.** coagulation of pedicle with endocoagulator.

Step 2

The ovary is grasped with locked clasping forceps and the ovarian hilum is precoagulated with the bipolar forceps or the bipolar button electrode (*Figs 15.63a, 15.63b*).

Step 3

The ovary is then removed by dissection with the hook scissors (*Fig. 15.63c*). Various laser modalities can be used if available.

Step 4

All other gonads to be removed have an extensive vascular hilum. These are best removed with dissection and ligation using endoloops applied to the residual vascular pedicle (*Fig. 15.63d*).

Step 5

It is essential that the ovary is dissected free of the pelvic sidewall. Removal of a totally adherent ovary merging into the pelvic sidewall and incorporating the ureter is best accomplished at laparotomy. In most cases, however, the ovary is first dissected free of all surrounding adhesions, keeping its pedicle mobile and well defined, thus permitting safe insertion of three ligatures around it. The significant part of this procedure is the careful dissection and mobilization of the ovary from surrounding structures. Customarily, to facilitate the dissection as at laparotomy, small pieces of ovarian tissues may be left in preference to traumatizing a major pelvic vessel or ureter.

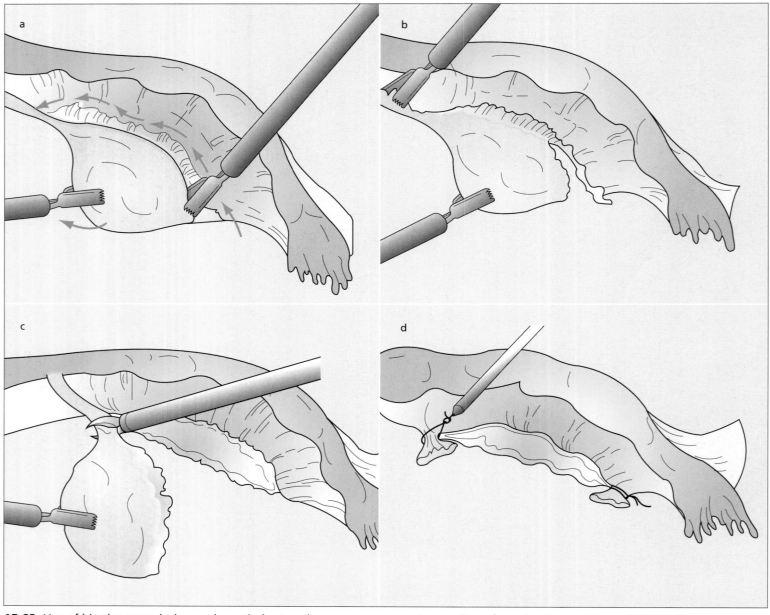

15.63 Use of bipolar coagulation and pre-tied suture loop:
a. precoagulation of ovarian ligaments and blood supply;
b. transection of ovarian vasculation and ligaments with hook scissors;
c. transection of ovarian ligament completes oophorectomy;
d. application of Roder endoloops to vascular pedicles in oophorectomy.

Step 6

Once the ovary has been fully mobilized, its pedicle is checked on each side. An endoloop is inserted through the ipsilateral portal. The claw forceps are passed through the endoloop and the ovary is grasped (*Fig. 15.64a*).

Step 7

The endoloop is then secured firmly around the gonadal base, attempting to secure as much of a pedicle as possible. The endoloop is transected (*Fig. 15.64b*).

Step 8

A second and a third endoloop are then placed in a similar fashion (*Fig. 15.64c*). The gonad is then removed, dissecting very close to the ovary using the hook scissors (*Fig. 15.64d*).

Step 9

Total hemostasis of the pedicle is checked and, when necessary, point coagulation or use of the bipolar forceps secures hemostasis of any minor vessels leaking through this pedicle (*Fig. 15.64e*).

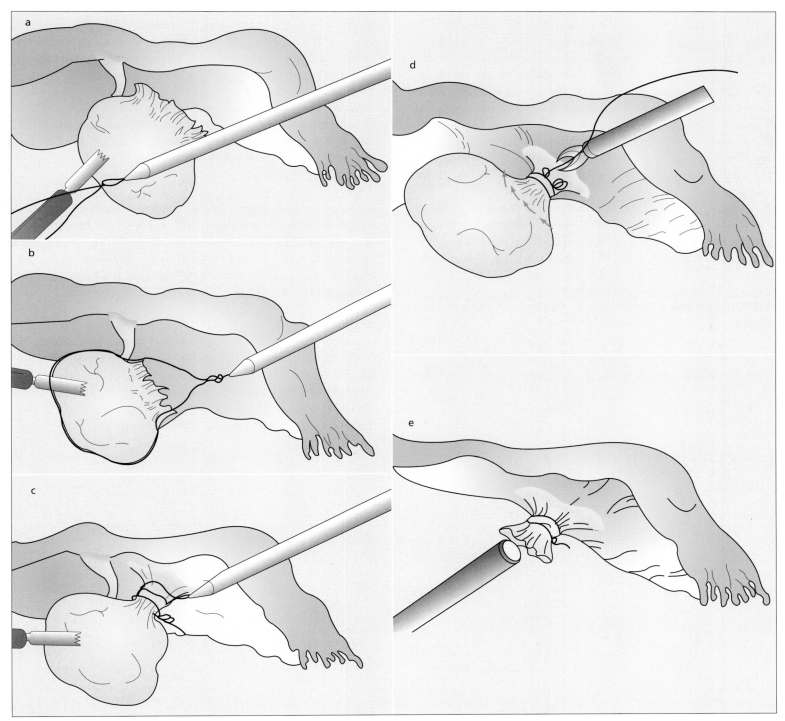

15.64 Use of pre-tied surgical loop for ovarian removal:
a. claw forceps grasp ovary after passage through endoloop;
b. endoloop is secured around ovarian base;
c. three ligatures are secured at ovarian pedicle;
d. intended line of incision is indicated;
e. completed operation with secure hemostatic pedicle.

Step 10

The ovary is held with the clasp forceps and the morcellator is placed through an 11-mm cannula. Sections of the gonad are then cut off in repetitive bites with the morcellator, which delivers the ovary through the cannula. Often the ovary is partially morcellated until a piece that will fit through the cannula is obtained. This piece is then carefully twisted into the cannula and removed. The peritoneal cavity is irrigated with 1–2 l of Ringer's lactate, absolute hemostasis is confirmed, and the fluid is then aspirated.

LAPAROSCOPIC APPENDECTOMY

Appendectomy can be performed during a nonfertility gynecologic laparoscopic procedure. The operation should be confined to a normal appendix being removed as in an incidental appendectomy or to one with chronic inflammation or endometriosis. Acute appendectomy can be completed laparoscopically in its earliest phase. Once the organ is friable or is potentially gangrenous or necrosed, or is significantly fixed and retrodisplaced, routine laparotomy and appendectomy should be carried out in the interests of reduction of morbidity and patient safety.

A routine right lateral 5-mm portal, together with a left 11-mm lower abdominal portal, are used to facilitate removal of the appendix after transection. The procedure requires two grasping forceps, hook scissors, a bipolar coagulator, and three chromic endoloops.

SURGICAL PROCEDURE
Step 1

The appendix is defined, then grasped by its tip with a grasping forceps and/or an endoloop secured around its distal portion (*Fig. 15.65a*).

Step 2

The organ is elevated so that the appendical artery and its corresponding fatty mesoappendix can be defined. The appendiceal artery is coagulated with a bipolar coagulator, and an endoloop can be placed around this stump and transected with the hook scissors (*Figs 15.65b, 15.65c*).

Step 3

The appendix is now dissected free from this fatty tissue and traced down to its base.

Step 4

An endoloop is secured around the base, tightly ligatured, and divided. The proximal appendiceal segment distal to this ligature is sterilized by coagulation with a bipolar forceps or the crushing endotherm apparatus until blanched.

Step 5

A second endoloop is placed on the proximal segment, a third distal to the site, and, including the site of coagulation and the appendix, is divided through this site (*Fig. 15.65d*).

Step 6

The remains of the stump are cleansed with alcohol or povodone–iodine on a small, lint-free cotton sponge held in a crocodile forceps (*Fig. 15.65e*). Hemostasis is checked. The operation can be terminated in this fashion, but preferably some of the fatty appendiceal tissue is placed over the stump or a purse-string suture is inserted on the bowel serosa.

Step 7

Three sutures are placed in the bowel serosa surrounding the appendiceal stump (*Fig. 15.65f*). The suture is then carefully approximated to bury the stump (*Fig. 15.65g*). The abdomen is liberally irrigated with 2–3 l of Ringer's lactate. This solution is then suctioned from the cul-de-sac with the patient in a slightly reversed, Trendelenburg/head-elevated position.

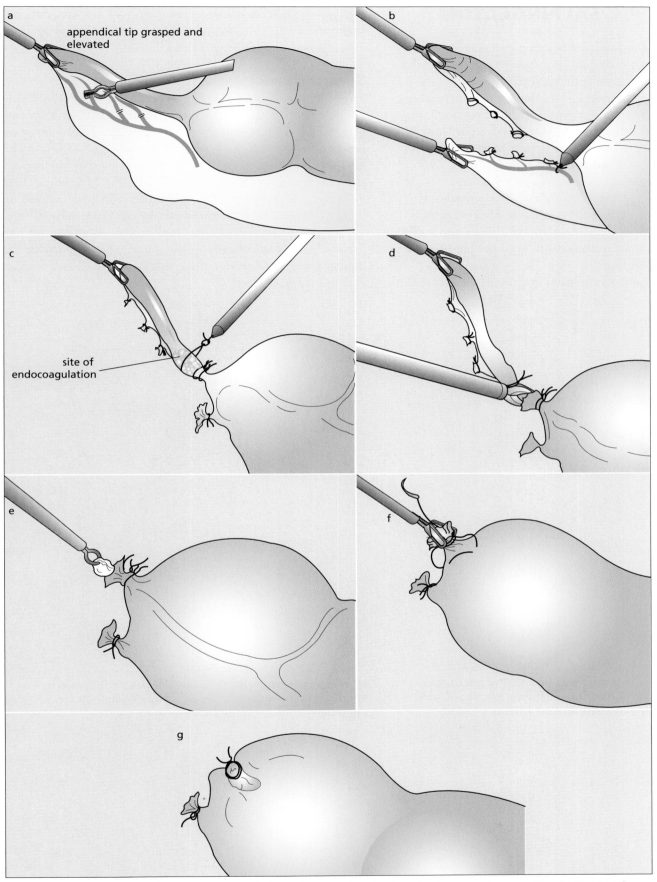

15.65 Laparoscopic appendectomy: **a.** coagulation of appendiceal artery; **b.** ligation of appendiceal artery and mesentery; **c.** appendix ligated with three endoloops, mesentery ligated, transected and removed; **d.** removal of appendix with hook scissors; **e.** cleansing of stump with alcohol on lint-free cotton sponge; **f.** purse-string suture on caecal serosa and direction for placement of appendiceal stump; **g.** closure of purse-string suture and burying of appendiceal stump.

LAPAROSCOPIC SALPINGECTOMY

Salpingectomy, partial or total, can be completed at laparoscopy. The primary and most common indication is removal of the oviduct for ectopic pregnancy in the multiparous patient who is not intent on future childbearing, or for isthmic ectopic pregnancy.

When the oviduct is extensively damaged and ruptured, but the patient is hemodynamically stable, salpingectomy may be necessary after acute torsion of this structure. In view of the risk of damage to the contiguous ovarian blood supply, hydrosalpinges are best treated by neosalpingostomy when a patient is being prepared for *in vitro* fertilization. If salpingectomy is contemplated for these hydrosalpinges in the patient intent on pursuing *in vitro* fertilization, it is the author's opinion that this should be completed at laparotomy, with maximal preservation of the gonadal blood supply.

Instrumentation required includes an irrigator, bipolar forceps,

the unipolar knife electrode, endoloops, hook scissors, optional fiberoptic or CO_2 lasers, and at least two lower abdominal cannulas, one being a large 11-mm cannula.

SURGICAL PROCEDURE

Five to 10 ml of a solution of vasopressin 5IU in 50 ml of saline is injected into the mesosalpinx using a protected 20-gauge endoscopy needle. The mesosalpinx swells and the vascular response renders the oviduct somewhat ischemic (*Fig. 15.66a*). The intended lines of dissection are precoagulated with the bipolar grasping forceps or button electrode (*Fig. 15.66b*). Once hemostasis is adequate, the section of oviduct is removed by precoagulation and dissection with the operating scissors (*Fig. 15.66c*). Any significant, isolated vessel noted within the mesosalpinx is specifically grasped and coagulated with the bipolar forceps. The distal tubal pedicle may be ligated with an endoloop (*Fig. 15.66d*).

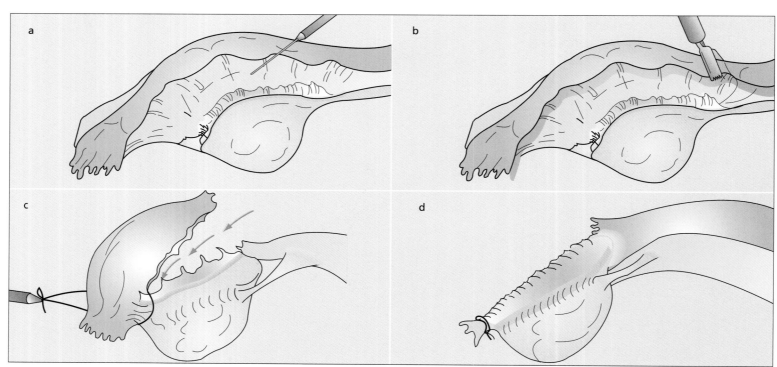

15.66 Laparoscopic salpingectomy: **a.** injection of mesosalpinx with vasopressin 5 ml in 50 ml of saline; **b.** precoagulation with bipolar grasping forceps and bipolar electrode; **c.** plane of incision with scissors, laser, or unipolar needle followed by endoligation of distal pedicle; **d.** complete salpingectomy operation.

An alternative technique for partial salpingectomy is similar to a Pomeroy sterilization. An endoloop can be inserted through the right lower abdominal portal and the mid-segment of oviduct can then be passed through the endoloop for ligation. At least two sutures are inserted, pushed down on the base with the plastic plunger, and transected (*Fig. 15.67a*). The oviduct is then divided using the operating scissors, fiberoptic laser, or CO_2 laser (*Fig. 15.67b*). Hemostasis is checked by liberal irrigation of the tubal stumps and, when necessary, coagulation is secured using endotherm or the bipolar coagulator. Total salpingectomy is never undertaken lightly in women considering future childbearing because of the possibility of damaging the ipsilateral ovarian blood supply. The oviduct is removed through the 11-mm cannula with a gentle, twisting and continual rotation of the grasping forceps.

In salpingectomy, care must always be exercised to avoid thermal damage to the underlying ureter at the site of the ovarian hilum and in the proximity of the infundibular pelvic ligament. Every effort must be made to preserve the blood supply of the ipsilateral gonad, thereby ensuring its normal postoperative function.

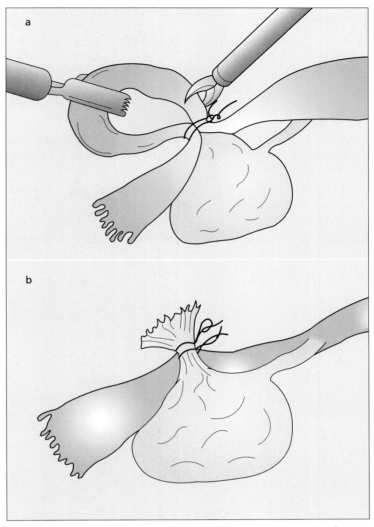

15.67 Laparoscopic partial salpingectomy: **a.** a segment of oviduct is doubly ligated using endoloops and transected with hook scissors; **b.** completed procedure of partial salpingectomy.

FURTHER READING

Adamson GD, Hurd SJ, Pasta DJ, Rodriquez BD. Laparoscopic endometriosis treatment: is it better? *Fertil Steril* 1993; 59:35.

The American Fertility Society. Revised American Fertility Society classification of endometriosis, *Fertil Steril* 1985; 43:351.

Bruhat MA, Manhes H, Mage G, LucPouly J. Treatment of ectopic pregnancy by means of laparoscopy. *Fertil Steril* 1980; 33:441.

Buttram VC Jr, Reiter RC. *Surgical Treatment of the Infertile Female.* Baltimore: Williams & Wilkins, 1985.

Chatman DL, Zbella EA. Biobsy in laparoscopically diagnosed endometriosis. *J Reprod Med* 1987; 32:855.

Confino E, Tur-Kaspa I, DeCherney AH, Corfman R, Coulam C, Robinson E, Haas G,

Katz E, Vermesh M, Gleicher N. Transcervical balloon tuboplasty: a multicenter trial. *JAMA* 1990; 264:2079.

Daniell JF, Kurtz BR, Gurley LD, *et al.* Laparoscopic presacral neurectomy vs neurotomy: Use of the argon beam coagulator compared to conventional technique. *J Gynecol Surg* 1993; 9:169–173.

Daniell JF, Meisel S, Miller W, Tosh R. Laparoscopic use of the KTP/532 laser in non-endometriotic pelvic surgery. *Colposc Gynecol Laser Surg* 1986; 2:107.

DeCherney A, Diamond M. Laparoscopic salpingostomy for ectopic pregnancy. *Obstet Gynecol* 1987; 70:948.

Johns A, Hardie R. Management of unruptured ectopic pregnancy with carbon dioxide laser. *Fertil Steril* 1986; 46:703.

Keye WR Jr, Hansen LW, Astin M, Poulson AM Jr. Argon laser therapy of endometriosis: a review of 92 consecutive patients. *Fertil Steril* 1987; 47:208.

Keye WR, Pouloun AM, Worley RJ: Application of simplified laser laparoscopy to preparation of the pelvis for in vitro fertilization. *J Reprod Med* 1985; 30:418.

Kresch AJ, Seifer DB, Sachs LB, *et al.* Laparoscopy in 100 women with chronic pelvic pain. *Obstet Gynecol* 1984; 64:672.

Levine RL. Economic impact of pelviscopic surgery. *J Reprod Med* 1985; 30(9):655.

Levy BS, Soderstrom RM, Dail DH. Bowel injuries during laparoscopy: Gross anatomy and histology. *J Reprod Med* 1985; 309:168.

Loffer FD. Outpatient management of ectopic pregnancies. *Am J Obstet Gynecol* 1987; 156:1467.

Martin DC, Diamond MP. Operative laparoscopy: Comparison of lasers with other techniques. *Curr Probl Obstet Gynecol Fertil* 1986; 9:563.

Nezhat C, Nezhat F. A simplified mehod of laparoscopic presacral neurectomy for the treatment of central pelvic pain due to endometriosis. *Br J Obstet Gynaecol* 1992; 99:659–663.

Novy MJ, Thurmond AS, Patton P, Uchida BT, Rosch J, Diagnosis of cornual obstruction by transcervical fallopian tube cannulation, *Fertil Steril* 1988; 50:434.

Olive DL, Haney AF, Endometriosis-associated infertility: a critical review of therapeutic approaches. *Obstet Gynecol Survey* 1986; 41:538.

Redwine DB. The distribution of endometriosis in the pelvis by age groups and fertility. *Fertil Steril* 1987; 47:173.

Reich H. Laparoscopic treatment of extensive pelvic adhesions, including hydrosalpinx. *J Reprod Med* 1987; 32:736.

Reich H, McGlynn F. Treatment of ovarian endometiomas using laparoscopic surgical techniques. *J Reprod Med* 1986; 31:577.

Reich H. New techniques in advanced laparoscopic surgery. In: Sutton C(ed.) Bailliere's Clinical Obstetrics and Gynecology, Philadelphia WB Saunders, 1989: 655.

Semm K. Course of endoscopic abdominal surgery. In: Friedrich ER, (ed.) *Operative Manual for Endoscopic Abdominal Surgery*, Chicago: Year Book 1987: 130.

Summit RL Jr, Stovall TG, Lipscomb GH, *et al.* Randomized comparison of laparoscopy-assisted vaginal hysterectomy in an outpatient setting. *Obstet Gynecol* 1992; 80:895–901.

INDEX